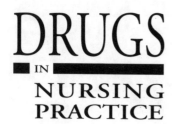

DRUGS
IN
NURSING
PRACTICE

For Churchill Livingstone

Commissioning editor: Ellen Green
Project development editor: Mairi McCubbin
Design direction: Judith Wright
Project manager: Valerie Burgess
Production desktop unit: Neil A. Dickson
Sales promotion executive: Hilary Brown

DRUGS
IN
NURSING
PRACTICE

An A-Z Guide

C. R. Henney RGN SCM
Formerly Research Officer (Nursing), Tayside Health Board and
Research Fellow, Dept of Pharmacology and Therapeutics, University of Dundee

R. J. Dow BSc MB MRCP(UK)
Vice-President and Programme Director, Syntex Pharmaceuticals, Research Park,
Heriot Watt University, Edinburgh
Formerly Senior Registrar, Department of Pharmacology and Therapeutics,
University of Dundee

A. M. MacConnachie BSc(Hons) MSc MRPS MCPP
Principal Pharmacist, Tayside Drug Information Service,
Dundee Teaching Hospitals National Health Service Trust, Dundee
Honorary Lecturer, Department of Clinical Pharmacology, University of Dundee
Part-time Lecturer in Nursing Studies, University of Abertay, Dundee

CHURCHILL LIVINGSTONE
EDINBURGH HONG KONG LONDON MADRID MELBOURNE NEW YORK AND
TOKYO 1995

CHURCHILL LIVINGSTONE
Medical Division of Longman Group Limited.

Distributed in the United States of America by Churchill
Livingstone Inc., 650 Avenue of the Americas, New York,
N.Y. 10011, and by associated companies, branches and
representatives throughout the world.

First published 1982
Second edition 1986
Third edition 1989
Fourth edition 1993
Fifth edition 1995

ISBN 0 443 052352

British Library of Cataloguing in Publication Data
A catalogue record for this book is available from the British
Library.

Library of Congress Cataloging in Publication Data
A catalogue record for this book is available from the Library
of Congress.

The
publisher's
policy is to use
**paper manufactured
from sustainable forests**

Produced through Longman Malaysia

Contents

How to use this book

This book is composed of five main sections:

1. Drug notes (arranged alphabetically by approved name)
2. Special notes
3. Appendices
4. Drug update
5. Drug indexes:
   Index 1 Approved and group names.
   Index 2 Proprietary and other common names.

DRUG NOTES

This is the major part of the text and consists of a description of drugs in common use listed in alphabetical order by approved name. When the nurse has found the individual drug about which information is required, a number of headings will appear as follows:

a. Presentation. This describes the various preparations which are available for each drug, e.g. tablets, injections, nasal spray, suppository, pessary, ointment etc.

b. Actions and uses. Knowledge of the actions and uses of the drug enables the nurse to monitor therapy more effectively in the patient, and therefore a brief description of pharmacological action for each drug is given. In this section the different methods of administration covering the various uses of the drug or drug groups are dealt with.

c. Dosage. The doses given in this book are those commonly ordered for the different types of presentation and mode of administration. The nurse should appreciate that the doctor is not bound to give this dose but may order more, or less, of any drug at his or her discretion. However, if the nurse finds that the dose of a drug given in this book deviates from that prescribed by the doctor, it is advisable to consider checking with the doctor that that particular dose really was intended. It should be remembered that doses for children are usually smaller than those for adults and this also applies to the elderly in the case of many drug groups.

d. Nurse monitoring. This section highlights the important contribution which nurses can make in achieving the most effective and safe use of drugs for their patients. It deals with possible unwanted side-effects of drugs and should be consulted to ascertain the symptoms and signs of adverse drug effects which may become manifest in the patient. The detection of the more serious of these may demand immediate action by the nurse, such as advising the patient to stop taking the drug and notifying the doctor. On other occasions the occurrence would only warrant the notification of the event to the doctor and in some instances would only require explanation to the patient, e.g. that the effect is not unexpected and has no serious significance. Lack of efficacy of a drug can constitute an adverse effect and may be related to inappropriate dose, an inappropriate drug or failure to comply with prescribing instructions. In all these circumstances the doctor should be notified.

e. General notes. Many modern drugs deteriorate, with potentially serious consequences for the patient, if the storage conditions are adverse. Both in hospital and in the community, the nurse has the best opportunity to monitor the storage conditions. This section provides the information which allows this to be done most effectively.

Where a large number of preparations belonging to a particular drug group exist, i.e. as with the beta-adrenergic receptor blockers, the major points on the drug group concerning (b) and (d) above are included under a group heading, i.e. 'beta-adrenergic receptor blockers', and thereafter, when individual members of this group appear in the text, readers are advised to refer back to the group heading.

SPECIAL NOTES

The second section of this book comprises the special notes. These deal with therapeutic topics of great importance to the nurse in everyday practice, and their contents are briefly as follows:

Note 1: Nursing aspects of intravenous therapy. This provides basic information on the types of intravenous infusion fluids available, and also gives practical guidance on common interactions either between drugs and intravenous infusion fluids or between combinations of drugs and intravenous infusion fluids.

Note 2: Intravenous (parenteral) feeding. This section outlines the therapeutic objectives of intravenous feeding and also gives practical guidelines as to how such a regime should be administered.

Note 3: Antibiotics and infectious diseases. This section gives a fuller outline of the action and use of antibiotics and sulphonamides. It includes a list entitled 'Common infections and the organisms which may cause them'. The purpose of this list is two-fold: if a nurse finds an infection described in the main text she/he will be able to obtain fuller information in the list as to the types of organisms which may cause that infection. Also, if an organism is referred to in the main text, the nurse may gain an idea of what types of infection that organism may cause by consulting this list.

Note 4: Drugs in breast milk. In recent times there has been a trend in favour of breast feeding. As many women who may wish to breast feed may be on coincident drug therapy, and also as many women already breast feeding may require to start drug therapy, it is essential that the nurse has some idea of which drugs are either safe or unsafe or whether, indeed, anything is known about the particular drug's excretion in breast milk, and its likely effect on the infant.

Note 5: Ophthalmic preparations. As there is a wide variety of ophthalmic preparations, an attempt has been made to summarise the various preparations available for problems which are suitably treated by topical application.

Note 6: Chronic cancer pain and its control. This is a major addition to the text which recognises the role played by nurses in promoting good pain assessment and analgesic drug therapy as a result. Chronic pain has all too often been poorly managed in the past but gradually pain management as practised in specialized units and hospices has had an increasing influence on the quality of care in the general hospital and community settings. The authors gratefully acknowledge the contribution by Dr Barbara Dymock and her nursing colleagues at Royal Victoria Hospital in Dundee in the preparation of this important new section.

Note 7: The acquired immune deficiency syndrome (AIDS): a guide for nurses. This section summarizes both the development and spread of AIDS and the measures required to minimize exposure and spread in hospitals. It also covers the advances which have been made in recent years in the prevention and treatment of various medical complications which occur in AIDS patients and contribute significantly to improved morbidity and mortality. The authors gratefully acknowledge the contribution to this Note made by Dr Tony France, a senior consultant in infectious diseases at Kings Cross Hospital in Dundee.

APPENDICES

The third section of the book comprises the appendices:

Appendix 1: The security and administration of medicines in hospitals. This deals with legal aspects of drug prescribing and the use of drug Kardexes.

Appendix 2: Metric weights and other measures. This section is included to allow nurses to refer to units of weights and measures with which they may not normally be familiar, and where possible methods of conversion to more commonly recognised units are given.

DRUGS UPDATE

The fourth section enables late entries to be included, in order to present the most up-to-date information available when the book goes to press.

DRUG INDEXES   APPROVED AND GROUP NAMES; PROPRIETARY AND OTHER COMMON NAMES

The two indexes included with this edition represent the fifth and final section of the book.

Index 1 Approved and group names This lists drugs by their official British or approved name, which is that used as the heading for each drug monograph in the text. If the reader locates a drug in this index, the page under which the appropriate monograph can be found is given as the first page referenced. Where approved named drugs are subsequently mentioned in the Special Notes and Appendices the corresponding page number(s) also appear in this index.

In addition, where several drugs of a particular group exists e.g. benzodiazepines, they are also discussed under a group heading in the text. The appropriate page number also appears under the group title.

Note that doctors are now actively encouraged to prescribe drugs by their approved name, with few exceptions.

Index 2 Proprietary and other common names The proprietary name of a drug denotes a trade name by which a given manufacturer's product can be identified e. g. Zantac = ranitidine, manufactured by Glaxo. Not surprisingly, it is this name that often appears in large or bold print in promotional material issued by the drug's manufacturer so that doctors may be influenced to prescribe using such names.

Other common names are those that may be assigned to a drug during its development and that are subsequently adopted, even after the drug comes to the market, for example, many people still recognise alteplase (proprietary name: Actilyse) as TpA. To assist the reader in locating the required drug, such common names have also been included where considered appropriate.

If a drug therefore does not appear in the first index it is likely that the proprietary or another common name has been used in its description. If so, by checking the second index the reader will be referred to the approved name of that drug, which can subsequently be located in the text.

Finally, it should be noted that numerous combinations of two or more drugs in a single tablet, capsule, etc. may exist with each combination described by a single proprietary name. It is not possible to cover all such combinations here and the reader must first determine what approved named drugs are included in such combinations and refer to each separately in the text.

Preface

We hope that **Drugs in Nursing Practice** will continue to serve as a pocket guide to those aspects of modern drug therapy which we believe are important to nurses in training and in day-to-day practice. The 5th edition of the book sees the introduction of up to 70 new drugs, the disappearance of over 30, and changes to a further 100 or more existing monographs, so emphasising the rapid rate of change which continues to take place in modern therapeutic practice. Also, it has become increasingly apparent since the last edition that the nurse's role has further developed, not only in supervising and monitoring the effects of drug prescribing, but even to the extent that nurse prescribing itself is soon to become a reality.

It was hoped to include in this edition a detailed account of the mechanism whereby nurse prescribing will proceed but this new and revolutionary development is not yet sufficiently advanced for us to do so. At the time of writing nurse prescribing is being piloted at one general medical practice in each of eight new regional health authorities in England and Wales from October 1994. Arrangements for Scotland and Ireland have not yet been announced. An early interpretation of how the new legislation might apply is given in 'Nurse Prescribing' on p. xiii.

A further change to take place in the United Kingdom during the 1990s has been the introduction of fundholding general practitioners and trust hospitals. Here the emphasis has been on transferring the cost of prescribing directly to predetermined budgets set for individual prescribers with the intention of increasing accountability for efficacy, safety and economy in prescribing. An interesting consequence has been the need to involve all health care professions more directly in monitoring outcome and improving communication with patients so that treatments are optimally used. The scope for nursing input here is obvious.

With regard to newer therapeutic groups in this edition, attention is drawn in particular to further developments in the treatment of infectious diseases and cancer chemotherapy as well as areas of general medical interest. A great deal of attention continues to focus on the human immunodeficiency virus and AIDS for which the availability of specific treatments or, better still, an effective vaccine, continues to elude medical researchers. Huge strides have however been made in the prevention and treatment of important AIDS-related diseases and the effects of widespread education of the general public in harm reduction methods have been manifest in a much lower number of reported cases than was originally feared by the mid-1990s. Accordingly the special Note addressing nursing aspects of HIV infection and AIDS has been substantially updated.

The special Notes on limited list prescribing and handling of cytotoxic drugs have been omitted. The former is now well established since it was introduced in 1985 and is unlikely to give rise to further confusion; the latter too has been widely discussed since 1982 and it is anticipated that by now all hospitals, where appropriate, will have in place guidelines on the safe handling of cytotoxic drugs. If in doubt check with the pharmacy department through which such guidance should be available and indeed in which cytotoxic chemotherapy is now often prepared in a safe and clean environment.

The opportunity has been taken to introduce a new Note which reviews the management of chronic pain, especially cancer pain, in the recognition that patients are increasingly able to receive high quality care at home supervised through the community nursing service. It is unfortunate that despite the availability of potent analgesics which, prescribed appropriately, can provide excellent control of severe and disabling chronic pain, we have often failed in the past to adequately treat patients with profoundly negative effects on quality of life. Developments within the hospice movement have now spilled over into community care with great effect, not least in the application of continuous analgesia and adjuvant therapy administered via the subcutaneous syringe driver.

Finally, an area in which there has been a notable development of nursing input is in the administration of intravenous therapy and it is clear that in many hospitals nurses outside intensive care units have become adept at administering drugs by this route to patients who already have intravenous access. As a result the Note on intravenous therapy has been suitably updated.

In closing, the authors look forward to the consolidation of recent changes which have promoted the nurse's role and the development of still newer initiatives in the field of drug therapy affecting nursing care. There should undoubtedly be sufficient advances to warrant further revision of **Drugs in Nursing Practice** in the years ahead.

April 1994   C.R.H., R.J.D., A.M.MacC.

Nurse prescribing

The publication of a **Nurse Prescribers' Formulary** — NPF pilot edition 1994 — heralds the beginning of nurse prescribing in the United Kingdom. The exercise, designated in the first instance a 'demonstration', commenced on 3rd October 1994 and was restricted to qualified nurses at eight GP practices in England and Wales, and selected qualified nurses employed by district health authorities and NHS trusts. The following is an early interpretation of how the new legislation might eventually apply. At the time of writing, however, it is recognised that some amendments or refinements will follow as the early demonstration progresses.

1. Nurse prescribing affects nurses in three professional categories who have successfully completed a prescribing training course, namely:
   a. general nurses
   b. those holding a district nursing qualification (paediatric specialists excepted) who are employed by health authorities or trusts, or fund-holding general medical practices
   c. registered health visitors employed as in the case of district nurses, above.

2. A new type of prescription has been introduced. For GP practice nurses this is a lilac-coloured FP10 (PN) form, and for community nurses or health visitors employed by a district health authority or NHS trust a green FP10 (CN) form.

3. Prescriptions issued by nurse prescribers are generally dispensed at neighbouring pharmacies but can also be dispensed at pharmacies anywhere within the UK. Pharmacists are able to authenticate any prescription by telephoning an automatic enquiry service inside normal office hours.

4. The first Nurse Prescribers' Formulary (NPF) has been published as an addendum to the 28th edition of the British National Formulary (BNF). It is the product of the BNF editorial committee in association with the Health Visitors Association and the Royal College of Nursing. Nurse prescribing applies only to products listed in the NPF.

5. NPF medicines and appliances include a range of products from the following categories.

Analgesics for minor pain

Asprin 300mg dispersible tablets.

Paracetamol 120mg and 250mg in 5ml oral liquid.

Paracetamol 500mg plain and soluble tablets.

Anthelmintics for pinworm, threadworm and roundworm infestation (enterobiasis)

Mebendazole 100mg (Ovex) tablets — sufficient for 1 or 2 doses.

Piperazine citrate (Pripsen) liquid and sachets.

Appliances

See Drug Tariff for further details.

Elastic hosiery and accessories.

Fertility (ovulation) thermometers.

Film gloves, disposable.

Hypodermic (U100 Insulin) syringes, carrying case, screw cap conversion needles, lancets, needle clipping device.

Incontinence appliances.

Ring pessaries.

Stoma appliances and related products.

Urethral catheters.

Urine sugar analysis equipment.

Catheter care solutions

Chlorhexidine (Uro-Trainer, Uriflex C).

Mandelic acid (Uro-Trainer).

Sodium Chloride (Uro-Trainer, Uriflex S).

Solution G/Suby G (Uro-Trainer, Uriflex G).

Solution R (Uro-Trainer, Uriflex R).

Head/body lice infestation

Carbaryl lotion and shampoo (Carylderm, Clinicide, Derbac-C, Suleo-C preparations).

Lindane (Quellada) lotion and shampoo.

Malathion lotion and shampoo (Derbac-M, Prioderm, Suleo-M).

Permethrin (Lyclear) cream and cream rinse.

Phenothrin (Full Marks) lotion.

Ointments, creams, and lotions

Aqueous cream.

Calamine preparations.

Clotrimazole (Canesten) cream.

Dimethicone (Conotrane, Savlon, Siopel, Vasogen) barrier creams.

Emulsifying ointment.

Hydrous (Lanolin) ointment.

Lignocaine gel (incl. with chlorhexidine) and ointment.

Magnesium sulphate paste.

Miconozole gel.

Povidone iodin (Betadine) aqueous solution.

Sterile Sodium Chloride solution.

Thymol glycerin comp.

Titanium ointment (Metosyn).

Zinc and Castor Oil cream.

Reagents

See Drug Tariff for further details.

Reagent tablets for detection of glycosuria and ketonuria.

Reagent strips for detection of glycosuria, ketonuria, proteinuria and blood glucose.

Rectal preparations and laxatives

Arachis oil enema.
Bisacodyl suppositories and tablets.
Docusate sodium preparations.
Glycerol suppositories
Ispaghula husk (Regulan, Fybogel).
Lactulose solution
Magnesium hydroxide mixture.
Phosphate enema.
Senna (Senokot) preparations.
Sterculia (Normacol and Normacol Plus granules).
Sodium citrate comp enema (Micolette, Micralax, Relaxit).

Wound care products

See Drug Tariff for further details.
Absorbent cottons/gauzes/plus viscose ribbon qauze.
Absorbent lint.
Arm slings.
Cellulose wadding.
Cotton conforming bandage.
Cotton crepe bandage.
Crepe bandage.
Dextranomer (Debrisan) paste/beads.
Elastic adhesive bandage.
Elastic web bandages.

Gauze and cellulose wadding tissue.
Gauze and cotton tissues.
Heavy cotton and rubber elastic bandage.
High compression bandages.
Knitted polyamide and cellulose contour bandage.
Knitted viscose primary dressing.
Multiple pack dressing 1 and 2.
Open-wove bandage.
Paraffin gauze dressing.
Perforated film absorbent dressing.
Polyamide and cellulose contour bandage.
Povidone iodine fabric dressing.
Skin closure strips.
Sterile dressing packs.
Stockinettes.
Surgical adhesive tapes.
Suspensory bandages, cotton.
Swabs.
Titanium dioxide elastic adhesive bandage.
Triangular bandage, calico.
Vapour-permeable adhesive film dressing.
Vapour-permeable waterproof plastic wound dressing.
Wound management (gel, colloid and foam) dressings.
Zinc paste bandages.

6. Patients continue to be liable to payment of prescription charges at the current rate unless there are recognised criteria for exemption from such charges.

At the time of going to press major progress in nurse prescribing is expected. Details of education and training leading to qualification as a nurse prescriber should be widely know and an extension of the service beyond the current 'demonstration' period developed. Given its successful introduction and honeymoon period, it is quite possible that the future will see an expanding Nurse Prescribing Formulary which includes an increasing range of medicinal prescription products.

Acknowledgements

The authors gratefully acknowledge the contributions of Dr Barbara Dymock and Dr Tony France (Dundee, Scotland) whose specialist comments in the areas of chronic pain control and the care of patients with HIV infection and AIDS (Notes 6 and 7, respectively) were invaluable in the preparation of the text.

DRUG NOTES
(arranged alphabetically by approved name)

A

ACARBOSE (Glucobay)

Presentation
Tablets—50 mg, 100 mg

Actions and uses
This drug is an intestinal alpha-glucosidase inhibitor. In the gut alpha-glucosidase is responsible for the 'digestion' of complex carbohydrates to monosaccharides which are then absorbed across the gut wall. Since the normal diet is full of complex carbohydrates, acarbose inhibits their utilization to the extent that it induces a 'low' carbohydrate diet. This makes it potentially useful as an adjunct to dietary therapy in type II (non-insulin dependent) diabetes mellitus.

Dosage
In adults: Initially 50 mg three times a day, either chewed with the first mouthful of food or swallowed whole directly before a meal. If there is an inadequate response after 1-2 months the dose may be doubled or re-doubled.

Nurse monitoring
1. This is a new drug unlike any other yet introduced and until experience dictates otherwise it should not be used in children or during pregnancy or in a breast-feeding mother.
2. It should not be used in patients with inflammatory bowel disease.
3. Retaining carbohydrate in the gut is likely to be associated with gas formation and flatulence, a feeling of fullness, abdominal discomfort and diarrhoea.
4. Since it reduces carbohydrate absorption it is likely that acarbose will be abused by patients as an aid to dieting to achieve cosmetic weight loss.

General note
Acarbose tablets may be stored at room temperature.

ACEBUTOLOL (Sectral)

Presentation
Capsules—100 mg, 200 mg
Tablets—400 mg

Actions and uses
Acebutolol itself is a cardioselective beta-adrenoreceptor blocking drug and therefore has the advantages described in the section on beta-blockers. It is metabolised in the body to another chemical which is, in fact, a non-selective drug which may explain why some patients are prone to develop side-effects equivalent to those seen in the non-selective beta-adrenoreceptor blocking group.

Dosage
Oral adult dose range is:
1. Hypertension: 400–800 mg daily in two divided doses. Occasionally up to 1200 mg may be required.
2. Angina pectoris: 200 mg twice daily. Occasionally 300 mg three times daily, with a maximum dose of up to 1200 mg per day.
3. Cardiac dysrhythmias:100–200 mg two-three times daily. Occasionally up to 1200 mg in divided doses may be necessary.

Nurse monitoring
See beta-adrenoreceptor blocking drugs.

General note
Acebutolol capsules and tablets are stored at room temperature.

ACE INHIBITORS (ACEIs)

A group of drugs which includes:
Captopril   Perindopril
Cilazapril   Quinapril
Enalapril   Ramipril
Fosinopril   Trandolapril
Lisinopril

Actions and uses

ACE is angiotensin-converting enzyme, a substance present in the circulation which promotes the formation of angiotensin. Angiotensin is normally produced in response to falling blood pressure and excess sodium loss when it causes profound vasoconstriction and sodium retention by the kidney so supporting the circulation. In hypertension and heart failure however it is often the case that ACE is overactive and causes unwanted vasoconstriction and sodium retention.

The ACEIs are a group of drugs which block the actions of ACE so producing vasodilatation and sodium excretion. In hypertension this leads to a reduction in peripheral vascular resistance and a corresponding fall in blood pressure. In heart failure it leads to an 'unloading' of the stressed myocardium by a reduction in congestion at the right side as well as a reduction in the energy required to eject blood from the left ventricle.

The ACE inhibitors are among the most important drugs used in the treatment of hypertension and heart failure.

Dosage

See individual drugs.

Nurse monitoring

1. Within a few hours of the administration of an ACEI there may be a sudden and precipitous fall in blood pressure, especially when patients have previously been treated with diuretics or are otherwise salt depleted. Patients should be therefore commenced on the lowest possible dose and carefully monitored during the first 24 hours of treatment.
2. The concentration of potassium in the blood may rise in patients receiving ACEIs particularly if they are already taking potassium supplements or potassium-sparing diuretics. A high blood potassium (hyperkalaemia) may cause dangerous cardiac arrhythmia.
3. All drugs of this type can produce a persistent dry cough (especially in women) which may be quite disabling in some patients. The reason appears to be that once ACE, which is also present in lung tissue, is blocked the formation of irritant substances called kinins follows. It may be possible to control the cough by using an anti-inflammatory drug such as ibuprofen or by the inhalation of sodium cromoglycate.
4. The use of an ACEI is associated with a reduction in filtration pressure in the kidney. Normally this has few consequences but in patients with renal impairment, particularly those with renal artery stenosis, renal failure may result. The monitoring of serum creatinine is advised so that early renal failure can be detected. Elderly patients in particular may have a degree of renal impairment.
5. Some ACEIs are excreted largely by the kidney and require to be given in reduced dosage if kidney function is impaired. Others are to a great extent excreted by the liver and may be preferred.

General note

See specific drugs.

ACEMETACIN (Emflex)

Presentation

Capsules—60 mg

Actions and uses

See the section on non-steroidal anti-inflammatory analgesic drugs.

Dosage

Adults only: Usually 60 mg twice daily but up to three times daily, if required.

Nurse monitoring
1. See the section on non-steroidal anti-inflammatory analgesic drugs.
2. As a new drug it is important that patients receiving acemetacin be closely monitored and that all possible adverse reactions be reported. Meanwhile, side effects attributed to indomethacin in particular (e.g. dizziness, tinnitus, etc), may be anticipated as well as those commonly reported for non-steroidal anti-inflammatory drugs.

General note
Acemetacin capsules may be stored at room temperature.

ACETAZOLAMIDE (Diamox)

Presentation
Tablets—250 mg
Capsules—250 mg sustained release
Injection—500 mg vials
Actions and uses
Acetazolamide inhibits the action of an enzyme called carbonic anhydrase and in so doing produces three major effects:
1. It increases urine output.
2. It decreases the flow of aqueous humour within the chamber of the eye thus reducing intra-ocular pressure.
3. By an unknown action in the brain it may reduce the frequency of seizures in epileptic patients.
In clinical practice this drug is now only used for the treatment of glaucoma.
Dosage
For the treatment of glaucoma:
Adults: 250 mg–1 g daily in divided doses or 250–500 mg daily as slow release capsules.

Nurse monitoring
1. Side-effects which occur most often in the initial stages of treatment include flushing, thirst, headache, drowsiness, dizziness, fatigue, paraesthesia, ataxia, hyperventilation and gastrointestinal upset (anorexia, nausea and vomiting).
2. Much more rarely hypersensitivity reactions may occur leading to skin, kidney and bone marrow damage. Acetazolamide is in fact a derivative of the sulphonamide group and affects the skin, kidney and bone marrow in the same way as described for Sulphonamides (q.v.).
3. Prolonged use may lead to stone formation in the kidneys with resultant ureteric colic.
4. The drug may produce an abnormality in blood biochemistry known as acidosis which can be potentially dangerous. Symptoms of this include altered consciousness—initially drowsiness and later coma and deep irregular breathing.

General notes
1. The preparation may be stored at room temperature.
2. Acetazolamide for intravenous injection is reconstituted with 5 ml of water for injection immediately before use.

ACETYLCYSTEINE (Fabrol, Parvolex)

Presentation
Injection—2 g in 10 ml
Sachets—200 mg (oral use)
Actions and uses
1. This substance is claimed to reduce the viscosity and tenacity of sputum and, therefore, may be used to good effect to aid the resolution of acute exacerbations of chronic bronchitis and chest infections associated with cystic fibrosis.
2. Acetylcysteine is a specific antidote to paracetamol which damages the liver in overdosage. It is administered intravenously in the treatment of paracetamol poisoning.

Dosage

1. Oral use: adults 1–2 sachets dissolved in water, three times daily. Children: under 2 years—one sachet daily; 2-6 years—one sachet twice daily; older children—as for adults.
2. Injection (to specifically treat paracetamol poisoning): initially, 150 mg/kg body weight by intravenous infusion over 15 minutes followed by an infusion of 50 mg/kg over 4 hours. Thereafter a dose of 100 mg/kg is administered in 1 litre over the next 16 hours. This provides a total dose of 300 mg/kg in 20 hours.

Nurse monitoring

1. When administered orally, side-effects are uncommon but include nausea, vomiting, heartburn, tinnitus, headache, and skin rashes (urticaria).
2. When administered by injection:
   a. Acetylcysteine is an effective antidote to paracetamol if administered up to 8-10 hours after poisoning. Its effectiveness rapidly diminishes thereafter. It is therefore important, if possible, to determine the time of poisoning in relation to hospital admission.
   b. Note that the drug is incompatible with rubber and metals and for this reason plastic cannulae are used when doses are administered.
   c. The drug is generally well tolerated but a few patients are hypersensitive and skin rashes may develop. Rarely, acute anaphylaxis has occurred.

General note

The drug should be stored in a cool place.

ACIPIMOX (Olbetam)

Presentation

Capsules—250 mg

Actions and uses

Acipimox is chemically related to nicotinic acid (a form of vitamin B$_3$ and has been produced as an effective, yet well-tolerated, lipid-lowering drug. Drugs of this type reduce raised cholesterol levels in hypercholesterolaemia and mixed hyperlipidaemia thereby reducing any associated coronary risk. Their action is exerted directly on liver synthesis of LDL-cholesterol and VLDL-cholesterol.

Dosage

The usual adult dose is 500–750 mg daily taken in 2 or 3 divided doses with meals.

Nurse monitoring

1. Nicotinic acid may produce severe gastrointestinal upset and, although derivatives such as acipimox are designed to reduce this risk, such an effect cannot be ruled out. It is therefore important to monitor patients for signs of gastrointestinal disturbances especially in those with a history of peptic ulcer disease.
2. Other side-effects common to nicotinic acid derivatives include flushing, nausea and diarrhoea.

General note

Acipimox capsules may be stored at room temperature.

ACITRETIN (Neotigason)

Presentation

Capsules—10 mg, 25 mg

Actions and uses

Acitretin is a chemical derivative of vitamin A and belongs to the family known as the retinoids. It is used in the treatment of severe psoriasis which is unresponsive to other first line drugs. Other uses include ichthyosis, a congenital skin disease characterized by hyperkeratinization, and Darièr's disease. The mechanism of action of acitretin and related vitamin A compounds lies in their antikeratitic (antimitotic) activity which results in inhibition of the abnormally rapid turnover of cells in the skin's thick outer keratin layer.

Dosage

Adults only: An initial dose of 25–30 mg is taken once daily for a few weeks then gradually adjusted according to the response. Up to 75 mg daily may be given but the lowest possible maintenance dose should be used.

Nurse monitoring

1. Treatment with acitretin is suppressive rather than curative and the patient should understand that long-term therapy is required.

2. Vitamin A derivatives are strongly teratogenic and fetal malform-ations are highly likely in the event of pregnancy. Pregnancy must be excluded in women of childbearing age at the outset and patients must be actively counselled thereafter to ensure that adequate contraceptive measures are always taken. Therapeutic abortion is offered if pregnancy occurs.
Furthermore, pregnancy must be avoided for at least 2 years after treatment is discontinued since acitretin metabolites are stored for prolonged periods in the body tissues.

3. It is important to note that treatment with acitretin must be arranged through a specialist clinic and supplies of the drug are restricted to hospitals only.

4. Vitamin A compounds are poorly tolerated by some patients (hence the need for careful dosage adjustment). Dryness of the skin, erythema, pruritus and alopecia are common and erosion of mucous surfaces is possible. Other side-effects include headaches, nausea, drowsiness, joint pain and myalgia.

5. Hepatotoxicity occurs and liver function tests should be carried out regularly to detect early liver damage. Concurrent use of hepatotoxic drugs and alcohol should be discouraged and treatment avoided in the event of existing liver impairment.

6. A further metabolic effect results in an unfavourable shift in the blood lipid profile and hyper-lipidaemia. This may have important consequences for patients who have a history of angina or myocardial infarction and other risk factors for coronary heart disease. Care is also required in patients with diabetes in whom glucose tolerance may be altered.

7. Abnormal bone formation and calcification of other tissues may occur during long-term use and should be monitored by occasional X-rays.

8. Acitretin must not be used in patients with renal failure.

General note

Acitretin capsules may be stored at room temperature and should be protected from light.

ACLARUBICIN (Aclacin)

Presentation

Injection—20 mg

Actions and uses

Aclarubicin is an anthracycline compound which is used as a cytotoxic drug. It potentially has actions and uses similar to those described for other anthracycline drugs including doxorubicin, daunorubicin, epirubicin and mitozantrone. At present, aclarubicin is indicated as alternative therapy in acute non-lymphocytic leukaemia where relapse or resistance to established cytotoxic drug regimes occurs.

Dosage

1. Adults and children: Initial regimens include:
   a. Rapid high dosage, e.g. up to 100 mg/m^2 body surface area for 3 doses.
   b. More prolonged use of lower dosage e.g. 25 mg/m^2 for 7 doses.

Doses are given on consecutive days.

2. For maintenance therapy, single doses of 25-100 mg/m² may be administered at intervals of 3-4 weeks.

Nurse monitoring
1. Aclarubicin may produce phlebitis. If it is administered via a peripheral vein it should first be diluted e.g. in 100 ml, and given over 30 minutes to 1 hour. Alternatively, it may be injected directly into a central line.
2. In common with other cytotoxic drugs of the anthracycline group, this drug is notably cardiotoxic and if total doses exceeding 400 mg/m² are administered cardiac status should be carefully monitored.

General notes
Aclarubicin powder for injection may be stored at room temperature, protected from light, for up to 3 years. After reconstitution the vial may be retained for 24 hours under refrigeration. If kept at room temperature it should be used within 6 hours.

The injection is reconstituted using water for injection or sodium chloride 0.9%. The latter should be used to administer intravenous infusions, since the drug may be degraded by solutions of low pH, typically associated with glucose injection.

ACRIVASTINE (Semprex)

Presentation
Capsules—8 mg

Actions and uses
This drug belongs to the antihistamine group (see antihistamines) but, being a new generation agent, is unlikely to produce significant sedation and drowsiness. Its licensed uses include the treatment of allergic rhinitis and urticaria.

Dosage
Adults: 8 mg three times daily.

Nurse monitoring
The group section under antihistamines should be consulted, but note that acrivastine is a relatively non-sedative drug.

General note
Acrivastine capsules may be stored at room temperature but should be protected from light.

ACROSOXACIN (Eradacin)

Presentation
Capsules—150 mg

Actions and uses
Acrosoxacin is a member of the quinolone group of antibiotics i.e. it chemically resembles ciprofloxacin, the first drug in this series. However, unlike ciprofloxacin, the uses of this drug are very narrow—restricted to the treatment of acute gonorrhoeal infection in both men and women. Because of its long-term action, single dose therapy is all that is required.

Dosage
Adults only: 300 mg is administered, under supervision, as a single dose.

Nurse monitoring
1. Compliance with drug treatment is a major problem in patients attending the genito-urinary clinic. For this reason, drugs which only require to be taken in one or two or otherwise few doses are favoured **but** supervision is recommended and dosing is preferably carried out before the patient leaves the clinic.
2. Since it is given as a single dose, acrosoxacin is unlikely to cause persistent side-effects. However, gastrointestinal upsets, headache, dizziness and drowsiness may be experienced, albeit short-lived.
3. Patients with liver and/or kidney impairment are more likely to report prolonged side-effects.

General note

Acrosoxacin capsules may be stored at room temperature but should be protected from light.

ACTINOMYCIN D (Cosmegen Lyovac)

(Also described as Dactinomycin)
Presentation

Injection—Vials containing 0.5 mg

Actions and uses

Actinomycin is a derivative of a group of antibiotics. A simplified version of its action is as follows: Every cell has in its nucleus two strands made up of proteins known as DNA. The DNA contains all the information necessary for cell duplication. When Actinomycin combines with DNA it blocks the process of cell duplication. This drug is used with some success in three rare conditions:

1. Wilms' tumour of the kidney
2. Choriocarcinoma
3. Testicular teratomas

There is evidence to suggest that the drug is more effective if patients receive concurrent radio-therapy.

Dosage

The dose depends on the type of tumour under treatment:

1. Adults:
   a. The usual adult dose is 0.5 mg by intravenous injection daily for courses up to 5 days in duration. These courses are repeated at intervals of several weeks.
   b. An alternative dose of 0.01 mg/kg body weight has been used.
2. Children:
   a. The usual dose by intravenous injection is 0.015 mg/kg daily for courses of up to 5 days in duration.
   b. An alternative regime is to give a total dose of 2.4 mg per ml² of body surface area over a period of 1 week

Nurse monitoring

1. The drug is always given by intravenous injection and is highly irritant if it escapes from the vein.
2. During the treatment course abdominal pain, anorexia, nausea and vomiting may occur.
3. Side-effects, which may be delayed for days or even weeks after finishing a course, include bone marrow depression with anaemia, leucopenia and thrombocytopenia and resultant increased risk of severe infection and haemorrhage. Ulcerative stomatitis and dysphagia, alopecia, erythema, fever, hypocalcaemia, myalgia, malaise and gastrointestinal symptoms can also occur.
4. Skin reactions may occur with this drug and these are more common at sites where simultaneous or prior irradiation has been given.
5. The drug should never be given to patients with chickenpox as a severe or fatal generalised reaction may result.
6. The drug should never be given during pregnancy.
7. Side-effects are particularly severe when given to children under the age of 1.
8. The nurse should be constantly aware that most cytotoxic drugs are irritant to the skin and mucous surfaces, and are in general very toxic. Great care should therefore be exercised when handling these drugs, and in particular spillage or contamination of personnel or the environment must be avoided. If cytotoxic drugs are handled regularly it is theoretically possible that repeated skin contact or inhalation may produce systemic toxic effects and in nurses who have developed hypersensitivity, severe local and general hypersensitivity reactions.

General notes

1. Solutions for injection are prepared by adding 1.1 ml water for injection to each vial to give a final solution containing 0.5 mg in 1 ml. This may be injected directly or via the drip tube of a 5% dextrose or 0.9% sodium chloride infusion. Any unused solution must be discarded.
2. Actinomycin D is very corrosive to skin and soft tissue and accidental leakage following intravenous injection may cause irritation, phlebitis and cellulitis.
3. Vials containing sterile powder for injection may be stored at room temperature under dry conditions.

ACYCLOVIR (Zovirax)

Presentation

Tablets—200 mg, 400 mg, 800 mg
Suspension—200 mg in 5 ml
Injection—250 mg, 500 mg vials
Eye ointment—3%
Cream—5%

Actions and uses

Acyclovir is an antiviral agent which has potent activity against herpes simplex virus (HSV) and is, to a lesser extent, active against herpes zoster virus (varicella) and possibly other viruses. In clinical practice it is used for the following:

1. Intravenously for the treatment of systemic infections due to herpes virus.
2. Intravenously for the prevention of systemic infections due to herpes virus following the appearance of oral and perioral herpetic lesions in immunosuppressed patients.
3. Orally for the treatment of HSV infections of the skin and mucous membranes, including genital herpes.
4. Orally for the treatment of shingles. Acute pain is alleviated and possibly also the pain associated with post-herpetic neuralgia.
5. Orally for the prevention of HSV infections in susceptible (immunocompromised) patients.
6. As ophthalmic ointment applied in the treatment of herpes simplex keratitis.
7. As topical cream, for the treatment of HSV infections of the skin, including genital herpes.

Dosage

1. Intravenous: Adults and children: By intravenous infusion, 5–10 mg/kg body weight is administered every 8 hours. Each infusion is administered slowly over a period of 1 hour.
2. Oral: Adults: 200 mg 5 times daily, usually for a period of 5 days for treatment of HSV infection.
3. Adults: 200 mg 4 times daily for prevention of HSV infection.
4. Doses of 2-4 times greater are used by the intravenous and oral routes for treatment of herpes zoster infection.
5. Ophthalmic: Adults and children: Ophthalmic ointment is applied 5 times daily at intervals of 4 hours with treatment continued for at least 3 days after healing takes place.
6. Cream: Adults and children: Apply to herpetic lesions 5 times a day and continue for at least 5 days after healing takes place.

Nurse monitoring

1. A reversible increase in blood urea and serum creatinine may occur after intravenous infusion. This effect is less marked if patients are well hydrated before treatment is administered.
2. Patients with severe renal impairment should receive a reduced dosage.
3. Acyclovir for infusion is irritant and inflammation and ulceration may occur at injection sites if leakage from the vein into the surrounding tissues occurs. Bolus injection or rapid infusions should therefore be avoided and patients should not take solutions prepared from injection vials by mouth.
4. Topical application may be associated with skin irritancy

which is usually described as a burning sensation.

5. The drug is only contraindicated in patients who have displayed previous hypersensitivity.

General notes

1. Preparations containing Acyclovir may be stored at room temperature.
2. Eye ointment should be discarded 1 month after opening.
3. Intravenous infusions are prepared in sodium chloride 0.9%, dextrose 5%, dextrose/saline mixtures or Hartmann's solution.

ADENOSINE (Adenocor)

Presentation
Injection—3 mg in 1 ml

Actions and uses
Adenosine is an anti-arrhythmic agent. When administered by rapid intravenous injection it slows conduction via the atrioventricular (A–V) node so interrupting re-entry circuits involving this pathway (including those associated with Wolff-Parkinson-White syndrome) and restoring sinus rhythm in patients with paroxysmal supraventricular tachycardia. A further use is in assisting interpretation of atrial activity in the ECG by transiently slowing the rate of cardiac conduction.

Dosage
1. Adults: 3 mg administered by rapid intravenous injection, i.e. over 2 seconds followed by further doses of 6 mg and 12 mg if arrhythmias are not abolished within 1-2 minutes.
2. Children: Doses of between 0.0375 and 0.25 mg (37.5 and 250 microgram)/kg body weight have been used as above.

Nurse monitoring

1. Facial flushing, chest tightness or dyspnoea, nausea, and lightheadedness are common side-effects. Others include sweating, palpitations, hyper-ventilation, headache, anxiety, burning sensation, bradycardia, chest pain, dizziness, arms, back and neck pain, and metallic taste.
2. Severe bradycardia has been reported. It is not reversed by Atropine administration and patients may require pacing.
3. Adenosine should be avoided in patients with 2nd or 3rd degree heart block and sick sinus syndrome (unless a functioning pacemaker is in situ).
4. Note that dipyridamole inhibits the inactivation of adenosine so potentiating its action. On the other hand, its activity is inhibited by theophylline and caffeine.

General note
Adenosine injection is for immediate use undiluted. Do not retain any residual solution.

ADRENALINE (Eppy, Simplene)

Note that the above named products are only two of the many forms in which this drug is administered. It is most often recognised by its approved name of adrenaline.

Presentation
Injection—1 in 1,000 = 0.1% solution or 1 mg in 1 ml
—1 in 10,000 = 0.01% solution or 0.1 mg in 1 ml (10 ml ampoule)

Eye Drops—0.5% and 1%

Actions and uses
Adrenaline is the hormone secreted by the adrenal medullary gland to 'boost' the sympathetic nervous system in times of stress. Once in the circulation, its effects are widespread and complex.
It increases cardiac output by stimulating the rate and force of contraction of the heart and

produces generalized vasoconstriction by its action on vascular smooth muscle. This is the basis for its use in cardiology and in acute anaphylaxis when circulatory support must be maintained. In the eye, adrenaline is only a weak mydriatic but it also reduces aqueous humor production and increases its outflow. Since it causes marked local vasoconstriction in the microcirculation, topical adrenaline solutions and ointments have been used to arrest bleeding.

In clinical practice adrenaline is used in:

1. Asystolic cardiac arrest in combination with calcium chloride to provoke ventricular fibrillation.
2. Anaphylactic shock or other manifestations of severe allergy.
3. Open angle (chronic simple) glaucoma.

Dosage

1. Acute coronary care: 10 ml of a 1 in 10,000 solution by intravenous injection.
2. Anaphylaxis and other allergic emergencies: 0.5–1 ml of a 1 in 1,000 solution by intramuscular injection. Some use the subcutaneous route but absorption from the site in shock is less predictable. Children: under 1 year—0.05 ml; 1-2 years—0.1 ml; 2-3 years—0.2 ml; 3-5 years—0.3 ml; 5-6 years—0.4 ml; 6-12 years—0.5 ml.
3. Glaucoma: One drop is instilled in the eye once or twice daily.

Nurse monitoring

1. Adrenaline is not used in heart failure or cardiogenic shock since it possesses both alpha and beta actions. The former carry a risk of precipitating cardiac arrhythmias. This is accepted in asystole however since it is intended that ventricular fibrillation (subsequently responsive to cardioversion) be produced.
2. Adrenaline injection may cause anxiety, tremors, dry mouth and cold extremities as well as tachycardia. It also raises blood pressure and its inadvertent

intravenous administration combined with a local anaesthetic has resulted in a precipitous rise in blood pressure and haemorrhage.
3. Adrenaline should be used with caution in situations where its stimulant action on the cardio-vascular system and endocrine function may pose problems e.g. ischaemic heart disease, hyperthyroidism, diabetes mellitus and hypertension.
4. Adrenaline applied to the eye may produce slight irritation.

General notes

1. Adrenaline eye drops may be stored at room temperature but must be protected from light. Any darkening in colour indicates light-accelerated degradation of the solution which should be discarded.
2. Eye drops, once open, can be used for 1 month in the community or 1 week in hospital wards.
3. Adrenaline injection solutions may be stored at room temperature but they too should be protected from light. Degradation may be detected as a slight pink discolouration of the solution.

ALCLOMETHASONE (Modrasone)

Presentation

Cream—0.05%
Ointment—0.05%

Actions and uses

See the section on corticosteroids. Alclomethasone is a mildly potent steroid for topical use only in the treatment of dermatoses.

Dosage

Cream and ointment should be applied to affected areas 2-3 times daily

Nurse monitoring

See the section on corticosteroids.

A

General note

Tubes of alclometasone cream and ointment are stored at room temperature. Dilution with other creams and ointments is not recommended.

ALCURONIUM CHLORIDE (Alloferin)

Presentation

Injection—10 mg in 2 ml

Actions and uses

Alcuronium is a muscle relaxant of the non-depolarizing type. Thus it reversibly paralyses skeletal muscle by competitive inhibition of acetylcholine, the transmitter substance released at the junction of the (motor) nerve and muscle fibre (motor end-plate receptor). Drugs of this type are used to produce muscle relaxation during surgical anaesthesia.

Dosage

1. Adults: Initially, 200–250 microgram/kg with incremental doses of 50 microgram/kg as required by intravenous bolus injection.
2. Children: over 1 month—125–200 microgram/kg.

Nurse monitoring

1. All patients must have their respiration assisted or controlled.
2. Muscle relaxants of this type are also used to produce paralysis in patients on assisted ventilation in ICUs.
3. Overdosage with muscle relaxant drugs of this type may result in paralysis of the respiratory muscles. If this occurs, an anticholinesterase such as neostigmine (which potentiates acetylcholine by blocking its inactivation) must be administered.

General note

Alcuronium injection may be stored at room temperature but must be protected from light.

ALFACALCIDOL (One-Alpha)

This drug is also known as One-Alpha Hydroxycholecalciferol.

Presentation

Capsules—0.25 microgram and 1 microgram
Solution—0.20 microgram in 1ml

Actions and uses

The actions and uses of alfacalcidol are in theory identical to all those described in the section on vitamin D, of which this drug is a highly active metabolite. In practice, however, alfacalcidol is used mainly for the treatment of renal osteodystrophy.

Dosage

For the treatment of renal osteodystrophy:

1. In adults and children over 20 kg body weight—1 microgram initially with subsequent adjustments according to clinical and biochemical response.
2. Children under 20 kg body weight—0.05 microgram/kg per day initially with subsequent adjustments according to clinical and biochemical response.

Nurse monitoring

The nurse monitoring aspects of this drug are identical to those described for vitamin D (q.v.). It is important to note that alfacalcidol is the most effective preparation of vitamin D and therefore requires careful monitoring as side-effects are more likely.

General note

The drug may be stored at room temperature.

ALFENTANIL (Rapifen)

Presentation

Injection—1mg in 2ml
—5mg in 1ml

Actions and uses

Alfentanil is a narcotic (morphine-like) analgesic which has a characteristically brief action i.e. approximately 30-45 minutes duration. It is widely used as an analgesic for short operative procedures e.g. in an out-patient setting when pain control can be readily adjusted by adjusting the rate of administration. Alfentanil is also used to enhance anaesthesia and reduce respiratory drive in ICU patients receiving assisted respiration.

An interesting development is the availability of alfentanil in transdermal patches which when applied to the skin release the drug at a slow but constant rate. It is thereafter gradually taken up by the skin circulation to provide a continuous background analgesia of 1-3 days duration. At the time of writing alfentanil patches are anticipated on the U.K. market within the following year.

Dosage

1. Administered by intravenous bolus injection with spontaneous respiration: 50–200 microgram with further doses of 50 microgram as required. Children: 3–5 microgram/kg with additional doses of 1 microgram/kg as required.
2. With assisted ventilation: 300–3500 microgram followed by 100–200 microgram as required. Children: 15 microgram/kg with additional doses of 1–3 microgram/kg as required.

Nurse monitoring

1. It is important to note that alfentanil is a potent respiratory depressant and patients not receiving assisted ventilation must be closely monitored.
2. It should be used with caution in situations where the occurrence of respiratory depression may pose a particular risk e.g. in myasthenia gravis, the elderly and debilitated, chronic respiratory disease, hypothyroidism, chronic liver disease, and obstetrics.
3. Other common side-effects include transient hypotension, bradycardia, nausea and vomiting.

General note

Alfentanil is a Controlled Drug and as such it must be stored in a locked cupboard, ordered by special requisition and its use recorded dose by dose, in line with current legislation.

ALGINIC ACID (Gastrocote, Gaviscon)

Presentation

Combined with various antacids in tablet, liquid and granular (sachet) form.

Actions and uses

Alginic acid forms a protective coating on the surface of gastric juice and therefore prevents reflux of gastric acid and bile into the oesophagus, and reduces the symptoms caused by such reflux. It should be used for the treatment of heartburn and dyspeptic pain when these are caused by hiatus hernia and reflux oesophagitis.

Dosage

1. Adults: 1–3 tablets or 10–20 ml (Gaviscon) after meals and at bedtime.
2. Children: one tablet or 5–10 ml liquid after meals and at bedtime.
3. Infants: a special formulation of infant Gaviscon is available for the very young. The dose is $1/2$–1 sachet mixed with water or with made up feeds.

Nurse monitoring

This drug is not associated with troublesome side-effects. It does however contain sugar and therefore if given to diabetics the amount of sugar in the preparation should be taken into account when formulating diabetic diets.

General note

Tablets, granules and liquid preparations containing alginic acid may be stored at room temperature. Tablets and granules should be thoroughly chewed before swallowing. The liquid may be diluted with up to an equal amount of water for ease of administration.

A

ALLOPURINOL (Zyloric)

Presentation

Tablets—100 mg, 300 mg

Actions and uses

If uric acid accumulates in excess in the blood, gout may be produced with subsequent arthritis, skin lesions and impairment of renal function. Increased blood urate occurs most commonly in patients suffering from classical gout and in patients with malignant disease who are treated with cytotoxic drugs or radiotherapy. In the latter case the increased urate is due to an increased destruction and turnover of cells. A less common cause of raised blood uric acid is diuretic therapy. Allopurinol may be used for the treatment of a raised blood uric acid. It acts by inhibiting one of the enzymes which take part in the production of uric acid from its constituent chemicals and it therefore reduces the total amount of uric acid produced.

Dosage

1. Adults:
   a. For the treatment of gout: Initially 100 mg once a day increasing to a maintenance dose of 300–900 mg per day in divided or single dosage.
   b. For treatment of hyperuricaemia in leukaemic patients: 200 mg three times a day for 3 days prior to treatment, then adjusted as required to a maintenance dose of 300 mg per day.
2. Children: Treatment of hyperuricaemia in leukaemia: Maintenance 20 mg/kg per day.

Nurse monitoring

1. When allopurinol treatment is commenced the blood urate is likely to fall. It has been found that any change in blood urate may lead to an acute attack of gout and therefore when allopurinol is commenced an anti-inflammatory analgesic drug is usually given concurrently for at least a month.

2. Side-effects which occasionally occur with this drug are nausea, vomiting and skin rashes. Rarely severe skin reactions, fever, joint pain and eosinophilia may occur.
3. Side-effects are more common in patients with kidney or liver disease and the dose should be reduced by an appropriate amount in patients with renal failure.
4. Allopurinol inhibits the liver metabolism of 6-mercaptopurine and azathioprine and the dosage of these drugs therefore has to be considerably reduced in such circumstances.

General note

Allopurinol tablets may be stored at room temperature.

ALTEPLASE (Actilyse, TpA)

Presentation

Dry powder for reconstitution. Vials containing 50 mg (equivalent to 29 million international units (i.u.)) or 20 mg (equivalent to 11.6 million i.u.).

Actions and uses

Actions and uses for alteplase are described in the section on thrombolytic drugs (q.v.).

Dosage

1. Adults: Acute myocardial infarction: a total dose of 100 mg alteplase (equivalent to 58 million i.u.) should be given intravenously over 3 hours as follows:

   a. An intravenous bolus over 1-2 minutes of 10% of the total dose.

   b. An infusion over the following hour of 50% of the total dose.

   c. An infusion over the subsequent 2 hours of 40% of total dose.

Note: Patients weighing less than 67 kg should receive a total dose of 1.5 mg/kg according to the above schedule.

1. Nurse monitoring notes for thrombolytic drugs (q.v.) apply to this drug.
2. The drug should be administered with great caution to patients with diabetes and severe renal failure.
3. There is no experience of the use of the drug in pregnancy. It is thus contraindicated.
4. Prior or concomitant administration of anticoagulants may increase the incidence of bleeding. Heparin has however been commonly administered in association with alteplase.

General notes
1. The drug should be stored below 25°C but reconstituted solution may be stored for up to 24 hours at 2-8°C and up to 8 hours at temperatures below 25°C. Vials should be kept in the original carton until preparation.
2. Prior to administration, the contents of a 50 mg injection vial should be dissolved in 50 ml water for injection (or a 20 mg vial dissolved in 20 ml water for injection). The contents of the reconstituted solution may be further diluted up to 1 in 5 with sterile sodium chloride intravenous infusion (BP 0.9% w/v). Water for injection or carbohydrate infusion solutions must not be used for this further dilution of alteplase.

ALLYLOESTRENOL (Gestanin)

Presentation
Tablets—5 mg
Actions and uses
1. The actions and uses of progestational hormones are described in the section on progestational hormones in Hormones (2).
2. In clinical practice this drug has three indications:
a. For the treatment of habitual abortion.
b. For the treatment of threatened abortion.
c. For the treatment of failure of nidation.

Dosage
1. For the treatment of habitual abortion—5–10 mg per day. Treatment may be continued for up to 16 weeks.
2. For the treatment of threatened abortion—5 mg three times per day for at least 5-7 days. If necessary daily dosage may be increased and the treatment period extended without risk.
3. For the treatment of failure of nidation—10–20 mg daily from the 16th to the 26th day of each cycle until conception is achieved. Thereafter 10 mg a day for at least 16 weeks.

Nurse monitoring
1. At the recommended doses no side-effects or other problems have been reported
2. In contrast to other pregnancy-maintaining progestational agents, virilisation of the fetus has not been reported with prolonged treatment.

General note
The drug may be stored at room temperature.

ALUMINIUM HYDROXIDE (Alu-Cap, Aludrox)

Presentation
Tablets—375 mg
Suspension/Gel—3.5–4.4% as aluminium oxide
Capsules—475 mg
Actions and uses
Aluminium hydroxide is an antacid used for the relief of dyspeptic pain and heartburn. Very high doses may in addition cure peptic ulcers, but few patients can tolerate the high doses required.
A further use of aluminium hydroxide is in chronic renal failure where there is reduced phosphate excretion by the kidney leading to high blood concentrations of phosphate.

Aluminium hydroxide binds to phosphate in the gut, reducing its absorption, and thus counterbalances the effect of the reduction in its excretion.

Dosage
1. For symptomatic relief of dyspeptic symptoms: 2 tablets or 10 ml suspension, 2-hourly if necessary. Alternatively 1 capsule may be taken regularly four times a day and at night on retiring.
2. For the treatment of hypophosphataemia in chronic renal failure: dosage should be individually determined.

Nurse monitoring
1. Constipation may occur. If used in combination with magnesium salts which tend to cause diarrhoea, this effect may be offset.
2. Neurological abnormalities may arise due to aluminium toxicity. This occurs only in patients with chronic renal failure who are taking very high doses.
3. Absorption and therefore clinical effectiveness of drugs such as salicylates, digoxin and antibiotics may be impaired.

General notes
1. Aluminium hydroxide preparations may be stored at room temperature.
2. Tablets should be chewed before swallowing and the suspension/gel thoroughly shaken before each dose is taken. Capsules are swallowed whole.

AMANTADINE (Symmetrel)

Presentation
Capsules—100 mg
Syrup—50 mg in 5 ml

Actions and uses
This drug was originally developed as an antiviral agent and was initially used for prophylaxis against and treatment of influenza. It still has a role in the treatment of herpes zoster. An additional benefit which was noticed in patients treated for infection was that it improves the symptoms of Parkinson's disease. The mechanism of action of this is unknown.

Dosage
1. Adults only:
   a. For Parkinson's disease: 100 mg once or twice daily.
   b. For the treatment of herpes zoster: 100 mg twice daily.
   c. For the treatment of influenza: 100 mg twice daily.

Nurse monitoring
1. This drug should be used with great caution in patients who have a past history of convulsion.
2. Side-effects involving the central nervous system may be severe and include: nervousness, insomnia, dizziness, convulsion, behavioural disturbance and hallucinations.
3. It should be noted that the beneficial effects of amantadine in the treatment of Parkinson's disease are short-lived, e.g. 4-6 weeks only.

General note
The drug may be stored at room temperature.

AMIKACIN (Amikin)

(See also Note 3, p. 362)

Presentation
Injection—500 mg in 2 ml
—100 mg in 2 ml

Actions and uses
Amikacin is an aminoglycoside antibiotic and its actions and uses are described in the section on these antibiotics. It may be effective in the treatment of infections due to gentamicin-resistant microorganisms.

Dosage
The dosage for adults and children is calculated on a basis of 15 mg/kg per day total, usually given in two divided doses by intramuscular or intravenous injections. Occasionally in adults as much as 500 mg 8-hourly may be given.

Nurse monitoring
1. The nurse monitoring notes for aminoglycoside antibiotics apply to amikacin.
2. Unlike gentamicin this drug may be given effectively by intravenous infusion in either normal saline, 5% dextrose or dextrose/saline mixtures.

General notes
1. The drug may be stored at room temperature.
2. The drug should never be mixed prior to administration with other antibiotics.

AMILORIDE (Midamor)

Presentation
Tablets—5 mg
Also combined with hydrochlorothiazide in Moduretic.

Actions and uses
Amiloride has a mild diuretic action. Its site of action is on the distal tubule where it inhibits active sodium reabsorption at the expense of potassium. It is of little use as a diuretic alone but it may be usefully combined with the thiazide and loop diuretics because of its potassium-conserving action. Amiloride is therefore used to prevent the hypokalaemia which is commonly encountered in patients treated with thiazide and loop diuretics alone. A more recent use is in aiding mucicilliary and cough clearance of sputum from the lungs of patients with cystic fibrosis, hence producing symptomatic improvement. Since amiloride can inhibit the active transport of sodium across membranes (the basis of its potassium-conserving diuretic action), it reduces the amount of sodium normally transported in excess across the airway epithelium which results in a thickened immobile mucus in patients with cystic fibrosis. Amiloride is administered by nebulizer for this purpose.

Dosage
1. The daily adult diuretic dose range is 5–20 mg taken as a single dose in the morning.
2. In cystic fibrosis doses of 3–4 ml of a 5 mmol/litre solution have been nebulized up to 4 times daily.

Nurse monitoring
1. Hyperkalaemia may occur, particularly in patients with impaired renal function. It is clinically undetectable, and extremely dangerous as it may lead to sudden death due to cardiac arrest.
2. Side-effects associated with oral therapy are as follows:
   a. Anorexia, nausea, vomiting, abdominal pain, constipation or diarrhoea
   b. Dry mouth, thirst, paraesthesia, dizziness, weakness, lethargy and muscle cramps
   c. Skin rashes, itching
   d. Mental confusion and visual disturbances.
3. In common with other diuretics, amiloride may alter blood glucose levels and therefore treatment requirements in diabetic patients may be altered.

General note
Amiloride tablets may be stored at room temperature. Nebulizer solutions should be freshly prepared and used within 1-2 weeks.

AMINOGLYCOSIDE ANTIBIOTICS

Amikacin
Gentamicin
Streptomycin
Tobramycin
Netilmicin
(See Note 3, p. 362 and Note 4, p. 366).

Presentation
See individual drugs.

Actions and uses
1. The aminoglycoside group of antibiotics has a predominantly bactericidal action, i.e. they kill bacteria present in body tissues.

They are effective against the following organisms:

a. Gram-negative pathogens including *E. coli*, proteus species and *Pseudomonas aeruginosa*
b. *Haemophilus influenza*
c. *Neisseria meningitidis.*

It is important to note that in recent years many organisms have developed resistance to drugs of this group.

These drugs are not sufficiently well absorbed to make oral administration effective. They can therefore only be given by the intravenous or intramuscular routes and because of this are reserved for the treatment of severe infections.

2. Superficial infections of the eye, ear and skin may be effectively treated by topical applications.

Dosage
See individual drugs.

Nurse monitoring

1. If excessive doses are administered, the 8th cranial nerve may be irreversibly damaged leading to deafness and difficulty with balance. High doses may also cause renal damage. These problems may nowadays be avoided by monitoring blood concentrations of the drug and adjusting doses appropriately. However, despite this the development of hearing or balance difficulties in a patient receiving aminoglycoside antibiotics should still be taken as an indication to stop the treatment.
2. Aminoglycoside antibiotics possess moderate muscle relaxant properties which may increase the effects of muscle relaxant drugs given during surgery.
3. The aminoglycoside, gentamicin, should always be given by bolus injection or rapid infusion and not by slow infusion as adequate blood levels cannot be maintained by the latter method of administration.

4. Aminoglycoside antibiotics are often given in combination with other antibiotics for the treatment of severe infections. It is important to note that they are chemically unstable and therefore may be rendered ineffective by mixing them before administration with other antibiotics, especially penicillin and cephalosporins.

General note
See individual drugs.

AMINOPHYLLINE (Phyllocontin)

Presentation
Tablets—100 mg
Tablets, slow release—100 mg, 225 mg, 350 mg
Injection—250 mg in 10 ml
Suppositories—5 mg, 50 mg, 150 mg and 360 mg

Actions and uses
Aminophylline produces three major effects which make it useful in clinical practice:

1. It produces relaxation of smooth muscle in the bronchi thus increasing airflow to the areas of oxygen exchange.
2. It stimulates the heart muscle and reduces congestion in the venous return to the heart.
3. It has a mild to moderate diuretic action.

It is used in the management of obstructive airways disease, e.g. asthma and chronic bronchitis, including status asthmaticus and in particular where respiratory disease is associated with heart failure, e.g. in cor pulmonale. It is also used in the management of apnoea in prematurity.

Dosage
1. Adults.
   a. Oral: 100–300 mg (conventional tablets) taken 3 or 4 times daily. Slow release tablets are used in a twice daily dosage of 225 mg to 450 mg.

b. Intravenous: 250 mg to 500 mg is administered very slowly (over 10-15 minutes) by bolus injection.
Alternatively, an intravenous infusion can be administered in sodium chloride 0.9% or dextrose 5% at a dosage of 500 microgram to 1 mg per kg per hour.

c. Rectal: One or two suppositories are inserted daily, usually at night for nocturnal wheezing.

2. Children:

a. Oral: Slow release tablets are used for older children 3-5 years or more, in a dose of 100–200 mg twice daily or as a single dose at bedtime for nocturnal wheeze.

b. Intravenous: A dose of 3 mg/kg body weight by bolus injection (over 15 minutes) is used. This may be followed if necessary by maintenance infusion at a rate of 800 microgram per kg per hour. Intravenous infusion has been administered in the management of apnoea in prematurity. Intramuscular injections have been given but this route is associated with extreme pain at the injection site.

c. Rectal: Up to 1 year—12.5–25 mg, 1-5 years—50–100 mg, 6-12 years—100-200 mg

Premature infants have received 5 mg suppositories on a 6-hourly basis for prevention of attacks of apnoea. Note that suppositories may be cut with a warmed knife to obtain non-standard dosages. Cuts should be made lengthwise to obtain quarter and half suppository quantities.

Nurse monitoring

1. The above dosages are for guidance only. In practice patients should have their blood theophylline (aminophylline is converted to theophylline) levels monitored. The precise dose is that which will maintain the blood theophylline level within the therapeutic range of 55–110 mmol/litre. Levels in excess of this range are associated with CNS toxicity.

2. It should be noted that certain factors may alter the theophylline blood level and might explain an apparent lack of effect or the sudden development of toxicity. Cimetidine, allopurinol and erythromycin may increase blood levels while barbiturates and cigarette smoking will reduce levels.

3. It is important to note that there is a major risk of very high (toxic) blood levels occurring rapidly after intravenous injection in patients already receiving aminophylline, theophylline or other drugs of this type by the oral or rectal routes. Intravenous injections should be avoided or given with extreme caution in these cases and it is important to determine in advance the patient's current drug therapy.

4. Gastrointestinal irritation is a major problem with oral therapy, particularly when conventional tablets are taken. It is much less likely if slow release tablets are used and patients who complain of dyspepsia may benefit from a change of theophylline preparation.

5. Suppositories are also irritant and frequently produce proctitis.

6. The other major side-effect which frequently occurs with blood levels in excess of the therapeutic range is CNS stimulation. This produces anxiety, confusion and restlessness and patients may complain of vertigo and show marked hyperventilation.

General notes

1. Preparations containing aminophylline may be stored at room temperature.

2. Suppositories must be kept in a cool place and not close to a radiator or other direct heat source since they are designed to melt at temperatures approaching body heat.

A

AMIODARONE (Cordarone X)

Presentation
Tablets—100 mg, 200 mg
Injection—150 mg in 3 ml

Actions and uses
Amiodarone is used for the treatment of cardiac dysrhythmias including paroxysmal supraventricular, nodal and ventricular tachycardias, atrial flutter and atrial fibrillation. It may be effective in dysrhythmias resistant to more commonly used drugs. It is thought to be of particular value in the treatment of paroxysmal arrhythmias associated with the Wolff-Parkinson-White syndrome.

Dosage
1. Adults:
   a. The initial loading regime is 200 mg 3 times a day for 1 week. This regime may be extended if a response is not achieved.
   b. To decide the maintenance dose the initial regime is gradually reduced until the lowest dose that will maintain control is obtained.

Nurse monitoring
1. During prolonged therapy patients have developed microcrystalline deposits of the drug in the cornea. These occasionally produce impairment of vision. Regular ophthalmic examinations are advised during prolonged treatment and should this side-effect arise, the drug should be stopped.
2. Peripheral neuropathy and tremor have occurred. These problems may be diminished or resolved by reduction in the dose but if they persist the drug should be withdrawn.
3. Photosensitivity and pigmentation of the skin may occur. Common side-effects include headaches, dizziness, nausea, vomiting and a metallic taste in the mouth. Sleep disturbance and nightmares also occur although these more frequently occur during the period of initial therapy and tend to diminish as maintenance doses are achieved.
4. The drug should be avoided or used with great caution in the following situations:
   a. Presence of sinus bradycardia or A-V block
   b. Where a patient has cardiac failure not controlled by digoxin and diuretic therapy
   c. Patients currently receiving beta-blockers or verapamil
   d. Those with a history of thyroid disease.
5. It is important to recognise that the drug may increase the serum level of digoxin in patients already receiving digoxin and the patient should therefore be carefully monitored for the side-effects which may arise.

General notes
1. The tablets may be stored at room temperature.
2. They should be protected from the light.

AMITRIPTYLINE (Tryptizol, Lentizol)

Presentation
Tablets—10 mg, 25 mg, 50 mg
Syrup—10 mg in 5 ml
Capsules—25 mg, 50 mg, 75 mg (all as sustained release)
Injection—10 mg in 1 ml

Actions and uses
Amitriptyline is a tricyclic antidepressant drug. Its actions and uses are described in the section on tricyclic antidepressant drugs.

Dosage
1. Orally for the treatment of depression: the usual dose range is 75–150 mg. The drug may be taken in three divided doses or as a single evening dose on retiring.
2. If given by the intramuscular or intravenous route: 20–30 mg four times daily is the usual required dose.
3. For the treatment of enuresis in children the following doses are administered:

a. Under 6 years: 10 mg in a single bed-time dose
b. 6-10 years: up to 20 mg in a single bed-time dose
c. 10-16 years: up to 50 mg in a single bed-time dose.

Nurse monitoring
As described in the section on tricyclic antidepressant drugs.

General notes
1. Preparations containing amitriptyline may be stored at room temperature.
2. The injection solution and syrup should be protected from light.
3. For ease of administration amitriptyline syrup may be diluted with Syrup B.P. before use but such dilutions must be used within 14 days.

AMLODIPINE (Istin)

Presentation
Tablets—5 mg, 10 mg

Actions and uses
Amlodipine is a calcium channel blocking drug (calcium antagonist) which possesses many of the properties described for nifedipine.

Dosage
Adults: a single daily dose of 5 mg which may be doubled depending upon the individual patient's response.

Nurse monitoring
The nurse monitoring section for Nifedipine applies to this drug.

General note
Amlodipine tablets may be stored at room temperature.

AMOXAPINE (Asendis)

Presentation
Tablets—25 mg, 50 mg, 100 mg, 150 mg

Action and uses
Amoxapine is an antidepressant which is chemically unrelated to the tricyclic antidepressants (e.g. amitriptyline, imipramine, etc; q.v.)

but nevertheless shares many of their properties. Like other antidepressants, it acts in the brain to boost levels of the neurotransmitter, noradrenaline. However, amoxapine also has central actions consistent with those of the neuroleptics or major tranquillisers and may therefore be of particular value in the treatment of psychotic depression which is unresponsive to an antidepressant drug alone.

Dosage
Adults: Initial doses of 100–150 mg daily are used and increased up to 300 mg depending upon clinical response. Amoxapine may be taken in divided doses throughout the day or if preferred as a single night-time dose.
Note: Lower doses are used in the elderly (see below).

Nurse monitoring
1. Nurse monitoring aspects for the tricyclic and related antidepressants (q.v.) also apply to this drug.
2. Lower initial doses are recommended for elderly patients e.g. 25 mg twice daily increased gradually over a period of one week to a maximum of 50 mg three times daily.
3. In common with other antidepressants, there may be a delay (though possibly as little as a few days only) before the benefits of treatment become apparent. Clinical improvement may continue for 1 month or more after treatment is started.
4. Early loss of efficacy, e.g. within 3 months of starting therapy, has been reported to occur in some patients treated with amoxapine. Regular supervision is essential in order to detect this, but non-compliance remains the likeliest cause of loss of effect.
5. Amoxapine should be avoided in patients who have sustained a recent myocardial infarction (e.g. within the previous 3-6 months), or in the presence of cardiac arrhythmias or heart block, mania, and severe liver disease.

General note

Amoxapine tablets may be stored at room temperature.

AMOXYCILLIN (Amoxil)

(See Note 3, p.362)

Presentation

Capsules—250 mg, 500 mg
Syrup—125 mg in 5 ml, 250 mg in 5 ml
Drops—125 mg in 1.25 ml
Injection—vials containing 250 mg, 500 mg and 1 g
Sachets—3 g

Actions and uses

Amoxycillin is an antibiotic of the penicillin group which has actions and uses identical to ampicillin (q.v.). It has an advantage over ampicillin when given by the oral route in that it is better absorbed from the gastrointestinal tract and may be given less frequently. By the parenteral route, however, it has little if any advantage over ampicillin.

Dosage

1. Oral:
   a. Adults and older children: 250–500 mg three times a day
   b. Children: 1-7 years—125–250 mg three times a day, less than 1 year—62.5 mg three times per day
2. Parenteral—The parenteral dosage is identical to the oral dosage.
3. Single (high) 3 g oral doses are available and may be repeated once at a 12-hourly interval. (These are used for short-term treatment of respiratory and urinary tract infections and prophylaxis of infective endo-carditis.)

Nurse monitoring

The nurse monitoring notes on ampicillin (q.v.) apply to this drug.

General notes

1. Preparations containing amoxycillin may be stored in dry powder form at room temperature.
2. When reconstituted with water for injection such solutions should be used immediately and any unused portion should be discarded.
3. Intravenous infusions should be given in 500 ml of sodium chloride 0.9%, dextrose 5% or dextrose/saline mixtures in the appropriate dose over 4-6 hours.
4. Syrup and suspension once prepared should be used within 7 days.

AMPHETAMINES AND RELATED DRUGS

Introduction

Because of the major problems of dependence and addiction associated with these drugs, discussion in this text will be restricted to an example of the group, namely dexamphetamine sulphate (Dexedrine).

Actions and uses

The amphetamines have two major clinical effects:

1. They produce a marked depression of appetite.
2. They produce a marked stimulation of neurological function.

In clinical practice they have only two indications:

1. For the treatment of narcolepsy
2. For the treatment of hyperkinetic states in children.

Dosage

1. For the treatment of narcolepsy: the recommended adult dose is 10 mg either in divided doses or as a single spansule in the morning. The dosage should be increased by 10 mg a day at weekly intervals to a maximum of 60 mg a day to obtain clinical response.
2. For the treatment of hyperkinetic states in children: Aged 3-5—2.5 mg a day increasing at weekly intervals by 2.5 mg, aged 6 and over—5–10 mg a day is recommended as a starting dose increasing by 5 mg at weekly intervals.

The usual upper limit of dosage for administration to children is 20 mg per day.

Nurse monitoring

1. The administration of amphetamines is associated with a serious risk of physical and psychological dependence. The administration of this drug is therefore entirely contraindicated other than for treatment of the conditions described above.
2. Side-effects include insomnia, restlessness, irritability, euphoria, tremor, dizziness, headache, dry mouth, anorexia, sweating, tachycardia, palpitations and moderate increase in blood pressure.
3. With higher doses symptoms of psychosis, indistinguishable from schizophrenia, may occur.
4. This drug should never be given to patients who are already receiving treatment with a monoamine oxidase inhibitor (q.v.) or in patients who have cardiovascular disease or hypertension or thyrotoxicosis.

General note

These drugs should be stored in a cool dry place and dispensed in moisture-proof containers. Restrictions on storage of 'controlled drugs' apply.

AMPHOTERICIN B (Ambisome, Fungilin, Fungizone)

Presentation

Tablets—100 mg
Suspension—100 mg in 1 ml
Lozenges—10 mg
Cream, ointment, lotion and oral (dental) paste—30 mg in 1 g
Pessaries—50 mg
Injection—50 mg vials
Vaginal cream—100 mg per 4 g application

Actions and uses

1. This drug is an effective antifungal agent useful against a wide variety of yeasts and yeast-like fungi including *Candida albicans*. It is important to note that absorption from the gut is negligible even with very large doses.
2. An intravenous preparation is available which is effective against cryptococcosis (Torulopsis), North American blastomycosis, the disseminated forms of candidosis, coccidiomycosis and histoplasmosis, and also aspergillosis and other extremely rare fungal infections.

Dosage

1. Ointment and cream preparations should be applied two to four times daily.
2. Lozenges are sucked four times daily.
3. Oral suspension should be applied four times daily.
4. Vaginal cream is inserted at night.
5. Pessaries should be inserted at night.
6. Tablets may be administered in a dose of one or two four times daily.
7. Parenteral therapy: For adults and children the total daily dose should be administered by slow intravenous infusion over a period of 6 hours. The dosage is calculated on the basis of initially 0.25 mg/kg body weight, gradually increasing to a level of 1 mg/kg body weight depending on individual response and tolerance.
8. Ambisome is a special formulation containing amphotericin in a fat emulsion carrier (liposome). This renders the drug much less toxic to the kidney and allows double and even treble the above dosage to be used in serious fungal infections unresponsive to conventional amphotericin doses.

Nurse monitoring

1. In treatment of the serious infections for which parenteral therapy is used, the duration of therapy may be extended to months and patients may require a great deal of psychological support.
2. Intravenous infusion may cause fever, rigor, headache, anorexia, weight loss, nausea, vomiting, malaise, painful muscles and joints, dyspepsia and cramping stomach pains, diarrhoea, anaemia and hypokalaemia.

3. The intravenous infusion may also cause irritation and thrombophlebitis at the injection site.
4. The intravenous infusion may cause renal failure, disturbance of cardiac rhythm, visual defects and convulsions.
5. The drug should be used with great caution in patients who are known to have kidney disease.
6. The drug should be used with great caution if other drugs known to damage the kidney are also being given, such as gentamicin or cephaloridine, and concurrent administration of corticosteroids is absolutely contraindicated.
7. Some gastrointestinal upset has followed the use of oral tablets which are otherwise without side-effects.
8. For intravenous infusions the final concentration of solutions for infusion must not exceed 0.1 mg in 1 ml.

General notes
1. Topical preparations, tablets and suspension may be stored at room temperature.
2. Powder for infusion should be refrigerated.
3. Ambisome brand of amphotericin is prepared under special conditions—seek advice from the Pharmacy.

AMPICILLIN (Penbritin)

(See Note 3, p. 362)
Presentation
Capsules—250 mg, 500 mg
Tablets—125 mg
Syrup and suspension—125 mg in 5 ml, 125 mg in 1.25 ml, dropper, 250 mg in 5 ml
Injection—Vials containing 250 mg and 500 mg
Actions and uses
Ampicillin is an antibiotic of the penicillin group. It is bactericidal, i.e. it kills cells present in the body. It does this by interfering with the synthesis of substances necessary to maintain the bacterial cell wall and therefore causes the cells to burst. It has a wider spectrum of antibacterial activity than Benzylpenicillin (q.v.) and is effective against Gram-positive and Gram-negative cocci and some Gram-positive and Gram-negative bacilli. It is therefore used for the treatment of ear, nose and throat infections, bronchitis, pneumonia, urinary tract infection, gonorrhoea, gynaecological infections, septicaemia, peritonitis, endocarditis, meningitis, enteric fever and gastrointestinal infections when they are caused by the above organisms.
Dosage
1. Oral:
   a. Adults and older children: 250-500 mg four times a day.
   b. Children: 1-7 years—125–250 mg four times a day. Children less than 1 year—62.5 mg four times per day
2. Parenteral: Parenteral doses are the same as for oral dose, although in severe illness higher doses may be used.
3. Ampicillin injection is occasionally used by local instillation either intrapleurally, intraperitoneally or intra-articularly. 500 mg in 5-10 ml of water for injection is given.

Nurse monitoring
1. It is important to note that ampicillin is an effective drug when taken orally.
2. Ampicillin is associated with a low incidence of the production of skin rashes.
3. The drug may produce serious effects in the few patients who are hypersensitive to it. These range from urticaria to anaphylactic shock.
4. Diarrhoea is a common problem with ampicillin.

General notes
1. Preparations containing ampicillin may be stored in dry powder form at room temperature.
2. When reconstituted with water for

injection such solutions should be used immediately and any unused portion should be discarded.

3. Intravenous infusions should be given in 500 ml of sodium chloride 0.9%, dextrose 5% or dextrose/saline mixtures in the appropriate dose over 4-6 hours.

4. Syrup and suspension once prepared should be used within 7 days.

AMSACRINE (Amsidine, m-AMSA)

Presentation
Injection—75mg ampoule

Actions and uses
Amsacrine is a cytotoxic drug which blocks the synthesis of DNA and hence cell proliferation by binding DNA through a mechanism known as intercalation. A toxic effect on the cell membrane is also likely to explain its action.

This drug has been used mainly in the treatment of acute leukaemia in adults either as remission induction or maintenance therapy.

Dosage
This is largely determined by specific indication and current schedules which are subject to change in line with existing knowledge. The existing schedule should be consulted for up-to-date details of dosage and route of administration. Courses of 90 mg–120/m^2 daily have been given for induction up to a total dose of 450 mg/m^2 and maintenance doses of about one-third of this used thereafter.

Nurse monitoring
1. Myelosuppression with pancytopenia leading to infection and haemorrhage is the major toxicity of this drug which limits the total dose that can be given. Treatment can be monitored by the use of a bone marrow biopsy.

2. Frequent side-effects include nausea (but not necessarily vomiting) and ulceration of the buccal mucosa and oesophagus.

3. CNS toxicity has resulted in generalized seizures requiring treatment with an anticonvulsant drug.

4. Amsacrine is also potentially toxic to the liver, kidney and heart and has produced jaundice, acute renal failure and cardiac failure and arrhythmias.

5. The incidence of alopecia with this drug is relatively high.

6. Severe local irritation and phlebitis results from extravasation of amsacrine and care is required when siting the needle: the infusion site should be closely examined during and following intravenous administration. Amsacrine must be diluted before use, see below.

7. The nurse should be constantly aware that most cytotoxic drugs are irritant to the skin and mucous surfaces and are in general very toxic. Great care should therefore be exercised when handling these drugs and, in particular, spillage or contamination of personnel or the environment must be avoided. If cytotoxic drugs are handled regularly it is theoretically possible that repeated skin contact or inhalation may produce systemic toxic effects and in nurses who have developed hypersensitivity, severe local and general hypersensitivity reactions.

General notes
1. Amsacrine may be stored at room temperature and should be protected from light.

2. Glass syringes only should be used when preparing intravenous infusions. The drug must be diluted in 500 ml glucose 5% and infused over 60-90 minutes. It must not be diluted in sodium chloride solutions.

3. Infusions must be used within 8 hours of preparation and be protected from light.

AMYLOBARBITONE (Amytal, Sodium Amytal)

Presentation
Tablets—15 mg, 30 mg, 50 mg, 100 mg and 200 mg
Tablets and capsules (as the sodium salt)—100 mg, 200 mg
Injection—250 mg, 500 mg (as the sodium salt)

Actions and uses
As described in the section on barbiturate drugs.
1. Amylobarbitone, base is used for day-time sedation.
2. The sodium salt of amylobarbitone, which has a slightly more rapid onset of action than the base, is taken at night as a hypnotic.

Dosage
1. For day-time sedation:
   a. 15–50 mg may be taken orally three or four times daily.
   b. Up to 500 mg may be given by the intramuscular route in adults.
   c. It is also possible to administer this drug by slow intravenous injection and up to 1 g may be given slowly.
2. For night sedation: Up to 200 mg may be administered as a single dose prior to retiring.

Nurse monitoring
As described in the section on barbiturates.

General note
Capsules and tablets containing amylobarbitone and amylobarbitone sodium may be stored at room temperature.

ANISTREPLASE (Eminase)

Presentation
Vials containing 30 units

Actions and uses
This drug, previously known as APSAC or Anisoylated Plasminogen Streptokinase Activator Complex, binds selectively to a preformed blood clot after which the strepto-kinase portion of the molecule is activated. Its actions and uses are described under thrombolytic drugs.

Dosage
Adults: A single daily dose of 5 mg which may be doubled depending upon the individual patient's response.

Nurse monitoring
1. The nurse monitoring notes for Thrombolytic Drugs (q.v.) apply to this drug.
2. The drug is contraindicated in pregnancy.
3. Early reactions include flushing, bradycardia and transient hypotension.
4. Allergic reactions include bronchoconstriction and anaphylaxis but are uncommon and usually reversible.
5. The most common complication associated with thrombolytic therapy is bleeding; this can be controlled by local pressure at the sites of intravenous cannulae.

General notes
1. The drug should be reconstituted by dissolving the contents of a 30 ml vial with 5 ml water for injection BP or normal sodium chloride injection BP 0.9% w/v. No other medication should be added to the vial or syringe containing eminase.
2. Reconstituted solution must not be administered by intramuscular injection or added to intravenous infusion fluids.
3. The drug must be stored at 2-8°C (not frozen). If removed from a refrigerator it must be used within 2-3 hours or discarded.
4. Reconstituted solution should be administered as soon as possible. If unused after 30 minutes the solution must be discarded.

ANTICONVULSANTS

The drugs used in the treatment of epilepsy include:
Carbamazepine
Clonazepam
Ethosuximide
Gabapentin
Lamotrigine
Methylphenobarbitone
Phenobarbitone
Phenytoin
Primidone
Sodium Valproate
Vigabratin

Presentation

See individual drugs.

Actions and uses

The epilepsies are a group of chronic disorders which may be classified as follows:

1. Grand mal epilepsy. In this the patient characteristically suffers repeated episodes of sudden loss of consciousness known commonly as a convulsion, accompanied by cessation of breathing, cyanosis, tongue-biting and rapid and irregular movements of the limbs. Patients frequently micturate during a convulsion and after the convulsion may remain unconscious for a number of hours and suffer headache on recovery.

2. Petit mal epilepsy. This is characterized by short periods wherein although the patient does not lose consciousness or develop abnormal muscular movement they actually lose awareness of their surroundings, noticed because their teachers or parents observe that they have periods of inattention.

3. Temporal lobe epilepsy. This form of epilepsy does not have a characteristic clinical presentation, but takes the form of paroxysmal episodes of alteration in behaviour or personality.

All forms of epilepsy are thought to be due to abnormal bouts of electrical activity in the brain. The anticonvulsants act by suppressing the abnormal activity and thus reducing the frequency.

Dosage

See individual drugs.

Nurse monitoring

1. Anticonvulsant therapy frequently has to be taken throughout life. The nurse may play an important role in emphasising, particularly to patients who are on successful therapy and who have therefore not had a fit for some time, that tablets should be regularly taken and dosage should only be altered after consultation with medical staff.

2. The second most important point to know about any anticonvulsant treatment is that it must not under any circumstances be suddenly stopped as this may precipitate the serious and life-threatening state of status epilepticus and the patient may suffer prolonged severe and repeated episodes of convulsions.

3. The nurse may also play an important role in detecting the adverse effects of anticonvulsant treatment which are due either to excessive dosage or to side-effects. These are discussed more fully under the specific drug headings.

4. It is important to note that a number of drugs may affect anticonvulsant control and frequency of convulsions and they should therefore be used with great caution in epileptic patients. These include phenothiazines (q.v.), tricyclic antidepressants (q.v.), isoniazid and lignocaine.

5. Epilepsy still carries, both with patients and the general public, an impression of abnormality which may lead to great social stress. The nurse may play an important role in encouraging a more enlightened approach to this illness in both patients and their relatives and the public in general.

6. Anticonvulsants can affect liver enzyme systems which are involved in the metabolism of many types of drugs. This may

A

lead to an alteration in the effect of other drugs given to patients already receiving anticonvulsants. Examples of this are with oral contraceptives which may be ineffective if anticonvulsants are being coincidentally administered. The dosage of anticoagulants may also have to be altered.

General note
See individual drugs.

ANTI-D IMMUNOGLOBULIN (Partobulin)

Presentation
Injection—1250 international units (i.u.) in 1 ml

Actions and uses
Anti-D immunoglobulin is administered to Rhesus negative women to prevent sensitization and formation of antibodies to fetal Rhesus positive cells which may mix with maternal blood during childbirth or abortion. In this way any subsequent child is protected from the danger of haemolytic disease of the newborn.

Dosage
1250 units is administered by intramuscular injection immediately or within 72 hours of childbirth or abortion. The same dose may be given at weeks 28 and 34 of pregnancy but this does not replace its use following birth.

Nurse monitoring
1. Rubella vaccination can be carried out at the same time anti-D is administered but different syringes and injection sites should be used and a test for rubella antibodies should follow 2 months or more later.
2. MMR vaccine should not be administered within 3 months of a dose of anti-D.

General note
This product has a shelf life of 3 years when stored in a refrigerator.

ANTIHISTAMINES

Introduction
This group of drugs comprises many different chemicals with a common action.

Actions and uses
Antihistamines block the effect at specific sites in the body of histamine, a chemical which is released in the body as part of the allergic or inflammatory response and which is therefore partly responsible for the production of inflammation, erythema and pruritus which accompany such reactions. The antihistamine group of drugs has in addition further effects on the autonomic nervous system and the central nervous system. In clinical practice they are used for the treatment of the following:
1. To suppress generalized minor allergic responses to allergens such as foodstuffs and drugs.
2. To suppress local allergic reactions, i.e. inflammatory skin responses to insect stings and bites, contact allergens, urticaria etc.
3. Orally and in eye drops for allergic ocular inflammatory conditions, e.g. due to hay fever and allergic rhinitis.
4. As nasal decongestants, e.g. in the treatment of allergic rhinitis and hay fever. They are also added to a few proprietary cough preparations because of their decongestant action.
5. In the treatment of nausea and vomiting, particularly motion sickness.
6. As an anti-pruritic agent.
7. They are also used for the treatment of vertigo and the symptoms of vertigo and nausea due to Menière's disease.

Dosage
See individual drugs.

Nurse monitoring
1. The older antihistamines have a sedative effect and may cause marked drowsiness, while some newer agents (e.g. astemizole, terfenadine) do not. In some

clinical situations sedative antihistamines are actually used for this effect, but where they are used for their other clinical effects, drowsiness may prove a troublesome side-effect and the nurse may contribute to patient management by re-emphasising the dangers of driving or using industrial machinery while receiving these drugs.
2. Common side-effects include headache, blurred vision, tinnitus, sleep disturbance, gastrointestinal upset and, in susceptible patients, urinary retention.
3. Topical applications of antihistamines may produce skin sensitization and subsequent eczematous and other eruptions.

General note
See individual drugs.

ASPARAGINASE

Presentation
Injection—10,000 units per vial
Actions and uses
Asparaginase is a cytotoxic drug. It is an enzyme obtained from cultures of Erwinia. It interferes with the synthesis of a specific amino acid required for the growth of malignant cells and therefore reduces the capacity of those cells to both grow and multiply. Its major use is in the induction of remission of acute lymphoblastic leukaemia. It has also been occasionally used in the treatment of acute myeloid leukaemia.
Dosage
It is important to note that a proportion of patients are hypersensitive to the drug and therefore all patients should receive an intradermal test dose of 50 i.u. and the injection site should be observed for 3 hours for signs of tissue reaction. If tissue reaction occurs this would be a contraindication to using the drug in its standard dosage. The usual initial dose is 200 units/kg body weight daily by slow intravenous injection or infusion over 20-30

minutes. Doses are then increased to a maximum of 1000 i.u./kg according to individual response. It is recommended that the course of treatment should be continuous as interruption and recommencement of treatment increases the risk of sensitivity reactions.

Nurse monitoring
1. As noted above all patients should receive an intradermal test dose prior to commencing full treatment.
2. Gastrointestinal side-effects include anorexia, nausea and vomiting.
3. Suppression of bone marrow function may result in anaemia and increased risk of infection due to suppression of white cell function.
4. In addition to bone marrow suppression which results in thrombocytopenia, levels of fibrinogen and clotting factors are also suppressed by this drug and therefore there is a marked risk of haemorrhage during treatment.
5. Impaired liver function, pancreatitis and hyperglycaemia have also been observed during treatment with this drug.
6. The nurse should be constantly aware that most cytotoxic drugs are irritant to the skin and mucous surfaces, and are in general very toxic. Great care should therefore be exercised when handling these drugs, and in particular spillage or contamination of personnel or the environment must be avoided. If cytotoxic drugs are handled regularly it is theoretically possible that repeated skin contact or inhalation may produce systemic toxic effects and in nurses who have developed hypersensitivity, severe local and general hypersensitivity reactions.

General notes
1. Vials for injection should be stored in a refrigerator.

2. The vials are reconstituted using the accompanying 10 ml sodium chloride 0.9% ampoules.

3. The prepared solution is administered by slow intravenous injection or as a rapid infusion (20-30 minutes) in 0.9% sodium chloride solution.

ASPIRIN (Platet, Solprin)

Presentation
Tablets—75 mg, 100 mg, 300 mg (including enteric-coated).

Actions and uses
1. Aspirin relieves pain and reduces inflammation in a variety of diseases affecting the joints, tendons, cartilages and muscles. To produce a significant anti-inflammatory effect in patients with chronic arthropathy very high regular doses are required.

2. Aspirin is an effective analgesic for minor painful disorders such as headache, toothache or muscle strain.

3. Aspirin may be used as an antipyretic to lower the temperature of fevered patients.

4. The antiplatelet action of aspirin has long been recognised and probably accounts for its major use today. Aspirin irreversibly blocks the synthesis of a prostaglandin, thromboxane A2, by the platelet in response to injury to the vascular epithelium. In the presence of this substance, platelets adhere to form a platelet plug which under normal circumstances reduces bleeding and promotes blood clotting. Aspirin is so potent in this respect that it can inhibit platelet aggregation and prevent clotting at very low concentrations. This has led to the widespread use of aspirin in the following situations:

   a. Prevention of stroke in patients with transient ischaemic attacks thought likely to be due to microembolization following platelet aggregation.

   b. Acute myocardial infarction in which aspirin adds considerably to the effectiveness of thrombolytic therapy in increasing survival.

   c. Primary prevention of myocardial infarction in patients with symptoms of coronary heart disease and secondary prevention of re-infarction and sudden death in the period following myocardial infarction.

   d. To improve prognosis after coronary artery by-pass graft surgery and vascular surgery of the lower limbs.

   e. Prevention of stroke in patients with non-rheumatic atrial fibrillation who are otherwise considered unsuitable for oral anticoagulant therapy.

Dosage
1. Adults:

   a. The usual adult anti-inflammatory dose range is 1200 mg to 4 g per day taken in divided doses, often with or after meals in an attempt to reduce gastric irritation.

   b. When used as an antithrombotic drug, single daily doses of 75 mg or 300 mg are taken.

Nurse monitoring
1. The nurse monitoring points described under non-steroid anti-inflammatory analgesic drugs are applicable to aspirin.

2. The use of aspirin in children is no longer recommended. This follows the observation that Reye's syndrome, a potentially fatal condition affecting the central nervous system, occurred in a number of young children with febrile illness who received aspirin. Although a clear association was not shown, safer alternatives now exist and should be used.

3. Toxic effects specific to aspirin are as follows:

a. Mild symptoms of intoxication include dizziness, tinnitus, sweating, nausea, vomiting, mental confusion.

b. More serious signs of toxicity include fever, ketosis, hyperventilation, respiratory alkalosis and metabolic acidosis. This may lead to shock, respiratory failure and coma.

c. It must be remembered that the early features of toxicity as described above may not occur in children who may present initially with the more serious effects described.

4. Aspirin is readily available in many 'over the counter' preparations. As it has serious potential side-effects the nurse should take every opportunity to advise the patient against taking aspirin for minor painful complaints and should encourage the use of other drugs such as paracetamol with less serious side-effects.

General notes

1. Aspirin tablets may be stored at room temperature but it is important to remember that they must be kept in a dry atmosphere since in a moist atmosphere the drug may be converted to acetic acid and may therefore be inactive. Drugs which have been inactivated in this way may be detected by their strong 'vinegary' smell.

2. Several forms of proprietary medicines which contain aspirin are included in a wide range of compound (mixed) preparations, many of which are bought over the counter as cold cures.

3. Because of the very high incidence of gastrointestinal upset associated with aspirin, it is almost always prescribed in soluble form. It is important to remember that the soluble form is not free from such effects.

ASTEMIZOLE (Hismanal)

Presentation

Tablets—10 mg
Oral suspension—5 mg in 5 ml

Actions and uses

Astemizole is an antihistamine and the actions and uses of these drugs in general are described in the antihistamine section. Note however that astemizole is long acting and lacks the marked sedative effect of the majority of drugs of this type. In practice, it is used in the management of hay fever, allergic rhinitis and allergic skin disorders.

Dosage

Adults: 10 mg taken once daily before one of the main meals.
Children (over 5 years): 5mg once daily as above.

Nurse monitoring

1. See the section on antihistamines.

2. During 1992 the Committee on Safety of Medicines drew attention to the possibility that serious cardiac dysrhythmias may arise in patients who receive excessive doses or in whom plasma concentrations are otherwise likely to be raised. The latter may arise if erythromycin is co-prescribed with astemizole. The drug is best avoided in patients with heart disease who may be predisposed to ventricular rhythm disturbances.

General note

Astemizole tablets and suspension may be stored at room temperature.

ATENOLOL (Tenormin)

Presentation

Tablets—25 mg, 50 mg, 100 mg
Injection—5 mg in 10 ml
Syrup—25 mg in 5 ml

Actions and uses

Atenolol is a cardioselective beta-blocking drug and its actions and uses are described in the section on beta-blockers.

Dosage
1. This drug is particularly long acting and single daily doses of 100–200 mg in adults are usually adequate.
2. By injection in cardiac dysrhythmias, 2.5 mg by slow intravenous injection (over $2^1/_2$ minutes) repeated after 5 minute intervals to a maximum total dose of 10 mg.

Nurse monitoring
1. See beta-adrenoreceptor blocking drugs.
2. Atenolol is a particularly useful drug in patients who have experienced central nervous system side-effects from other beta-blockers such as nightmares and hallucinations.

General note
Atenolol may be stored at room temperature.

ATRACURIUM (Tracrium)

Presentation
Injection—25 mg in 2.5 ml
—50 mg in 5 ml
—250 mg in 25 ml

Actions and uses
Atracurium is a muscle relaxant of the non-depolarizing type. Thus it reversibly paralyses skeletal muscle by competitive inhibition of acetylcholine, the transmitter substance released at the junction of the (motor) nerve and muscle fibre (motor end-plate receptor).
Drugs of this type are used to produce muscle relaxation during surgical anaesthesia.

Dosage
Adults and children: Initially 300–600 microgram/kg followed by 100–200 microgram/kg as required by bolus intravenous injection. May also be administered by intravenous infusion at a rate 5–10 microgram/kg/minute (300–600 microgram/kg/hour).

Nurse monitoring
1. All patients must have their respiration assisted or controlled.
2. Muscle relaxants of this type are also used to produce paralysis in patients on assisted ventilation in ICUs.
3. Overdosage with muscle relaxant drugs of this type may result in paralysis of the respiratory muscles. If this occurs, an anticholinesterase such as neostigmine (which potentiates acetylcholine by blocking its inactivation) must be administered.

General note
Atracurium injection should be stored in a refrigerator and protected from light.

ATROPINE

Introduction
Atropine is the main component of the belladonna alkaloids, a family of complex chemicals found widely in nature but notably in the deadly nightshade plant. Hyoscine (scopolamine) is chemically closely related to atropine and the same considerations apply to both drugs in clinical practice. Atropine is generally in use as atropine sulphate and hyoscine as hyoscine hydrobromide.

Presentation
Injection—600 microgram in 1 ml; 500 microgram in 5 ml; 1 mg in 10 ml
Eye drops and ointment—1%

Actions and uses
Atropine blocks the actions of the neurotransmitter, acetylcholine, at nerve endings (muscarinic sites) in the parasympathetic nervous system. This action is often referred to as 'anticholinergic' or more accurately 'antimuscarinic' which denotes the precise site of acetylcholine blockade. Atropine has several uses in clinical practice:
1. It increases heart rate by blocking the restraining effects of the vagus nerve on the sinus node

and for this reason is used in the treatment of sinus bradycardia, especially if complicated by hypotension following myocardial infarction. It may also be administered in asystolic cardiac arrest unresponsive to DC shock therapy.

2. It reduces bronchial and salivary secretions and is used in pre-operative medication to inhibit excess of these secretions in response to intubation and some inhalation anaesthetics.

3. In the eye, atropine dilates the pupil and causes prolonged paralysis of the ciliary muscle i.e. it is a mydriatic and long acting cycloplegic, and is used for refraction procedures and in the treatment of iridocyclitis. Homatropine may also be used for this indication.

4. It reduces gut motility and may be used as a gastrointestinal antispasmodic (gastrointestinal sedative) in irritable bowel syndrome and diverticular disease, though hyoscine and other synthetic antimuscarinic drugs are more often used. Atropine is also combined with diphenoxylate in the antidiarrhoeal preparation, Lomotil.

5. It reduces gastric acid secretion and may be used to relieve dyspeptic symptoms, usually in antacids sold over the counter which contain atropine in the form of belladonna extract. However, antimuscarinics are now rarely used to treat peptic ulcer.

6. Atropine is often given at the same time as a cholinesterase inhibitor e.g. neostigmine when it is used to reverse the effects of certain muscle relaxant drugs administered during surgery. Atropine prevents bradycardia and excessive salivation which might otherwise occur in response to the anticholinesterase agent.

7. For similar reasons to 6. above, atropine is administered in emergencies associated with organophosphorus poisoning.

These agents are commonly used as pesticides in agriculture and are potent and irreversible inhibitors of acetylcholinesterase. If swallowed, inhaled or absorbed in quantity through the skin, widespread and often fatal overstimulation of the sympathetic nervous system results. Organophosphorus agents also form the main group of chemical (non-biological) warfare nerve gases.

Dosage

1. Cardiac arrhythmias:
   a. Sinus bradycardia—300 microgram repeated if required.
   b. Asystolic cardiac arrest—single dose of 3 mg by slow intravenous injection.

2. Pre-operative medication:
   a. Adults—300–600 microgram 30 minutes to 1 hour before induction anaesthesia. Usually by intramuscular injection.
   b. Children—20 microgram/kg as above.

3. Ophthalmology: Single drop 1 hour before refraction. Used daily in uveitis.

4. Control of side-effects to neostigmine when used to reverse the effects of muscle relaxant drugs in surgery—600 microgram to 1.2 mg by intravenous injection at the same time that neostigmine is administered.

5. Organophosphorus poisoning: 2 mg by intravenous (if severe poisoning) or intramuscular (less severe poisoning) injection, repeated until the skin becomes flushed and dry, the pupils are dilated and tachycardia occurs.

Nurse monitoring

1. The side-effects of atropine can be summed up as a representation of parasympathetic underactivity or resultant unrestrained sympathetic activity.

2. They include typically dry mouth, flushing, dry skin, swallowing difficulty due to reduced oesophageal motility, tachycardia and palpitations, dilatation of the pupil and loss of accommodation, raised intraocular pressure, urinary retention, and constipation.
3. It follows that the elderly, in particular, may be vulnerable to the above effects. Caution is warranted in patients with dysphagia, reflux oesophagitis, myocardial insufficiency, glaucoma, lower GI obstruction, and prostatic hypertrophy.

General note
Preparations containing atropine are stored at room temperature.

AURANOFIN (Ridaura)

Presentation
Tablets—3 mg
Actions and uses
Auranofin is a gold salt used in the treatment of active rheumatoid arthritis which is progressive and unresponsive to other first line treatments. It is one of a number of agents which collectively are termed 'disease modifying' although its precise mechanism of action is unknown (its antirheumatic action was discovered by accident). Gold salts inhibit production of the inflammatory mediator prostaglandins, but they also bind to products of the immune response such as immunoglobulins and complement and in doing so may modify the autoimmune process which underlies rheumatoid arthritis.

Dosage
Adults only: Initially, 3 mg twice daily or 6 mg as a single daily dose is given for up to 6 months and the response is then assessed. Thereafter, the dose may be increased to 3 mg three times daily but treatment should be discontinued if there is no response within a further 3 months.

Nurse monitoring
1. It is important that patients realise that there may be a delay of 1-2 months before a response is achieved in order that good compliance is maintained during the early treatment period.
2. Gold salts are poorly tolerated by many patients and some adverse reactions are particularly severe. For example it is estimated that as many as 5% will experience a severe reaction so that close support and careful monitoring of the patient is therefore essential.
3. Diarrhoea, nausea and abdominal pain are common. The incidence of diarrhoea may be reduced by combined use of dietary fibre supplement (e.g. bran) which bulks the stool.
4. Adverse effects which must be reported immediately include oral ulceration (a possible sign of haematological toxicity), altered (metallic) taste sensation, bleeding, skin reactions, peripheral neuritis, breathlessness, alopecia, and jaundice.
5. Regular blood counts are recommended.
6. Contraindications to auranofin include existing liver and kidney impairment, exfoliative dermatitis, systemic lupus erythematosus, a history of blood disorders suggestive of bone marrow aplasia, pulmonary fibrosis, and enterocolitis.
7. Auranofin must not be administered during pregnancy.

General note
Auranofin tablets may be stored at room temperature.

AZAPROPAZONE (Rheumox)

Presentation
Capsules—300 mg
Tablets—600 mg
Actions and uses
See the section on non-steroidal anti-inflammatory analgesic drugs.

This drug is generally reserved for the treatment of acute gout.

Dosage

The initial adult dose is 1200 mg daily taken in two to four divided doses. Once adequate clinical effect has been obtained, the dose is reduced to the minimum that will continue to keep the patient comfortable.

Nurse monitoring

1. See the section on non-steroidal anti-inflammatory analgesic drugs.
2. It should be noted that this drug is particularly likely to interact with warfarin so increasing the possibility of haemorrhage. Reduced daily doses of warfarin may therefore be required if azapropazone is commenced in an anticoagulated patient and close monitoring of the prothrombin time is essential for the first 48 hours.

General note

Azapropazone capsules may be stored at room temperature.

AZATADINE (Optimine)

Presentation

Tablets—1 mg
Syrup—0.5 mg in 5 ml

Actions and uses

Azatadine is an antihistamine. The actions and uses of antihistamines in general are described in the antihistamine section. Azatadine is used specifically:

1. To suppress generalized minor allergic responses to allergens such as foodstuffs and drugs.
2. To suppress local allergic reactions, i.e. inflammatory skin responses to insect stings and bites, contact allergens, urticaria etc.
3. Orally for other allergic conditions, e.g. hay fever and allergic rhinitis.

Dosage

1. Adults: 1–2 mg b.d.
2. Children: 6-12 years—1 mg b.d.

Nurse monitoring

See the section on antihistamines.

General note

The drug may be stored at room temperature.

AZATHIOPRINE (Imuran)

Presentation

Tablets—25 mg, 50 mg
Injection—Vials containing 50 mg

Actions and uses

Azathioprine is slowly converted in the body to its active derivative 6-mercaptopurine. It has the following actions:

1. It suppresses the immune response after organ or tissue transplantation and therefore prevents tissue rejection and enhances the survival and function of transplanted organs.
2. It is also used in a number of other diseases where it appears to alter the disease process producing an improvement in symptoms. Examples of such diseases are rheumatoid arthritis, systemic lupus erythematosus and Crohn's disease.

Dosage

1. For immunosuppression after organ transplantation: The recommended dose is 1–4 mg/kg body weight daily (average 2.4 mg/kg).
2. For the treatment of the other diseases mentioned above: It is usually given in a dose range of 1–2.5 mg/kg.
3. It may be given by intravenous injection at the above doses for short periods when oral treatment is unsuitable.
4. The combination of azathioprine with a corticosteroid drug usually permits the use of lower doses of both drugs while maintaining their clinical effect.

Nurse monitoring

1. Azathioprine commonly causes gastrointestinal upset and symptoms include anorexia, nausea, vomiting and diarrhoea.

2. It depresses the bone marrow and seems particularly to affect white cell function leading to an increased risk of infection. Patients suffering from acute infection therefore should never be given the drug. Infections by bacteria, fungi, protozoa and viruses which do not normally occur in healthy adults may occur in patients on this drug.
3. It should be used with caution in patients who have existing liver disease and cases of hepatitis and biliary stasis have been reported. Despite this it is worth noting that it is actually used in the treatment of active chronic hepatitis.
4. The drug has been shown to cause fetal abnormality if taken either during pregnancy, or by the father prior to conception. It is important therefore to encourage patients to take adequate contraceptive measures.
5. Serious toxic effects will occur when the drug tends to accumulate in the body. This will occur in two instances:
   a. In patients with reduced renal function.
   b. In patients who are also taking allopurinol which inhibits the body's capacity to metabolise azathioprine. In such cases the dose of azathioprine should be reduced accordingly.

General notes
1. Azathioprine tablets and injection should be stored at room temperature.
2. Injection solutions are prepared by adding not less than 5 ml water for injection to each 50 mg vial.
3. Solutions are alkaline and very irritant to the venous tract. They should be injected slowly, preferably via the drip tubing of a running 5% dextrose or 0.9% sodium chloride infusion.
4. Any unused solution should be discarded immediately.

AZELASTINE (Rhinoplast)

Presentation
Metered nasal spray—0.1%

Actions and uses
Azelastine is an antihistamine. The actions and uses of antihistamines in general are described in the antihistamine section. Azelastine is used specifically as a local nasal decongestant in the treatment of perennial and seasonal allergic rhinitis.

Dosage
One metered dose (0.14 ml) sprayed into each nostril twice daily.

Nurse monitoring
Azelastine administered locally may produce mild irritation to the nasal mucosa and taste disturbance but is otherwise well tolerated.

General note
Azelastine metered aerosol may be stored at room temperature. As with all pressurized devices it must not be incinerated when discarded.

AZITHROMYCIN (Zithromax)

(See also Note 3, p. 362)

Presentation
Capsules—250 mg
Suspension—200 mg in 5 ml

Actions and uses
Azithromycin is an antibiotic of the erythromycin group which has a notably long action (once daily dosing is permissible) and good tissue penetration. It is somewhat less active than erythromycin against Gram-positive bacteria but has enhanced activity against certain Gram-negative organisms. Azithromycin is indicated for the treatment of infections of the upper and lower respiratory tract, skin and soft tissues, otitis media and genital infections due to *Chlamydia trachomatis*.

Dosage
1. Adults: Usually a short course (e.g. 3 days) of 500 mg once daily. In genital chlamydial infections, as a single dose of 1 g.

A

2. Children: Over 6 months—10 mg/
   kg once daily for 3 days; 15-25 kg
   weight—200 mg once daily for
   3 days; up to 35 kg—300 mg once
   daily for 3 days; up to
   45 kg—400 mg once daily for 3
   days.

Nurse monitoring
The nurse monitoring section for
erythromycin also applies to this
drug with the additional comment
that gastrointestinal upsets are less
likely or less severe.

General note
Azithromycin capsules and powder
for suspension may be stored at
room temperature.

AZLOCILLIN (Securopen)
(See Note 3, p. 362)
Presentation
Injection—0.5 g, 1.0 g, 2.0 g vials
and 5 g infusion pack
Actions and uses
Azlocillin is a member of the
penicillin group of antibiotics. It has a
much wider spectrum of activity than
the parent drug, benzylpenicillin. Its
indications are for the treatment of
bacterial infection in any tissue of
the body when the organism has
been shown to be sensitive to it.
It is of particular interest to note
that this drug is useful in the
treatment of serious infections due
to Pseudomonas species which
are frequently resistant to other
antibacterial drugs.
Dosage
1. Adults: 2–5 g every 8 hours
   according to the severity of the
   infection.
2. Children: for premature infants
   and children under 3 kg: 50 mg/kg
   body weight every 12 hours;
   under 3 months—0.15–0.25 g
   every 8 hours; 3 months to 1
   year—0.25–0.5 g every 8 hours;
   1-2 years—0.5 g every 8 hours; 2-
   6 years—0.5–1 g every 8 hours; 6
   years and over—1–3 g every
   8 hours.
N.B. Doses below 2 g are administered by intravenous bolus injection.

Higher doses should be given by
rapid intravenous infusion over 20-
30 minutes. Solutions for injection
should be prepared in a concentration of 10% in water for injection.

Nurse monitoring
See benzylpenicillin.

General notes
1. The drug may be stored at room
   temperature.
2. 10% solution for injection should
   be prepared immediately before
   use and any remaining solution
   discarded.

AZTREONAM (Azactam)
(See Note 3, p. 362)
Presentation
Injections—500 mg, 1 g and 2 g in
            15 ml
            —2 g in 100 ml for
            intravenous infusion
Actions and uses
Aztreonam is a monocyclic beta-
lactam antibiotic which in effect
means that, while it shares some
features in common with the
penicillins and cepahalosporins, it
also has important structural
differences. For this reason it can be
safely used as an alternative to
penicillins and cephalosporins for
patients who are allergic to these
drugs but who nevertheless require
a drug of that type. The antibiotic
spectrum of aztreonam is however
restricted to the Gram-negative
organisms, *E. coli, Klebsiella sp.*,
and occasionally pseudomonas,
*Proteus mirabilis, Serratia
marcescens* and *Neisseria
gonorrhoea*: it is also effective in the
treatment of ampicillin-resistant
Haemophillus influenzae infections.
Typical infections which may
respond to aztreonam include the
infections of the lower urinary and
respiratory tracts, bacteraemia,
septicaemia, venereal disease,
skin and soft tissues, intra-
abdominal and gynaecological
infections.

Dosage

Adults: Usually 4 g daily in 3-4 divided doses but up to 8 g daily may be given.

Nurse monitoring

1. Intramuscular injections may be given up to total doses of 1 g above which the intravenous route is recommended.
2. For intramuscular injection each 500 mg is prepared by addition of 1.5 ml water for injection or sodium chloride 0.9% Injection. The dose is administered into deep, large muscle, e.g. lateral thigh.
3. For bolus intravenous injection add 6-10 ml water for injection to each 1 g or 2 g vial and administer slowly over 3-5 minutes.
4. Intravenous infusions are administered over 20-60 minutes as a 2% solution. If dilution is required, this may be administered in standard sodium chloride or glucose solutions or mixtures thereof.
5. The common side-effects of aztreonam are similar to those reported with the penicillins, e.g. allergic skin reactions, local reactions or pain at the injection site and gastrointestinal upsets. Also blood disorders and jaundice have been reported.
6. The clotting time should be closely monitored in patients also treated with oral anti-coagulant drugs such as warfarin.
7. The dose of aztreonam should be halved for patients with moderate renal failure (creatinine clearances 10-30 ml/minute) and reduced to 1/4 for those with severe renal failure (< 10 ml/minute).

General notes

1. Aztreonam injection may be stored at room temperature.
2. Reconstituted solutions remain stable if stored in a refrigerator for up to 24 hours.

B

BACAMPICILLIN (Ambaxin)

(See Note 3, p. 362)

Presentation
Tablets—400mg

Actions and uses
Bacampicillin is an ampicillin ester i.e. a chemical form of ampicillin which is well absorbed so producing rapid high blood levels of ampicillin to which it is subsequently converted. Bacampicillin is used in the treatment of respiratory tract infections, skin and soft tissue infection and UTI but its major use is as a single large dose in the treatment of gonorrhoea when the high levels of ampicillin which result are especially advantageous.

Dosage
1. Adults:
   a. General use: 400–800 mg two or three times daily.
   b. Gonorrhoea: 1.6 g (with probenecid 1 g) as a single dose.

Nurse monitoring
See the section on ampicillin

General note
Bacampicillin tablets are stored at room temperature.

BACLOFEN (Lioresal)

Presentation
Tablets—10 mg
Liquid—5 mg in 5 ml

Actions and uses
Baclofen is used in the treatment of chronic severe spasticity of voluntary muscle. Spasticity is a disorder associated with increased muscle tone but loss of muscle power as a result of damage to corticomotorneurone pathways in the brain and spinal cord. Baclofen reduces spasticity and flexor spasms by enhancing the activity of an inhibitory pre-synaptic neurotrans-mitter, gamma amino butyric acid (GABA) in the spinal cord and by its depressant effect in the CNS. Examples of conditions in which a spastic state may develop include cerebral palsy, post-meningitis and stroke, multiple sclerosis and spinal injury.

Dosage
1. Adults: Initially, 5 mg three times a day increased gradually (e.g. at 3 day intervals) by 5 mg three times day until a response is obtained. Up to 100 mg daily may be required.
2. Children: Over 10 years—0.75–2 mg/kg/day (maximum 2.5 mg/kg/day) or 2.5 mg four times daily increased gradually to a main-tenance dose of 10–20 mg daily (1-2 years), 20–30 mg (2-6 years) or 30–60 mg (6-10 years).

Nurse monitoring
1. The list of possible side-effects with this drug is extensive and is the reason for careful dosage adjustment initially. Patients may be tempted to discontinue therapy and must be warned against doing so abruptly.
2. Baclofen is a CNS depressant and frequently causes sedation or drowsiness. Patients may also complain of nausea and light-headedness.

3. Other CNS side-effects include ataxia, dizziness, confusion, headaches, hallucinations, euphoria, depression, insomnia, tremors and (with very high doses) convulsions. Paraesthesia, muscle pain and weakness may develop.
4. Other side-effects include visual, G.I. and urinary disturbances, sweating, skin rashes and altered liver function. Even a paradoxical *increase* in spasticity rarely occurs.
5. The elderly patient may be particularly susceptible to the above range of side-effects. Clearly, baclofen must also be used with caution in those with a history of epilepsy, stroke and psychiatric disturbance. Dosage adjustment may be required for patients with liver and/or kidney impairment.
6. Baclofen is contraindicated in patients with active peptic ulcer disease.

General note
Baclofen tablets and liquid are stored at room temperature.

BARBITURATES

Amylobarbitone
Butobarbitone
Methohexitone
Methylphenobarbitone
Phenobarbitone
Quinalbarbitone
Thiopentone

Actions and uses
Barbiturates are drugs which depress the function of the brain. This leads to a number of potential uses:
1. To induce sleep
2. To produce day-time sedation
3. As anaesthetics
4. As anticonvulsants.
The very potent short-acting drugs are used as intravenous anaesthetics. Intermediate acting barbiturates readily produce sleep when taken as single night time doses. Phenobarbitone is specially useful as an

anticonvulsant. As it has a cumulative action it is not recommended for production of sleep.
Dosage
See individual drugs.

Nurse monitoring
1. Perhaps the most important point to make about barbiturates is that prolonged use can cause physical dependence and addiction. Obviously when used as an anticonvulsant phenobarbitone is an acceptable form of treatment but there are now available alternative drugs for the induction of sleep and it is not recommended that patients receive barbiturates for this purpose. As many patients receive sleeping tablets on repeat prescriptions there may be a significant number of patients in the community who still receive barbiturates for this purpose. The nurse may play an important role by helping to identify these patients and bringing them to the notice of the doctor.
2. It is extremely dangerous suddenly to stop barbiturate treatment in any patient who has been on such treatment for a prolonged period of time. Epileptic fits and convulsions may be precipitated. The nurse may play an important role by ensuring that patients are aware of this danger.
3. Doses of barbiturates given at night to produce sleep, although effective for this purpose, often lead to 'hangover' symptoms and confusion the following day particularly in elderly patients. The nurse may play a useful role in identifying this adverse effect.
4. Barbiturate drugs depress respiratory, neurological and cardiovascular function. This is particularly important in the following instances:
   a. Patients with severe respiratory disease may have their respiratory function further

depressed by administration of
barbiturates. This may lead to
death.
b. Depression of CNS function by
barbiturates may be accentu-
ated by the coincident ingestion
of alcohol. All patients must be
warned of the dangers of taking
alcohol with barbiturates.
5. Gastrointestinal upset frequently
occurs with oral administration.
6. When given intravenously severe
depression of respiration,
hypotension, coughing, sneezing
and laryngeal spasm may occur.
The accidental injection of
barbiturate drugs into arteries
has caused arterial spasm with
resultant gangrene and loss of
the affected limb.

General note
See specific drugs.

BECLOMETHASONE (Becotide, Propaderm, Beconase)

Presentation
Inhalation—metered aerosol 50 and
100 microgram per dose.
'Rotacaps'—100 and 200 microgram
Nasal spray—50 microgram per
metered dose
Cream—0.025%, 0.5%
Ointment—0.025%

Action and uses
Beclomethasone is a corticosteroid
(see the section on corticosteroids)
used primarily in three situations:
1. It is administered topically for the
treatment of inflammatory skin
conditions such as psoriasis,
eczema and dermatitis.
2. It is administered by inhalation for
the management of asthma.
3. It is instilled nasally in the
management of allergic rhinitis
and hay fever.

Dosage
1. Topical use: apply sparingly twice
daily.
2. By inhalation:
a. Adults: on average 100
microgram (two puffs) three or
four times daily. Up to 800

microgram may be given in
severe cases.
b. Children: usually receive half
the adult dose and the
maximum daily dose by
inhalation recommended is 500
microgram. It is worth noting
that capsules containing dry
powder (Rotacaps) may be
more acceptable to younger
patients.
3. For nasal instillation: one
metered dose (50 microgram) is
instilled four times daily.

Nurse monitoring
See the section on corticosteroids.
It is worth noting that whatever the
route of administration, sufficient of
this drug may be absorbed to
produce the systemic effects
described in the section mentioned
above.

General notes
1. Preparations containing
beclomethasone may be stored at
room temperature.
2. In common with other pressurised
containers, metered aerosols and
nasal sprays should not be
punctured or incinerated after use.
3. If necessary beclomethasone
cream may be diluted with
cetomacrogol cream, Formula A,
or the ointment with white soft
paraffin.

BENDROFLUAZIDE (Neo-Naclex)

Presentation
Tablets—2.5 mg, 5 mg

Actions and uses
See the section on thiazide and
related diuretics.

Dosage
1. Adults. The daily adult dose range
is 2.5–10 mg which may be taken
as a single morning dose since
the duration of action of
bendrofluazide is approximately
24 hours.

2. Children: Up to 5 years—1.25 mg;
5 years plus—2.5 mg.

Nurse monitoring
See the section on thiazide and
related diuretics.

General note
Bendrofluazide tablets may be
stored at room temperature.

BENORYLATE (Benoral)

Presentation
Tablets—750 mg
Suspension—4 g in 10 ml
Actions and uses
1. See the section on aspirin.
2. Benorylate is converted in the
blood to aspirin and paracetamol.
It may therefore occasionally be
used successfully in patients who
are unable to tolerate aspirin due
to its gastric irritant effect.
Dosage
1. Adults: The average adult dosage
is 1.5 g (tablets) three times a day
or 4 g (10 ml suspension) twice
daily.
2. Children: Up to 1 year—25 mg/kg
body weight up to four times daily;
1-2 years—250 mg up to four
times daily; 2-6 years—500 mg up
to three times daily; 6-12 years—
500 mg up to four times daily.
It must be remembered that as this
compound is converted to aspirin it
should be used with great care in
children and should really only be
given to children under the age of 1
under strict medical supervision.

Nurse monitoring
1. The nurse monitoring notes for
aspirin (q.v.) are applicable to
this drug.
2. It is also converted to
paracetamol; the nurse monitoring notes for paracetamol (q.v.)
are also applicable.

General note
Benorylate tablets and suspension
may be stored at room temperature.

BENPERIDOL (Anquil)

Presentation
Tablets—0.25 mg
Actions and uses
Benperidol is a neuroleptic drug
which has many of the actions and
uses described for haloperidol. It has
a particular use in the management
of patients displaying unusual sexual
behavioural disturbances.
Dosage
Adults: The standard dose is 0.25–
1.5 mg daily, though up to 9 mg daily
has been used in schizophrenia.

Nurse monitoring
See the section on haloperidol.

General note
The drug may be stored at room
temperature.

BENZATHINE PENICILLIN (Penidural)

(See Note 3, p. 362)
Presentation
Suspension—229 mg in 5 ml
(equivalent to benzylpenicillin
300 000 units in 5 ml)

Actions and uses
Benzathine penicillin has identical
actions and uses to those described
for benzylpenicillin (q.v.). It is used
either alone or in combination with
benzylpenicillin and procaine
penicillin G and its advantage is that
it has a prolonged duration of action.
The indications for its use are
identical to those described for
benzylpenicillin.
Dosage
1. Adults: Orally 10 ml syrup
(equivalent to 600 000 units of
benzylpenicillin) three to four
times per day
2. Children: Orally 5 ml syrup
(equivalent to 300 000 units of
benzylpenicillin) three to four
times per day.

> **Nurse monitoring**
> See the section on benzylpenicillin.

General note
The oral preparation may be stored at room temperature.

BENZHEXOL (Artane)

Presentation
Tablets—2 mg and 5 mg
Syrup—5 mg in 5 ml

Actions and uses
Benzhexol has a number of actions known as 'anticholinergic effects' including the potential to relax muscle and abolish rigidity and tremor. This makes it useful for the treatment of Parkinson's disease and it is often given to psychiatric patients treated with phenothiazine tranquillizers who may develop this as a side-effect of their phenothiazine therapy.

Dosage
Adults: 6–16 mg daily in three divided doses.

> **Nurse Monitoring**
> 1. The drug's anticholinergic actions produce dry mouth, blurred vision, constipation and urinary retention.
> 2. Further common adverse effects include dizziness, nervousness and nausea.
> 3. Mental confusion and agitation are less common problems.
> 4. The drug should be used with caution in patients with:
>   a. Glaucoma
>   b. Gastrointestinal obstruction
>   c. Prostatism.

General note
The drug may be stored at room temperature.

BENZODIAZEPINES AND RELATED DRUGS

Bromazepam
Chlordiazepoxide
Clobazam
Clonazepam
Diazepam
Flunitrazepam
Flurazepam
Lorazepam
Medazepam
Nitrazepam
Oxazepam
Potassium clorazepate
Temazepam

Actions and uses
Benzodiazepines are sedative drugs. They have this effect by their action on a specific area in the brain known as the limbic system. This area of the brain is thought to be concerned with the control of emotion. The advantage that benzodiazepines have over other central nervous system sedative drugs such as barbiturates, is that they do not have a general depressant effect on cerebral function and therefore are not as dangerous. As well as their sedative effect certain of this drug group have other uses. These are as follows:
1. Nitrazepam and temazepam have a marked sedative effect and may be taken at night to induce sleep.
2. Clonazepam has a specific anti-convulsant action and is taken orally in the treatment of epilepsies.
3. Chlordiazepoxide has a specific indication for the control of delirium tremens in alcoholic patients.
4. Diazepam is particularly useful for intramuscular or intravenous administration as it provides sufficient sedation to relieve either acute anxiety or to allow minor practical procedures such as dental surgery or endoscopy. Diazepam is also useful in the treatment of status epilepticus and tetanus when it may be given by the intramuscular or intravenous route.

Dosage
See individual drugs.

> **Nurse monitoring**
> 1. When given during the day for their sedative and anxiolytic action the sedative effect may occasionally be excessive

leading to drowsiness and may be accompanied by an inability to walk properly without staggering. These effects are seen particularly when alcohol is taken in addition to the drugs. Patients must therefore be encouraged not to consume alcohol while taking these drugs and in addition they should be warned about the potential dangers of excess sedation when driving or operating machinery.

2. The drugs of this group which are given at night as hypnotics can produce effects lasting into the following day which are known as hangover effects. These are symptoms of drowsiness, lethargy and headache and may, especially in elderly patients when high dosage has been given, cause frank confusion. Patients themselves may not notice effects of over-sedation and nurses can play an important role in detecting such effects.

3. Occasionally when these drugs are given an unusual or paradoxical reaction may occur and the patient may become agitated, excited and may even experience hallucinations.

4. Drugs of the benzodiazepine group, even when taken in massive overdosage orally, rarely produce profound neurological depression. This makes them preferable to barbiturates. However, it must be stressed that when given intravenously for short-term sedation they may still cause respiratory depression and therefore should never be given intravenously unless facilities for resuscitation are available.

5. These drugs are not recommended for regular use in pregnancy.

6. Nursing mothers should be warned that if they take benzodiazepines while breast feeding the drug will be excreted in their milk and may lead to marked sedation of their children.

7. Side-effects of this group of drugs include gastrointestinal upset, blurred vision, dry mouth and headache.

8. Benzodiazepine dependence and addiction: During the past 10 years or more it has become apparent that drugs of this group may produce marked dependence when taken continuously for prolonged periods. This has, at least in part, resulted from overuse, often inappropriately for assumed anxiety.
Benzodiazepine dependence is now widespread and occurs in patients who are not otherwise considered to be regular drug abusers. Doctors are now requested to prescribe such drugs on a limited basis only (i.e. for 2-3 weeks). The symptoms of drug withdrawal are complex and may be difficult to interpret. They include anxiety, restlessness and agitation, sleep disturbances, hallucinations and even convulsions. Once detected, it is important that patients receive reassurance and support in attempting to 'wean off' the habit. This is often a prolonged and painstaking process and requires specialist psychiatric support for many.

General note
 See specific drugs.

BENZTROPINE (Cogentin)

Presentation
 Tablets—2 mg
 Injection—1 mg in 1 ml
Actions and uses
 1. Benztropine is an anticholinergic drug which has actions and uses identical to those described for benzhexol (q.v.).
 2. Benztropine is also used in clinical practice for emergency treatment of acute dystonic reactions such as torticollis and oculogyric crises.
Dosage
 1. For the treatment of Parkinsonism: The adult dose is 1–6 mg

per day as a single dose at bedtime. The dose may alternatively be divided and given two or three times a day.
2. For the emergency treatment of acute dystonic reactions: 1–2 mg is given by intramuscular or intravenous injection.

Nurse Monitoring
Nurse monitoring aspects of benzhexol (q.v.) apply to this drug.

General notes
1. The drug may be stored at room temperature.
2. Solution for injection should be protected from light.

BENZYLPENICILLIN (Crystapen G)

(See Note 3, p.362)
N.B. Also referred to as penicillin G available as the potassium or sodium salt.

Presentation
Tablets—250 mg
Syrup—125 mg in 5 ml
            250 mg in 5 ml
Injection—1 mega unit (600 mg) vials
Eye drops and ointment—various strengths

Actions and uses
Benzylpenicillin was the first of the penicillin group of antibiotics and has a bactericidal action, i.e. it kills bacterial cells in the body. It does this by interfering with the synthesis of bacterial cell walls causing them to burst. It has a narrow antibacterial spectrum. The microorganisms streptococci, pneumococci, meningococci and gonococci are usually sensitive to this drug. Nowadays staphylococci are only rarely sensitive. It therefore has the following clinical uses:
1. In the treatment of infections caused by the above organisms as outlined in Note 3.
2. In the treatment of venereal disease, both syphilis and gonorrhoea.
3. In the treatment of gonococcal infection of the eye in the newborn (ophthalmia neonatorum).

Dosage
N.B. One mega unit is equivalent to one million units or 600 mg of penicillin.
1. Oral:
   a. Adults—250–500 mg four times a day.
   b. Children—125–250 mg four times a day.
   c. Infants—62.5–125 mg four times a day.
The drug should preferably be given 1 hour before meals.
2. Parenteral:
   a. Adults: 600–1200 mg 4 times daily. The drug may be given by intramuscular or intravenous bolus injection or intravenous infusion. By the intravenous route at least 1 minute should be taken for each 300 mg injected.
   b. Children aged 1 month to 12 years: 10–20 mg/kg body weight in total in 24 hours, usually divided into four doses.
   c. Neonates (less than 1 month): 30 mg/kg per day in total in divided doses, usually twice daily in the first few days of life and then 3-4 times daily.
3. Topical applications (eye drops and ointment): The doses of these vary widely depending on the condition treated.
4. Intrathecal route: Rarely benzylpenicillin is given intrathecally for the treatment of bacterial meningitis. Injection of an excessive dose by this route is highly dangerous and in many centres it is now felt that intravenous dosage is quite adequate, and intrathecal therapy unnecessary. Maximum doses recommended are as follows:
   a. Adults: 6 mg dissolved in 10 ml of sodium chloride or 10 ml of the patient's CSF. The usual daily dose is 6 mg but on occasions up to 12 mg may be used.
   b. For infants and children: 0.1 mg/kg body weight is suitable.

The concentration of penicillin in the injection should not exceed 0.6 mg/ml.

5. Intra-ocular: In certain eye infections $1/2$ to 1 mega unit may be given by subconjunctival injection.

N.B. It is important to note that the above dosages are only an outline and under certain circumstances much higher doses may be given. Examples of this are in bacterial endocarditis in adults where up to 12 mega units may be given parenterally per day and in neonatal meningitis when the systemic dosage may be 60–90 mg/kg per day in total.

Nurse monitoring

1. Penicillins are most noted for their production of adverse effects in patients who are hypersensitive to the drug group. The effects produced may range from skin rash and urticaria to anaphylactic shock. Patients with a history of penicillin allergy should never be given penicillin under any circumstance by any route.
2. As allergy to penicillin can be so dangerous the nurse may play an important role in the management of these patients by ensuring that their allergy once identified is recorded on patients' Kardexes and in their notes, and brought to the attention of the medical staff.
3. Although oral preparations of penicillin G are available it is important to note that they are not particularly effective.
4. Oral penicillins may commonly produce mild diarrhoea.
5. If very high doses are given haemolytic anaemia and convulsion may occur.

General notes

1. Preparations containing benzylpenicillin may be stored at room temperature.
2. Solutions for injection should be prepared as follows:

a. Intramuscular injection: Add 1.6–2 ml of water for injection to each 1 mega unit vial.
b. Intravenous injection: Dissolve 1 mega unit in 4–10 ml water for injection (note that the maximum infusion rate by intravenous bolus injection is 300 mg/minute).
c. Intravenous infusion: The dose to be given is added to 500 ml of 0.9% sodium chloride or 0.5% dextrose of dextrose/saline mixture and infused over 4-6 hours.

3. Solutions containing benzylpenicillin should be used immediately as they quickly deteriorate. Intravenous infusions must never be stored for any length of time. However, buffered solutions, once prepared, may last for 3 days at room temperature or up to 2 weeks in a refrigerator.

BEPHENIUM (Alcopar)

Presentation

Granules—2.5 g

Actions and uses

This antihelminthic drug is used in the treatment of:

1. Hookworm (ancylostomiasis)
2. Roundworm (ascariasis)
3. Trichostrongyliasis.

Dosage

1. For adults and children over 10 kg body weight—2.5 g
2. Children under 10 kg body weight—1.25 g.

Nurse monitoring

1. The required dose should be mixed in water or a sweet liquid and drunk immediately.
2. In the presence of heavy infestation it is recommended that the treatment be repeated after 3 days.
3. No purgation is necessary.
4. Gastrointestinal upset may occur including nausea, vomiting, abdominal pain and diarrhoea.

B

General note
The drug may be stored at room temperature.

BETA-ADRENORECEPTOR BLOCKING DRUGS (Beta-blockers)

Acebutolol
Atenolol
Betaxolol
Bisoprolol
Carteolol
Celiprolol
Esmolol
Labetalol
Metipranolol
Metoprolol
Nadolol
Oxprenolol
Pindolol
Propranolol
Sotalol
Timolol
Xamoterol

Actions and uses
The sympathetic nervous system is activated at two distinct receptor sub-types termed alpha- and beta-adrenoreceptors. The latter are further sub-divided into:
1. beta$_1$ receptors
2. beta$_2$ receptors
Simulation of beta$_1$ receptors leads to an increase in heart rate and cardiac output. Stimulation of beta$_2$ receptors causes dilation of the small airways in the lung and dilation of small arteries and arterioles. Beta-adrenoreceptor blocking drugs block the effect of the sympathetic nervous system and therefore potentially produce a reduction in heart rate, cardiac output and blood pressure and may potentially cause bronchoconstriction and vasoconstriction. The group as a whole may be distinguished on the basis of three pharmacological effects:
1. Cardioselectivity
2. Partial agonist activity
3. Membrane stabilizing activity.
By far the most important clinical effect is cardioselectivity. Drugs which are non-selective block sympathetic stimulation at both beta$_1$ and beta$_2$ sites and are therefore

likely to produce unwanted side-effects of bronchospasm and vasoconstriction. Cardioselective drugs tend to block the beta$_1$ (cardiac) sites rather than the beta$_2$ (peripheral) sites and therefore are less likely to cause side-effects. In summary, beta-blockers may be used for:
1. The prevention of angina pectoris
2. The management of hypertension
3. The control of cardiac dysrhythmias
4. A few specialist uses include treatment of anxiety, prevention of migraine and control of portal hypertension. Seek further advice on these.

Dosage
See individual drugs.

Nurse monitoring
1. Any patient treated with a beta-blocker may develop heart failure and therefore all patients should be observed for the development of symptoms and signs indicative of this problem.
2. Many diabetics recognise the early symptoms of a hypoglycaemic attack by noticing sweating, tremor and tachycardia. They may prevent the development of a full-blown attack by taking sugar. If diabetics are given beta-blockers these early symptoms may not be felt and hypoglycaemic coma may follow. Thus beta-blockers must be used with great caution in diabetic patients. There is some evidence that cardioselective beta-blockers are less likely to have this effect and therefore if beta-blockers must be used in diabetic patients a cardioselective preparation should be chosen.
3. As mentioned above, beta-blocking drugs may cause bronchospasm and vasoconstriction. Non-selective beta-blockers are therefore definitely contra-indicated in patients with asthma or peripheral vascular disease. Cardioselective beta-blockers are less likely to exacerbate

B

bronchospasm and peripheral vascular disease but patients given these drugs who have these problems must always be carefully observed in case even the cardioselective drugs cause an exacerbation of symptoms.

4. Gastrointestinal side-effects of nausea, vomiting and diarrhoea occur commonly and may be reduced if the drug is taken just before meals.

5. Central nervous system effects include dizziness, drowsiness, lassitude, depression, insomnia, nightmares and hallucinations. These effects are more likely to be seen in lipid soluble beta-blockers such as propranolol and it is worth noting that atenolol is the least lipid soluble preparation available and therefore may be the preparation of choice in patients who suffer these symptoms severely.

6. Other side-effects include skin rashes, pruritus, and flushing.

7. It is important that the nurse remembers that beta-blockers will by definition produce a slow pulse and pulse rates below 50 per minute are not an indication to stop the drug unless symptoms suggest heart failure is present. A useful point to note is that pulse rates of less than 50 per minute are often acceptable as long as they can be shown to rise after exercise.

General note
See individual drugs.

BETAHISTINE (Serc)

Presentation
Tablets—8 mg, 16 mg
Actions and uses
Betahistine is an antihistamine. The actions and uses of antihistamines in general are described in the section on antihistamines. In clinical practice betahistine is used in the treatment of vertigo and the symptoms of vertigo and nausea due to Menière's disease.

Dosage
Adults: 8-16 mg taken three times daily.

Nurse monitoring
See the section on antihistamines.

General note
The drug may be stored at room temperature.

BETAMETHASONE (Betnelan, Betnesol, Bextasol, Betnovate)

Presentation
Tablets—0.5 mg (plain and soluble)
Injection—4 mg in 1 ml
Inhaler—100 microgram per dose
Ointment, cream and application—0.1 % (also combined with antibiotic)
Rectal—ointment 0.05% and suppositories 0.5 mg
Eye, ear and nose drops—0.1 %
Eye ointment—0.1 %
Actions and uses
See the section on corticosteroids.
Dosage
Doses vary considerably with the nature and severity of the illness being treated and it is not therefore appropriate to quote specific instances.

Nurse monitoring
See the section on corticosteroids.

General notes
1. Preparations containing betamethasone may be stored at room temperature.

2. The injection solution should be protected from light and as with other pressurized inhalers, aerosols should never be punctured or incinerated after use.

3. Intravenous injections are given slowly over 30 seconds to 1 minute.

4. If given by intravenous infusion, normal saline or 5% dextrose solutions can be used as diluents.

BETAXOLOL (Betoptic, Kerlone)

Presentation
Tablets—20 mg
Eye drops—0.5%

Actions and uses
Betaxolol is a cardioselective beta-blocking drug and its action and uses are described in the section on beta-adrenoreceptor blocking drugs. In clinical practice, it has two major uses:
1. As an antihypertensive agent.
2. In the treatment of glaucoma (ocular hypertension) some beta-blockers applied to the eye lower intraocular pressure by causing a reduction in aqueous humor production.

Dosage
1. Hypertension: 10–20 mg daily as single dose.
2. Glaucoma: 1 drop instilled in eye twice daily.

Nurse monitoring
1. See beta-adrenoreceptor blocking drugs.
2. Note also that systemic side-effects may be associated with the use of eye drops, after absorption of the drug across the cornea.
3. Application of betaxolol to the eye may be associated with minor irritation or discomfort.

General note
Betaxolol tablets and eye drops may stored at room temperature. Eye drops, once opened, have a relatively short life due to the risk of bacterial contamination during use. Normally eye drops of any kind should not be used after 1 week for a hospitalized patient or after 4 weeks for others.

BETHANECHOL (Myotonine)

Presentation
Tablets—10 mg and 25 mg

Actions and uses
Many functions of the body including the rate at which the heart beats, the cardiac output, the amount of respiratory secretion, the degree of muscle tone in the bronchi (airway), the movement of gut wall and the function of the bladder are controlled by the autonomic nervous system.

This system is divided into two parts known as the sympathetic and parasympathetic systems. Their interrelation is a complex process and is beyond the bounds of this text. Bethanechol stimulates the parasympathetic segment of the autonomic nervous system. Its useful effects are as follows:
1. It may effect the contraction of bladder muscle so promoting micturition and is used where normal control of bladder function has been lost resulting in urinary retention.
2. It stimulates gastric peristaltic waves and has been used in the management of various gastrointestinal disorders including post-operative abdominal distension and megacolon.

Dosage
Orally: 5–30 mg three or four times daily.

Nurse monitoring
1. The other effects of stimulating the parasympathetic section of the autonomic nervous system are in fact this drug's side-effects. They include:
   a. Reduction of heart rate and cardiac output
   b. Peripheral vasodilation
   c. An increase in respiratory secretions and constriction of the bronchi.
2. The drug should be used with great care in patients who have suffered from asthma, chronic obstructive lung disease, or those with urinary or gastrointestinal obstruction.
3. The drug should never be given to patients who have heart disease.

4. If this drug is given to a patient who has normal sensation to the bladder but has difficulty with passing water, if micturition does not occur severe discomfort will be produced and facilities for catheterization should be available.

General note
Bethanecol tablets may be stored at room temperature.

BETHANIDINE (Esbatal)

Presentation
Tablets—10 mg, 50 mg
Actions and uses
See the section on guanethidine.
Dosage
1. Initially adults are commenced on 10 mg three times a day with increments of 5–10 mg three times daily as required until effective control of hypertension is achieved. Up to 200 mg per day may be necessary in total.
2. Children's doses are: Less than 1 year—2.5 mg; 1-6 years—5 mg; 7 years plus—5–10 mg. These doses are taken three times a day. Children's doses likewise may be increased about 20 times these values to achieve the required effect.

Nurse monitoring
See the section on guanethidine.

General note
Bethanidine tablets may be stored at room temperature.

BEZAFIBRATE (Bezalip)

Presentation
Tablets—200 mg, 400 mg (slow release)
Actions and uses
This drug is a member of the fibrate group of lipid lowering drugs and as such it is similar to clofibrate. The exact mechanism of action of these agents is unknown: they reduce both triglyceride and low-density lipoprotein (LDL-cholesterol) levels so favourably influencing the LDL to HDL cholesterol profile. Bezafibrate is used in the treatment of certain of the familial hyperlipidaemias and hyperlipid-aemias associated with coronary risk in patients who fail on diet alone. It is occasionally necessary to combine therapy with other types of lipid lowering drugs.
Dosage
Adults only: 200 mg three times daily or 400 mg slow release tablet once daily at night or in the morning.

Nurse monitoring
1. Dosages are best taken with or immediately after meals to minimize the severity of gastrointestinal upsets.
2. Skin rashes and muscle pain may occur especially in patients with impaired kidney function and treatment should be avoided if this is severe.
3. All drugs of the fibrate group enhance warfarin and may produce bleeding in patients already receiving anticoagulant therapy. Close monitoring of prothrombin time is especially important in this group.

General note
Bezafibrate tablets may be stored at room temperature.

BIPERIDEN (Akineton)

Presentation
Tablets—2 mg
Injection—5 mg in 1 ml
Actions and uses
Biperiden is an anticholinergic agent used in the treatment of extrapyramidal symptoms associated with antipsychotic drug therapy and other types of parkinsonism. In this respect it resembles benzhexol and procyclidine.

Dosage

Adults: Usually 2 mg three times daily which may be reduced during maintenance therapy. In an acute situation 2.5–5 mg and up to 20 mg in one day may be given by intramuscular or slow intravenous injection.

Nurse monitoring

As described for benzhexol and procyclidine.

General note

Biperiden tablets and injection are stored at room temperature.

BISACODYL (Dulcolax)

Presentation

Tablets-5 mg
Suppositories—5 mg and 10 mg

Actions and uses

The general actions of laxatives are discussed in the section on laxatives. Bisacodyl is a member of group 1, i.e. it has an irritant action on the gut wall. It is used for the treatment of constipation.

Dosage

1. Adults: 10 mg orally at night or one 10 mg suppository inserted each morning.
2. Children: one 5 mg suppository inserted each morning.

Nurse monitoring

Bisacodyl's irritant effect on the gut wall may lead to cramping abdominal pain, otherwise there are no specific problems with this drug.

General notes

1. Preparations containing bisacodyl may be stored at room temperature.
2. It is important that suppositories are not stored in a warm area, e.g. above or near a radiator, since they will readily melt.

BISOPROLOL (Emcor, Monocor)

Presentation

Tablets—5 mg, 10 mg

Actions and uses

Bisoprolol is a beta-blocking drug which is reported to have a degree of cardioselectivity which is far in excess of other so-called cardioselective beta-blockers. With this in mind, the reader is referred to the general account of beta-adrenoreceptor blocking drugs (q.v.).

Dosage

Bisoprolol has a long duration of action and is required to be taken once daily only. The usual dose lies in the range 5–20 mg for treatment of either angina pectoris or hypertension.

Nurse monitoring

1. The nurse monitoring aspects described under beta-adrenoreceptor blocking drugs apply.
2. Note that although a very high degree of cardioselectivity is claimed for bisoprolol, it should nonetheless be used with caution in patients with asthma and chronic severe obstructive airways disease.

General note

Bisoprolol tablets may be stored at room temperature.

BLEOMYCIN

Presentation

Injection—ampoules containing 5 and 15 mg

Actions and uses

Bleomycin is a cytotoxic drug derived from a family of antibiotics which have been found to have this action. It has a mode of action similar to that of actinomycin (q.v.). It is used in the treatment of the following conditions:

1. Squamous cell carcinomas, i.e. in the mouth, nose, throat and oesophagus.
2. Hodgkin's disease and other lymphomas.

3. Testicular teratoma.
4. Bleomycin has also been used in melanoma and carcinoma of the thyroid, lung and bladder.

Dosage

Bleomycin may be used alone but is usually given in combination with other cytotoxic drugs. It may be administered by various routes including intramuscular, intravenous, intra-arterial, intrapleural or intraperitoneal injection. It has also been injected directly into tumours.

1. Adult doses: These vary widely according to the age of the patient, the route used and the type of tumour being treated. It is usually given by intravenous or intramuscular injection and twice weekly doses of 30 mg for 5 weeks are used.
2. Doses for children are calculated upon body surface area.

Nurse Monitoring

1. It is interesting and important to note that bleomycin in contrast to most other cytotoxics has little or no harmful effect on the bone marrow.
2. Gastrointestinal symptoms such as anorexia, nausea and vomiting may occur during treatment and stomatitis often occurs.
3. Because the drug is irritant, local reactions and thrombophlebitis.
4. Most patients develop skin lesions after receiving full courses. These skin lesions include hyperkeratosis, impaired nail formation, reddening and peeling of the skin and alopecia.
5. Interstitial pneumonia may develop during treatment and if the drug is continued fatal pulmonary fibrosis may result. This effect limits the total dose given to any one patient to 300 mg at a maximum.
6. If patients are known to have impaired renal function reduced dosages are used.

7. It is important to note that when bleomycin is to be given, intra-muscular injections may be prepared using a 0.1 % lignocaine solution. Local pain may be considerably reduced by this action.
8. The nurse should be constantly aware that cytotoxic drugs are very toxic and therefore must be handled with great care. Spillage and contamination of the skin of the patient or nurse may lead to a degree of absorption of the drug which, if chronically repeated, may be harmful. The skin may also be sensitized to the drug making it, in some cases, impossible for the nurse to continue working with the drug since hypersensitivity reactions may result.

General notes

1. Bleomycin injection may be stored at room temperature. It is stable for up to 3 years and an expiry date is printed on the label of individual ampoules.
2. Any solution remaining after injection should be immediately discarded.
3. Recommended diluent is 0.9% sodium chloride.
4. Bleomycin solutions should not be mixed with other drugs, except where lignocaine is added for intramuscular injection.

BRETYLIUM TOSYLATE (Bretylate)

Presentation

Injection—100 mg in 2 ml

Actions and uses

Bretylium tosylate has a suppressant effect on the heart muscle and its conducting tissues and can be used to treat ventricular dysrhythmias. It is now rarely used as first choice but may be considered for patients in whom resistance to first line drugs such as lignocaine, mexiletine, disopyramide or beta-blockers occurs.

Dosage

Bretylium is given intramuscularly. Intravenous injection confers no advantage and may produce more serious side-effects. The adult dosage is 5 mg/kg body weight given at intervals of 6-8 hours.

Nurse monitoring

1. The nurse will virtually never see this drug used outside coronary care or other intensive care units and even in these specialist units it will be used only rarely, if at all.
2. The patient should be in the supine position during treatment as the drug produces hypotension.
3. The development of nausea or vomiting is an indication to reduce the dosage or withdraw the drug altogether.

General note

Bretylium tosylate injection should be stored in a refrigerator.

BROMAZEPAM (Lexotan)

Presentation

Tablets—1.5 mg, 3 mg

Actions and uses

Bromazepam is a member of the benzodiazepine group (q.v.) used for the treatment of severe anxiety, especially that associated with insomnia.

Dosage

Adults only: The lowest effective dose, usually in the range 3–18 mg daily in three divided doses. A lower starting dose of 1.5 mg is appropriate for frail or elderly patients in whom high doses should be avoided.

Nurse monitoring

See the section under benzodiazepines.

General note

Bromazepam tablets are stored at room temperature.

BROMOCRIPTINE (Parlodel)

Presentation

Tablets—1 mg, 2.5 mg
Capsules—5 mg, 10 mg

Actions and uses

Bromocriptine inhibits the release of the hormones prolactin and growth hormone normally produced in the pituitary gland which lies within the brain. This makes it useful in clinical practice in a number of situations:

1. For the treatment of acromegaly (a disease caused by excess secretion of growth hormone, usually by a tumour of the pituitary associated with excessive growth of facial bones, hands and feet, headache, sweating, hypertension, heart disease and chest disease).
2. For the inhibition of puerperal lactation.
3. For the treatment of infertility in females when this is found to be associated with an excess production of prolactin.
4. The drug is used for the treatment of galactorrhoea (production of milk by the breast) when this is shown to be due to an excess production of prolactin.
5. Since bromocriptine exerts its action by stimulating receptor sites which respond to the natural substance, dopamine, i.e. it exerts a dopaminergic action, this effect in a specific area of the brain (the extrapyramidal system) which coordinates movement, produces benefit in symptoms associated with Parkinson's disease.
   Parkinson's disease is characterized by a lack of dopamine in the brain.

Dosage

1. For the treatment of acromegaly: The dosage is adjusted according to response, monitored both clinically and by measuring blood levels of growth hormone. It is worth noting that acromegalics require fairly high doses for effective treatment.

2. For the inhibition of puerperal lactation: 2.5 mg twice daily.
3. For the treatment of infertility: Initially 2.5 mg once or twice a day is given and the dose is gradually increased until menstruation or pregnancy is achieved.
4. For the treatment of galactor-rhoea: Initially 2.5 mg once or twice a day with gradual increments in the dose until galactorrhoea ceases..
5. In the treatment of Parkinson's disease (usually in conjunction with Levodopa): A daily dose ranging from 10-100 mg may be used depending upon the balance between patient response and the occurrence of unwanted side-effects. Daily doses are achieved by the use of gradual dosage increments following an initial low dose until the optimum is reached in the individual.

Nurse monitoring
1. Perhaps the most important problem with this drug is that it produces nausea. This can be minimized by commencing with a very low dose and building up the dose slowly and by starting therapy on a once daily basis at night. However, despite this nausea remains a major problem.
2. Other less common side-effects include: postural hypotension, dizziness, headache, vomiting and constipation.
3. Rare side-effects include drowsiness, confusion, agitation, hallucination, dyskinesia, dry mouth and leg cramps.
4. Note that side-effects are considerably more likely to occur with high doses such as those used in the treatment of Parkinson's disease.

General note
The drug may be stored at room temperature.

BROMPHENIRAMINE (Dimotane)

Presentation
Tablets—4 mg, 12 mg (slow release)
Elixir—2 mg in 5 ml
Actions and uses
Brompheniramine is an antihistamine. The actions and uses of antihistamines in general are discussed in the antihistamine section. Brompheniramine is specifically used:
1. To suppress generalized minor allergic responses to allergens such as foodstuffs and drugs.
2. Orally for allergic conditions, e.g. hay fever and allergic rhinitis.
3. As a nasal decongestant, e.g. in the treatment of allergic rhinitis and hay fever. It is also added to a few proprietary cough preparations because of its decongestant action.
Dosage
1. Adults:
   a. Standard tablets: 4–8 mg 4-hourly.
   b. Slow release tablets: 12–24 mg twice a day.
2. Children: Less than 3 years—1 ml syrup/kg per day; 3-6 years one-quarter of adult dose; 6-12 years—one-half of adult dose.

Nurse monitoring
See the antihistamines section.

General note
The drug may be stored at room temperature.

BUDESONIDE (Pulmicort, Rhinocort)

Presentation
Pressurized Inhaler—50 and 200 microgram per dose
Dry Powder Turbohaler—100, 200 and 400 microgram per dose
Nebulizer Solution—250 and 500 microgram ampoules
Nasal Spray—50 microgram per pressurized metered dose, 100 microgram aqueous pumped dose.

Actions and uses

Budesonide is a corticosteroid for local use which shares the anti-allergic and anti-inflammatory properties of beclomethasone. It is used in the prophylactic treatment of asthma (in which inflammation and allergy underlies bronchial hyper-responsiveness) and perennial and seasonal rhinitis.

Dosage

1. Asthma
   a. Inhalation: Regular twice daily (morning and night-time) inhalation in doses ranging from 50–400 microgram with lower doses for children. Dry powder inhalation in double these doses. The dose is that which enables good control of chronic asthma and reduces the need for regular or frequent use of bronchodilator inhalers (e.g. salbutamol, terbutaline).
   b. In acute or severe chronic asthma: Respirator solution may be nebulized e.g. 0.5–2 mg (adults) or 0.5–1 mg (children) according to response.
2. Seasonal and perennial rhinitis
   a. Intranasal use: 1-2 applications into each nostril twice daily.

Nurse monitoring

1. See the section under corticosteroids.
2. It should be noted that overuse of the above products may result in systemic steroid effects but in practice only local problems are encountered.
3. Oral thrush and dysphonia can be minimized by using the pressurized inhaler in combination with the spacing nebuhaler device. Rinsing the mouth after use should also be encouraged.
4. Patients should realize that they must use steroid inhalers regularly. They may not appreciate their important effects on asthma progression and rely too much on symptomatic control with a bronchodilator alone.

General notes

1. Budesonide preparations are stored at room temperature.
2. Pressurized devices must not be incinerated after they are apparently empty.
3. Ampoules are **not for injection**.

BUMETANIDE (Burinex)

Presentation

Tablets—1 mg, 5 mg
Injection—1 mg in 4 ml, 6.25 mg in 25 ml

Actions and uses

Bumetanide has a mode of action and uses identical to those described under frusemide (q.v.).

Dosage

Bumetanide is 40 times more potent than frusemide, i.e. 1 mg bumetanide produces the same effect as 40 mg of frusemide. Recommended doses are therefore 1/40th of those discussed under frusemide.

Nurse monitoring

The nurse monitoring notes for thiazide diuretics are applicable to bumetanide. It should be noted that problems with transient deafness do not seem to occur with bumetanide as they do with frusemide.

General notes

1. Bumetanide tablets and injection are stored at room temperature. The injection solution is sensitive to light and is therefore packed in amber coloured ampoules.
2. Unlike frusemide, bumetanide is stable in dextrose solutions and dextrose 5% injection may be used as a diluent before infusion. The standard dose by intravenous infusion is 2–5 mg in 500 ml of diluent given over a period of 30-60 minutes.

BUPIVACAINE (Marcain)

Presentation
Injection—Plain 0.25% and 0.5%
        —With adrenaline 0.25%
          and 0.5%

Actions and uses
This potent local anaesthetic drug has a much longer duration of action than lignocaine. It is used in minor surgical and obstetric procedures to produce extradural block, digital block, nerve plexus block and pudendal block.

Dosage
Individual doses vary considerably with the type of procedure and the patient response. It is recommended that the maximum dosage in any 4-hour period should be 2 mg/kg body weight.

Nurse monitoring
The nurse monitoring aspects of the local anaesthetic, lignocaine (q.v.) apply to this drug.

General note
The drug may be stored at room temperature.

BUPRENORPHINE (Temgesic)

Presentation
Injection—0.3 mg in 1 ml, 0.6 mg in 2 ml
Tablets, sublingual—0.2 mg

Actions and uses
This narcotic analgesic (opioid) drug has a moderate analgesic action and is now subject to the legal requirements of 'controlled drugs'. It is used for the treatment of conditions associated with moderate to severe pain.

Dosage
1. Adults:
    a. By injection: 300–600 microgram (0.3–0.6 mg) every 6-8 hours by intramuscular or slow intravenous injection.
    b. Oral: 200–400 microgram (0.2–0.4 mg) dissolved under the tongue every 6-8 hours or as required for pain.

2. Children
    a. By injection (over 6 months only): 3–9 microgram/kg body weight 6-8 hourly by slow intravenous or intramuscular route.
    b. Oral (over 16 kg body weight only): 100 microgram (16–25kg), 200 microgram (25–37.5kg), 300 microgram may be given to heavier children.

Nurse monitoring
1. The problem of addiction with continued use is now established with this drug.
2. The drug is therefore now subject to the legal requirements of 'controlled drugs'.
3. Constipation and suppression of cough may occur.
4. With excessive dosage there is a risk of prolonged sedation and respiratory depression. Treatment with repeated doses of the opioid antagonist naloxone may be required.

General note
Buprenorphine may be stored at room temperature and should be protected from light.

BUSERELIN (Suprefact)

Presentation
Injection—1 mg in 1 ml
Nasal spray—100 microgram, 150 microgram/dose

Actions and uses
Buserelin is a chemical analogue of the hypothalamic hormone gonadotrophin releasing hormone (GnRH), also known as LHRH (luteinising hormone releasing hormone) or gonadorelin. It acts by downregulating the release of pituitary gonadotrophins (it induces a desensitization to gonadotrophin release) with consequent suppression of pituitary gonadal function. Buserelin has three main uses.

1. It is used in the treatment of advanced prostatic cancer (stages C or D) when suppression of testosterone is required (such tumours are testosterone dependent): its action has been described as equivalent to a 'medical castration'.
2. It inhibits ovarian secretion of sex steroids and it is used therefore in the treatment of endometriosis.
3. It is used at specialist fertility clinics to desensitize the pituitary and so facilitate induction of ovulation by administered gonadotrophins.

Dosage

1. Prostatic cancer: At the start of therapy, a series of subcutaneous injections, the usual dose is 500 microgram, is given 8-hourly for 1 week. This is followed by intranasal maintenance therapy with one application (100 microgram) into each nostril 6 times daily to coincide with the three main meals.
2. Endometriosis: One application (150 microgram) is sprayed into each nostril 3 times daily commencing on the first or second day of menstruation and continued for a maximum treatment duration of 6 months.
3. Anovulatory infertility: One application (150 microgram) is sprayed into each nostril 4 times daily commencing in early follicular phase (day 1) or, provided pregnancy is first excluded, in midluteal phase (day 21) and continued until suppression of pituitary function is achieved (usually after 2-3 weeks).

Nurse monitoring

1. The effectiveness of treatment is highly dependent upon good patient compliance and patients require careful instruction in the use of maintenance therapy. For example, in prostatic cancer six daily doses are administered as follows: dose 1 (before breakfast), dose 2 (after breakfast),

doses 3 and 4 (before and after the mid-day meal), doses 5 and 6 (before and after the evening meal).
2. Since in prostatic cancer buserelin affects only testosterone-dependent tumours it should not be used if orchidectomy has been carried out. Also failure to obtain a response (measured by falling testosterone levels) within 6 weeks on full doses indicates the presence of an insensitive tumour and buserelin therapy should be stopped.
3. A high proportion of patients experience an initial flare-up in their condition associated with a transient rise in testosterone levels, accompanied by increased bone pain, at the start of therapy. To offset this, an anti-androgen (cyproterone acetate) may be administered concurrently, starting a few days before buserelin therapy and continued for about 3 weeks thereafter.
4. Buserelin must not be used during pregnancy, breast-feeding or in patients with undiagnosed vaginal bleeding.
5. Common side-effects include hot flushing, loss of potency and libido, breast swelling and tenderness. Occasionally patients may complain of nasal irritation when on maintenance therapy.

General note

Buserelin injection and nasal spray should be stored at room temperature. The nasal spray, once started, is used for 7 days then discarded and replaced.

BUSPIRONE (BuSpar)

Presentation
Tablets—5 mg
Actions and uses
Buspirone is an anxiolytic and antidepressant which appears to combine the effects of the

benzodiazepines and tricyclic and related antidepressants though its precise mechanism of action is unknown. It is used in the treatment of anxiety, particularly that in which depression is an associated finding.

Dosage
Adults: Usually 5 mg taken 2-3 times daily but up to a maximum dose of 45 mg daily may be required.

Nurse monitoring
1. Side-effects commonly experienced during the early period of treatment include nausea, headache, dizziness or lightheadedness, and irritability. Tachycardia, palpitations, sweating, confusion and fatigue are also reported.
2. The nurse monitoring section for tricyclic antidepressants should also be consulted.

General note
Buspirone tablets may be stored at room temperature.

BUSULPHAN (Myleran)

Presentation
Tablets—0.5 mg, 2 mg

Actions and uses
Busulphan is a cytotoxic drug which is converted in the body to a highly reactive product which in turn binds irreversibly to substances in cells which are essential for cell growth and division. The process of growth and division is therefore blocked by this action. Rapidly dividing cells such as tumour cells and cells of the bone marrow are more likely to be affected by this drug than slowly dividing cells. In practice busulphan has the following uses:
1. It is used in the treatment of chronic myeloid leukaemia.
2. It is used in the treatment of primary polycythaemia.

Dosage
The average adult dose is 2–4 mg daily taken for a period of 6 months when an optimum response is usually achieved. If treatment is stopped at this stage relapse often occurs 6-18 months later. Patients are therefore usually continued on maintenance doses ranging from 0.5–3 mg per day and with maintenance therapy the disease may be controlled for longer periods of time, i.e. 2 years or more. This regime is not used in the treatment of children.

Nurse monitoring
1. Excessive bone marrow depression may occur and thrombocytopenia with resultant haemorrhage is particularly common. Anaemia and infection due to suppression of white cell production also occur.
2. If patients are given this drug for several years pulmonary fibrosis may develop. This may present as progressive breathlessness on exertion or may be detected on routine X-ray examination. If this side-effect is noticed at an early stage and the drug is stopped then stoppage of the drug and a course of steroid therapy may reverse the process. If the effect is not recognised progressive irreversible fibrosis with respiratory failure and death will follow. It is important, therefore, that all staff involved in the care of patients on this treatment should observe the patient for development of such symptoms.
3. Other side-effects include skin pigmentation which may be extensive and especially affects light exposed areas, pressure areas, skin creases, axillae and nipples. Amenorrhoea, testicular atrophy and gynaecomastia may also occur.
4. Adrenal gland insufficiency (Addison's disease) has been reported as a rare complication of this treatment.
5. The nurse should be constantly aware that most cytotoxic drugs are irritant to the skin and mucous surfaces, and are in general very toxic. Great care should therefore be exercised

when handling these drugs, and in particular spillage or contamination of personnel or the environment must be avoided. If cytotoxic drugs are handled regularly it is theoretically possible that repeated skin contact or inhalation may produce systemic toxic effects and in nurses who have developed hypersensitivity, severe local and general hypersensitivity reactions.

General note
Busulphan may be stored at room temperature.

BUTOBARBITONE (Soneryl)

Presentation
Tablets—100 mg
Actions and uses
Butobarbitone is a barbiturate drug (q.v.). Its main use is as a hypnotic drug but occasionally it is used as a day-time sedative.
Dosage
1. For hypnosis: 100–200 mg on retiring.
2. For day-time sedation: 100 mg twice daily.

Nurse monitoring
See the section on barbiturate drugs.

General note
Butobarbitone tablets may be stored at room temperature.

BUTRIPTYLINE (Evadyne)

Presentation
Tablets—25 mg, 50 mg
Actions and uses
Butriptyline is a tricyclic antidepressant drug. Its actions and uses are described in the section on tricyclic antidepressant drugs.
Dosage
The average oral dosage for the treatment of depression is 25 mg three times a day. It may be increased if required to a maximum of 150 mg per day in total.

Nurse monitoring
See the section on tricyclic antidepressants.

General note
Butriptyline tablets may be stored at room temperature.

C

CALCIFEROL

Calciferol is a mixture of ergo-calciferol and cholecalciferol.

Presentation

Tablets—10 000 units/tablet, 50 000 units/tablet

Oral solution—3000 units in 1 ml and 400 000 units/ml (Sterogyl)

Injection—300 000 units in 1 ml

Actions and uses

The actions and uses for calciferol are identical to those described in the section for vitamin D.

Dosage

1. For the treatment of vitamin D deficiency states (q.v.): Initially 500-5000 units of calciferol per day depending on the severity of the deficiency state and the age of the patient. The dose should thereafter be carefully monitored by regular estimation of blood calcium and assessment of clinical improvement and should be tailored to suit the needs of the individual patient.

2. For the treatment of resistant rickets and hypoparathyroidism: Much higher doses of between 50 000 to 150 000 units per day are necessary.

Nurse monitoring

The nurse monitoring notes on vitamin D (q.v.) are applicable to this drug.

General note

The drug may be stored at room temperature.

CALCIPOTRIOL (Dovonex)

Presentation

Ointment—0.005%

Actions and uses

Calcipotriol is a chemical derivative of vitamin D which has been shown to reduce plaque formation in psoriasis. It is used in mild to moderate psoriasis which affects up to 40% of the body skin area.

Dosage

Ointment is applied to the affected area twice daily.

Nurse monitoring

1. It is recommended that application be restricted to 100 g weekly and that application to the face be avoided.

2. Since it is a vitamin D analogue, calcipotriol should not be used in patients with hypercalcaemia.

3. The effects of large quantities of topical vitamin D in pregnancy and lactation are unknown and calciptriol should therefore be avoided in these situations.

4. A degree of irritation is reported which may be more marked when applied to the face. Perioral lesions in particular may occur.

General note

Calcipotriol ointment may be stored at room temperature.

CALCITONIN (Calcitare)

Presentation

Injection—160 units

Actions and uses

A form of calcitonin derived from pig (porcine) thyroid tissue. In this form it is more immunogenic than salmon calcitonin (see salcatonin q.v.) which is therefore generally preferred. Calcitonin is a hormone secreted by the thyroid and parathyroid glands which regulates bone turnover. It does so by lowering plasma calcium and phosphate levels, and by antagonizing the actions of para-thyroid hormone on bone. In particular, calcitonin:

1. Inhibits the activity of bone cells called osteoclasts which continu-ously digest bone tissue releasing free calcium and phosphate.
2. Promotes the renal excretion of calcium and phosphate.
3. Inhibits the activation of vitamin D and hence calcium absorption from the gut.

It is used in conditions associated with rapid bone turnover including Paget's disease (to relieve pain and neurological complications), post-menopausal osteoporosis, hyper-calcaemia of malignancy, and for pain relief in metastatic disease of the bone.

Dosage

Administration is usually by subcuta-neous (occasionally intramuscular) injection.

1. Paget's disease in adults: Ranges from 80 units on alternate days to 160 units daily as a single dose or in 2-3 divided doses.
2. Hypercalcaemia: Based on 4 units/kg and increased according to response.

See salcatonin for details of other indications.

Nurse monitoring

1. As described above, calcitonin is to some extent immunogenic and injections may be poorly tolerated by some patients in whom it causes nausea, vomiting, flushing, diarrhoea, tingling sensation and skin rashes. Anaphylaxis has occurred.

2. As a result of the above, patients may be assessed for likely allergy by prior skin prick or scratch testing.
3. If used to arrest the rate of bone turnover in osteoporotic women it is important that supplementary calcium and vitamin D be given also.

General notes

1. Porcine calcitonin is supplied as a dry powder which must be reconstituted with a special gelatin diluent with which it is provided.
2. Dry powder ampoules may be stored at room temperature but solution, once prepared, should be used within 24 hours. If refrigerated however, solutions can be stored for 7 days.

CALCITRIOL (Rocaltrol)

This drug is also known as 1, 25-dihydroxycholecalciferol.

Presentation

Capsules—0.25 microgram and 0.5 microgram

Actions and uses

The actions and uses of calcitriol are identical to those described in the section for vitamin D.

Dosage

For the treatment of renal osteo-dystrophy:

1. In adults and children over 20 kg body weight the initial dose recommended is 1 microgram with subsequent dosage adjusted according to clinical and bio-chemical response.
2. Children under 20 kg body weight: 0.05 microgram/kg per day with subsequent adjustments in dosage according to clinical and biochemical response.

Nurse monitoring

The nurse monitoring aspects of this drug are identical to those described for vitamin D in general (q.v.)

General note

The drug may be stored at room temperature.

CAPREOMYCIN (Capastat)

Presentation
Injection—1 mega unit (equivalent to 1 g) vials

Actions and uses
Capreomycin is a drug which has been found to be useful in the treatment of tuberculosis due to the organism *Mycobacterium tuberculosis*. It is, however, because of its severe side-effects (see below) reserved for use in patients who either cannot tolerate more commonly used drugs or where culture tests indicate that the organism has become resistant to the more commonly used drugs.

Dosage
Adults: 1 mega unit (1 g) daily by intramuscular injection.

Nurse monitoring
1. Patients undergoing treatment for tuberculosis receive their drugs for considerable periods of time. The nurse may play an important role in reminding patients that their drug therapy must be taken regularly for as long as recommended by medical staff, whether or not they themselves feel that they have recovered.
2. This drug is associated with a number of potentially serious side-effects and its use is limited to the situations described above.
3. Painful hardening of the skin at injection sites is common and therefore frequent variation of injection site is recommended.
4. Widespread metabolic disturbance may occur involving protein, calcium and potassium metabolism in the body.
5. Progressive damage to the liver and kidney may occur.
6. Severe neurological side-effects including vertigo, tinnitus and deafness (which may be occasionally irreversible) may occur.
7. Hypersensitivity reactions including skin rash, fever, eosinophilia may occur.
8. The drug should be used with caution in patients with reduced renal or liver function or where other drugs which are known to be potentially ototoxic (i.e. aminoglycoside antibiotics (q.v.) are to be used.
9. It is usually recommended that liver function, renal function, blood calcium, potassium levels and auditory function be regularly monitored during treatment.

General notes
1. Vials of capreomycin should be stored in a cool place, preferably a refrigerator.
2. The injections are prepared by the addition of 2 ml sodium chloride 0.9%.

CAPTOPRIL (Acepril, Capoten)

Presentation
Tablets—12.5 mg, 25 mg, 50 mg

Actions and uses
See section on ACE inhibitors.

Dosage
Range: 25–50 mg twice daily.

Nurse monitoring
See section on ACE inhibitors

General note
Captopril tablets may be stored at room temperature.

CARBAMAZEPINE (Tegretol)

Presentation
Tablets—100 mg, 200 mg and 400 mg
Chewable tablets—100 mg, 200 mg
Controlled-release tablets—200 mg, 400 mg
Liquid—100 mg in 5 ml
Suppositories—125 mg, 250 mg

Actions and uses
Carbamazepine has two main uses:
1. It is an anticonvulsant drug and the actions and uses of anticonvulsants in general are described in the section on anticonvulsants.

2. It has been found to be an effective analgesic for treating the pain associated with trigeminal neuralgia.

Dosage

1. For the treatment of epilepsy: It is advised that a gradually increasing dosage regime is used and this should be adjusted to suit the needs of the individual patient.

    a. Adults: Oral—Initially 100–200 mg once or twice daily followed by a slow increase until the best response is obtained. This usually occurs when the patient is receiving 800–1200 mg in total per day but in some instances 1600 mg daily may be necessary.

    Rectal—Using the oral dose as a guide with 125 mg and 250 mg rectally corresponding to 100 mg and 200 mg orally respectively (i.e. an increase in dose of 25% to account for slightly poorer absorption from the rectum).

    b. Children: Less than 1 year—100–200 mg per day given in divided doses; 1-5 years—200–400 mg per day given in divided doses; 5-10 years—400–600 mg per day in total given in divided doses; 10-15 years—600–1000 mg per day given in divided doses.

The above doses are maintenance doses. Initial doses should be considerably smaller.

2. For the treatment of trigeminal neuralgia: The individual dosage requirements of carbamazepine vary considerably depending on the age and weight of the patient. An initial dose of 100 mg per day is recommended. Under normal circumstances, 200 mg 3-4 times daily is sufficient to maintain a pain-free state and in rare instances a total dose of 1600 mg per day may be necessary.

Nurse monitoring

1. The nurse monitoring aspects of anticonvulsant drugs in general are discussed in the section on anticonvulsants.

2. Drowsiness and dizziness are common at the start of treatment especially if the initial dose is high or is subsequently increased too quickly.

3. Dry mouth, diarrhoea, nausea and vomiting are common side-effects.

4. Unusual side-effects include skin rash, light-sensitive dermatitis, jaundice, leucopenia and aplastic anaemia.

5. Suppositories have been only relatively recently introduced. They are especially useful to cover periods when the oral route is unavailable e.g. due to severe nausea and vomiting or in the peri-operative period.

6. Rectal carbamazepine is reported occasionally to produce local irritation.

7. Carbamazepine is a potent inducer of the liver microsomal enzyme system and as such it may increase the rate of metabolism of other drugs taken concurrently. Interactions of this type occur with the following drugs which are extensively metabolized by the liver: corticosteroids, cyclosporin, other anticonvulsants, theophylline, thyroxine and warfarin. It may be necessary to review the dosage of such drugs to avoid a loss of effect if one is already being prescribed for a patient commenced on carbamazepine.

General note

All forms of the drug may be stored at room temperature.

CARBENICILLIN (Pyopen)

(See Note 3, p. 362)

Presentation

Injection—vials containing 1 g and 5 g powder.

Actions and uses

Carbenicillin is a member of the penicillin group of antibiotics which has been found to be particularly useful against *Pseudomonas aeruginosa* and Proteus species.

These two groups of organisms are particularly resistant to most antibiotics. Carbenicillin therefore is used for the treatment of bacteraemia, septicaemia, endocarditis, meningitis, infected burns and infected wounds when they are caused by these organisms.

Dosage

Carbenicillin is given by slow intravenous injection (over 3-4 minutes) or by rapid intravenous infusion (over 30-40 minutes using the special infusion pack) or by the intramuscular route. Dose ranges are as follows:

1. Adults.
   a. Intramuscular: 1–2 g 4 to 6-hourly.
   b. Intravenous bolus or intravenous infusion: 5 g 4 to 6-hourly.
2. Children:
   a. Intramuscularly: 50–100 mg/kg body weight in total daily given in 4-6 divided doses.
   b. Intravenously: 250–400 mg/kg body weight in total daily given in 4-6 divided doses.

Nurse monitoring

1. The nurse monitoring notes for all penicillins as described under benzylpenicillin (q.v.) apply to Carbenicillin.
2. It is important to note that carbenicillin is used for the treatment of severe infections by organisms normally resistant to most other antibiotics. It is important therefore to ensure that the dosage given is adequate and appropriate for the patient and condition under treatment. Treatment with lower dosage may lead to failure to eradicate the infection and acquisition of resistance to the drug by the organism. Dosages should never be lower than those recommended except in the situation where the patient under treatment has impaired renal function.

General notes

1. Carbenicillin injection should be stored in a cool place, preferably a refrigerator.

2. To prepare injections or infusion:
   a. For intramuscular use: add 2 ml water for injection to each 1 g vial.
   b. For intravenous use: dilute initially by adding 5 ml to each vial and after dissolution further dilute to 20 ml prior to administration.
   c. Intravenous infusions are prepared by mixing the contents of each vial with the 50 ml of diluent provided. This may be further diluted in 0.9% sodium chloride, 5% dextrose or dextrose/saline mixtures.

CARBENOXOLONE (Biogastrone, Pyrogastrone)

Presentation

Tablets—50 mg

Also combined carbenoxolone and antacid tablets.

Actions and uses

Carbenoxolone is effective in healing gastric ulcers and oesophageal irritation and ulceration. It is postulated to do this by the following mechanisms:

1. It increases mucus production which in turn protects gastric mucosa from damage.
2. It reduces the back diffusion of hydrogen ions from the stomach contents into the mucosa, again protecting the mucosa from damage.
3. It increases the life span of gastric epithelial cells. The drug is taken as conventional tablets for the treatment of gastric ulcer.

Dosage

Gastric ulcer: 100 mg three times daily after meals for 1 week, followed by 50 mg three times daily until the ulcer has healed.

Oesophageal irritation/ulceration: 1-2 Pyrogastrone tablets chewed 3 times daily after meals. Treatment course up to 2 months.

Nurse monitoring

1. The principal problem with carbenoxolone is that it causes sodium and water retention with consequent oedema, hypertension and hypokalaemia. It must therefore be used with great caution in patients with hypertension, heart disease, renal or liver dysfunction.
2. It should be remembered that hypokalaemia is particularly dangerous in patients taking digoxin or other cardiac glycosides and this constitutes a relative contraindication for the coincident use of these two drugs.

General note

Preparations containing carbenoxolone may be stored at room temperature.

CARBIMAZOLE (Neo-Mercazole)

Presentation

Tablets—5 mg

Actions and uses

Carbimazole inhibits the production of thyroxine by the thyroid gland. This action is shared by its active metabolite, methimazole. Both these drugs are therefore termed anti-thyroid drugs and are used in the treatment of thyrotoxicosis. They may be used on their own for prolonged periods in the treatment of this disease or they may be given for a short period in thyrotoxic patients prior to surgery.

Dosage

1. Adults: Initially a high dose is used in order to render the patient euthyroid (i.e. to produce a normal thyroid function). 30-60 mg is usually given for the first month. After this the dose is gradually reduced to maintain the patient in a clinically and biochemically euthyroid

state. The total daily dosage is usually taken in three divided doses.
2. Children: An average daily dose for children is 5 mg three times per day initially reducing to doses as determined by the clinical and biochemical state of the patient.

Nurse monitoring

1. A rare but extremely important adverse effect of this drug is the production of bone marrow depression. Depression of white cell function leads to an increased liability to infection and this side-effect often manifests itself as a throat infection. All patients receiving this drug should therefore be warned to report immediately the development of a sore throat and the drug should be stopped while blood tests are performed. The nurse may play an important role by emphasising the importance of reporting this development to the patient.
2. Other side-effects include nausea, headache, arthralgia, gastrointestinal upset, skin rash and uncommonly hair loss.
3. If carbimazole is given to a pregnant patient adverse effects on the thyroid function of the developing fetus may occur. It is therefore particularly important to achieve the correct dosage in pregnant patients.
4. As the drug is actively secreted in breast milk, mothers receiving this drug should be advised not to breast feed.

General note

Tablets containing carbimazole may be stored at room temperature.

CARBOPLATIN (Paraplatin)

Presentation

Injection—50 mg in 5 ml, 150 mg in 15 ml, 450 mg in 45 ml

Actions and uses
Carboplatin is a platinum-containing cytotoxic drug which is similar to cisplatin and the section under cisplatin should be read. It is mainly used in the treatment of advanced ovarian carcinoma and small cell carcinoma of the lung.

Dosage
This is largely determined by specific indication and current schedules which are subject to change in line with existing knowledge. The existing schedule should be consulted for up-to-date details of dosage and route of administration. Doses in the region of 400 mg/m² body surface area have been used.

Nurse monitoring
See the section under cisplatin.

General note
Carboplatin injection may be stored at room temperature. Infusions are prepared in glucose 5% or sodium chloride 0.9% injection diluted to concentrations as low as 0.5 mg in 1 ml.

CARBOPROST (Hemabate)

Presentation
Injection—250 microgram in 1 ml
Actions and uses
Carboprost is a prostaglandin derivative used to treat post-partum haemorrhage which is unresponsive to first line treatment with ergotamine and oxytocin.

Dosage
250 microgram by deep intramuscular injection repeated as required at intervals as short as 15 minutes and up to 90 minutes. A maximum of 12 mg (48 doses) may be given.

Nurse monitoring
1. Carboprost injection may produce nausea, vomiting, diarrhoea, flushing and bronchospasm. Other adverse effects include a raised blood pressure, pulmonary oedema, chills and sweating, dizziness, and erythema,
2. It must be avoided in acute pelvic inflammatory disease, and cardiac, pulmonary, and hepatic disease. Caution is necessary in patients with a history of glaucoma, asthma, hypertension, anaemia, jaundice, diabetes, epilepsy, and uterine scars since excessive dosage may cause uterine rupture.

General note
This drug has a 3 year shelf life when stored in a refrigerator.

CARMUSTINE (BiCNU)

Presentation
Injection—100 mg (plus ethanol diluent 3 ml)
Actions and uses
Carmustine is a cytotoxic drug of the nitrogen mustard group which arrests cell proliferation and growth by a chemical binding (alkylating) action on DNA and other cellular substances which are essential for cell division to proceed. Its main use is in the treatment of myeloma, lymphoma and brain tumours but the uses of cytotoxic drugs do vary from time to time.

Dosage
This is largely determined by specific indication and current schedules which are subject to change in line with existing knowledge. The existing schedule should be consulted for up-to-date details of dosage and route of administration. Courses of 200 mg/m² either as a single dose or a series of daily doses have been used and repeated several weeks later.

Nurse monitoring
1. Delayed myelotoxicity is the most common and serious adverse effect of this drug. Anaemia, leucopenia and, in particular, thrombocytopenia may develop up to 6 weeks after the drug has

been administered and is dose-related.

2. Carmustine causes frequent nausea and vomiting within 2 hours of dosing and lasting for about 4-6 hours.

3. Adverse effects are also reported on the liver (raised liver enzymes), lung (pulmonary infiltration/fibrosis) and kidney (renal failure).

4. Carmustine causes a burning irritation at the injection site and extravasation must be avoided. If administered too rapidly there may be intense flushing lasting for several hours.

5. The nurse should be constantly aware that most cytotoxic drugs are irritant to the skin and mucous surfaces and are in general very toxic. Great care should therefore be exercised when handling these drugs and, in particular, spillage or con-tamination of personnel or the environment must be avoided. If cytotoxic drugs are handled regularly it is theoretically possible that repeated skin contact or inhalation may produce systemic toxic effects and in nurses who have developed hypersensitivity, severe local and general hypersensitivity reactions.

General note

Carmustine injection must be stored in a refrigerator. It is reconstituted using the ethanol diluent supplied and further diluted in 500 ml glucose 5% or sodium chloride 0.9% injection. The infusion, once prepared, may be stored under refrigeration for 48 hours before use. It must be protected from light and rapidly degrades at room temperature.

CARTEOLOL (Teoptic)

Presentation
Eye drops—1%, 2%

Actions and uses

Carteolol is a beta-blocking drug and it has the actions and uses of other drugs described in the section on beta-adrenoreceptor blocking drugs. In practice, however, carteolol is only used in the form of eye drops for the treatment of ocular hypertension and chronic open-angle glaucoma: topical beta-blockers lower raised intraocular pressure by an unknown mechanism which is associated with a reduction in aqueous humour production.

Dosage

Glaucoma: One drop is instilled in the affected eye twice daily, therapy being initiated with 1% strength drops and increased in time as necessary.

Nurse monitoring

1. Despite the fact that this drug is administered externally, sufficient may be absorbed from the cornea to produce systemic side-effects in susceptible patients (see beta-adrenoreceptor drugs). Thus patients with obstructive airways disease (particularly asthmatics) and those with uncontrolled heart failure should not be treated with beta-blocker eye drops.

2. Other patients in whom carteolol must be used with caution include those with sinus bradycardia and 2nd or 3rd degree heart block.

3. Carteolol eye drops may cause stinging of the eye on application and should be avoided if the patient uses soft contact lenses.

General note

Carteolol eye drops may be stored at room temperature. They have a relatively short life during use when a risk of bacterial contamination after opening exists and normally eye drops of any kind should not be used after 1 week for a hospitalized patient or after 4 weeks for others.

CEFACLOR (Distaclor)

(See Note 3, p. 362)
Presentation
Capsules—250 mg
Syrup—125 mg in 5 ml, 250 mg in 5 ml
Actions and uses
This drug is a member of the cephalosporin group of antibiotics and its actions and uses are described in the section dealing with the group. Cefaclor is a 1st Generation cephalosporin. It may be given orally.
Dosage
1. Adult: 250 mg to 500 mg 8-hourly.
2. Children: 20 mg/kg body weight daily in total given in three divided doses.

Nurse monitoring
See the section on cephalosporins.

General notes
1. The drug may be stored at room temperature.
2. Once prepared the syrup should be refrigerated and used within 14 days.

CEFADROXIL (Baxan)

(See Note 3, p. 362)
Presentation
Capsules—500 mg
Suspension—125 mg in 5 ml, 250 mg in 5 ml, 500 mg in 5 ml
Actions and uses
This drug is a member of the cephalosporin group of antibiotics and its actions and uses are described in the section dealing with the group. Cefadroxil is a 1st Generation cephalosporin.
Dosage
1. Adults: 1 g twice daily (or once daily for urinary tract infection).
2. Children: Under 1 year old—25 mg/kg body weight in total daily in 2 divided doses; 1-6 years old—125–250 mg twice daily; over 6 years old—250–500 mg twice daily.

Nurse monitoring
See the section on cephalosporins.

General notes
1. The drug may be stored at room temperature.
2. Once prepared the suspension is stable if stored at room temperature for 7 days (or 14 days if refrigerated).

CEFAMANDOLE (Kefadol)

(See Note 3, p. 362)
Presentation
Injection—500 mg and 1 g in 10 ml vials, 2 g in 100 ml vials
Actions and uses
This drug is a member of the cephalosporin group of antibiotics and its action and uses are described in the section on cephalosporins. Cefamandole is a 2nd Generation cephalosporin.
Dosage
1. Adults: The dose range is 500 mg–2 g 4 to 8-hourly by intravenous injection or deep intramuscular injection. Intravenous bolus injections are given slowly over 3-5 minutes or alternatively by infusing in 0.9% sodium chloride, 5% dextrose or dextrose/saline mixtures.
2. Children: The dose range is 50–100 mg/kg body weight in total daily either 4-8 hourly by deep intramuscular injection or intravenous bolus injection or intravenous infusion.

Nurse monitoring
See the section on cephalosporins.

General notes
1. The drug should be stored at room temperature.
2. After reconstitution, vials should be stored in a refrigerator and must be discarded if unused after 96 hours.
3. Prolonged storage at room temperature will generate carbon dioxide gas within the vial and create increased pressure.

4. The drug should be reconstituted as follows:
   a. For intramuscular injection: add 3 ml water for injection or 0.9% sodium chloride to each 1 g.
   b. For intravenous injection: after reconstitution the drug should be diluted to 10 ml and given over a period of 3-5 minutes.
   c. If given by continuous intravenous infusion, the drug may be diluted in any common infusion solution and administered over the appropriate time.

CEFOTAXIME (Claforan)

(See Note 3, p. 362)

Presentation
Injection—500 mg, 1 g and 2 g vials

Actions and uses
This drug is a member of the cephalosporin group of antibiotics and its action and uses are described in the section on cephalosporins. Cefotaxime is a 3rd Generation cephalosporin.

Dosage
1. Adults: 2–12 g daily in total in 2, 3 or 4 divided doses depending upon the nature and severity of infection. May be administered by intramuscular and intravenous injection or by intravenous infusion.
2. Children: 100–200 mg/kg body weight in total daily in 2-4 divided doses.

Nurse monitoring
See the section on cephalosporins.

General notes
1. The drug should be stored at room temperature.
2. It should be reconstituted as follows:
   a. For intravenous or intramuscular injection, add 2 ml water for injection to 500 mg vial, 4 ml to 1 g vial and 10 ml to 2 g vial. Lignocaine 1% may be used in place of water for injection if pain on injection is a problem.
   b. For intravenous infusion, dissolve in 100 ml sodium chloride 0.9%, dextrose 5% or dextrose/saline mixtures and administer over 20–60 minutes.
3. After reconstitution, intramuscular and intravenous injections should be administered immediately and any drug remaining should be discarded. Solutions for infusion should be discarded after 24 hours.

CEFOXITIN (Mefoxin)

(See Note 3, p. 362)

Presentation
Injection—1 g and 2 g vials

Actions and uses
This drug is a member of the cephalosporin group of antibiotics and its actions and uses are described in the section on cephalosporins. Cefoxitin is a 2nd Generation cephalosporin.

Dosage
1. Adults: 1–2 g may be given every 8 hours by intramuscular or intravenous bolus injection or intravenous infusion in all common infusion fluids.
2. Children: 80–160 mg/kg body weight in total daily given in 4 or 6 divided doses.

N.B. The intramuscular injection may be reconstituted with 0.5% or 1 % lignocaine to reduce pain at the injection site.

Nurse monitoring
See the section on cephalosporins.

General notes
1. The drug should be stored in a refrigerator.
2. Reconstituted solutions for injection must be used within 24 hours if kept at room temperature or 1 week if refrigerated.
3. To prepare an injection:
   a. For intramuscular use: add 2 ml diluent to each 1 g vial.
   b. For intravenous use: add 10 ml diluent to each 1 g vial.
4. Intravenous injections should be given slowly over 3-5 minutes.

CEFSULODIN (Monaspor)

(See Note 3, p. 362)

Presentation

Injection—500 mg and 1 g vials

Actions and uses

This drug is a member of the cephalosporin group of antibiotics and its actions and uses are described in the section on cephalosporins. Cefsulodin is a 3rd Generation cephalosporin.

Dosage

1. Adults: 1–4 g daily in 2-4 divided doses, administered by intra-muscular and intravenous injection or by intravenous infusion.
2. Children: 20–50 mg/kg body weight in 2-4 divided doses.

Nurse monitoring

See the section on cephalosporins.

General notes

1. The drug should be stored at room temperature.
2. It should be reconstituted as follows:
   a. For intramuscular injection, add 3 ml of 0.5% lignocaine injection to each vial (500 mg or 1 g).
   b. For intravenous injection, add 5 ml to 500 mg vial or 10 ml to 1 g vial of water for injection.
   c. For intravenous infusion, dissolve in 100 ml sodium chloride 0.9%, dextrose 5% or dextrose/saline mixtures and administer over 30-60 minutes.
3. Intramuscular and intravenous injections should be prepared immediately before administration. Infusions should be used within 12 hours if stored at room temperature or 24 hours if refrigerated.

CEFTAZIDIME (Fortum)

(See Note 3, p. 362)

Presentation

Injection—500 mg, 1 g and 2 g vials

Actions and uses

This drug is a member of the cephalosporin group of antibiotics and its actions and uses are described in the section on cephalosporins. Ceftazidime is a 3rd Generation cephalosporin.

Dosage

1. Adults: 1–6 g daily in 2 or 3 divided doses, administered by intramuscular and intravenous injection or by intravenous infusion.
2. Children: 30–100 mg/kg body weight in 2 or 3 divided doses.

Nurse monitoring

See the section on cephalosporins.

General notes

1. The drug should be stored at room temperature.
2. It should be reconstituted as follows:
   a. For intramuscular injection, add 1.5 ml to 500 mg and 3 ml to 1 g vial of water for injection or sodium chloride 0.9% injection.
   b. For intravenous injection, add 5 ml diluent to 500 ml vial and 10 ml to 1 g and 2 g vials.
   c. For intravenous infusion, dissolve in 50 ml sodium chloride 0.9%, dextrose 5% or dextrose/saline mixtures and administer over 20-30 minutes.
3. Carbon dioxide gas is formed during the mixing of ceftazidime injection creating an increase in the internal pressure of the vial.
4. Prepared solutions for injection may be stored for up to 18 hours at room temperature if not immediately used.

CEFTIZOXIME (Cefizox)

(See Note 3, p. 362)

Presentation

Injection—500 mg, 1 g and 2 g vials

Actions and uses

This drug is a member of the cephalosporin group of antibiotics and its actions and uses are described in the section on cephalosporins. Ceftizoxime is a 3rd Generation cephalosporin.

Dosage
1. Adults. 1–9 g daily in 2 or 3 divided doses, administered in intramuscular or intravenous injection or intravenous infusion.
2. Children: 30–150 mg/kg body weight daily in 2-4 divided doses.

Nurse monitoring
See the section on cephalosporins.

General notes
1. The drug should be stored at room temperature.
2. It should be reconstituted as follows:
   a. For intramuscular and intravenous injections, add 2 ml to 500 mg vial, 3 ml to 1 g vial and 6 ml to 2 g vial of water for injection.
   b. If intramuscular injections are very painful, the injection may be prepared using 0.5% lignocaine injection.
   c. Intravenous infusions are prepared in 50–100 ml sodium chloride 0.9%, dextrose 5% or dextrose/saline mixtures and administered over 20-30 minutes.
   d. Solutions for injection or infusion should be used within 8 hours of preparation if stored at room temperature.

CEFTRIAXONE (Rocephin)

(See Note 3, p. 362)
Presentation
Injection—250 mg, 1 g, 2 g vials
Actions and uses
This drug is a member of the cephalosporin group of antibiotics and its actions and uses are described in the section on cephalosporins. Of particular interest is the much longer shelf life of ceftriaxone compared to other cephalosporins which enables it to be used in a single daily dosage regimen. Although it has a relatively broad spectrum, ceftriaxone has notable antistaphylococcal activity which reflects its use in the treatment of infections of skin and soft tissue, bone, lower respiratory tract and septicaemia, and for surgical prophylaxis to prevent post-operative wound infections. It is also of potential value in treating meningitis and gonorrhoea but is much less useful in the treatment of pseudomonal infections.

Dosage
1. Adults:
   a. Usually by intravenous infusion, 1–4 g administered once daily depending upon the severity of infection and response to treatment.
   b. Lower doses e.g. 1 g can be administered by intramuscular injection in less severe infections.
   c. Single doses of 250 mg are effective for the treatment of gonorrhoea.
   d. For surgical prophylaxis a single dose of 1 g is administered, by the intravenous route immediately prior to surgery.
2. Children: Over 6 weeks only: 20–50 mg/kg body weight daily as above up to 80 mg/kg in severe infections e.g. meningitis.

Nurse monitoring
The nurse monitoring section under cephalosporins applies to this drug.

General notes
1. Powder in vials for reconstitution is stored at room temperature.
2. Intravenous infusions are administered in 100 ml sodium chloride 0.9% or glucose 5% or 10% minibags over 30 minutes. Alternatively, the drug can be administered as a slow bolus dose via the drip tubing of a running intravenous fluid. **Do not** mix with calcium-containing salts.

CEFUROXIME (Zinacef, Zinnat)

(See Note 3, p.362)
Presentation
Tablets—250 mg
Injection—250 mg, 750 mg, 1.5 g

Actions and uses
This drug is a member of the cephalosporin group of antibiotics and its actions and uses are described in the section on cephalosporins. Cefuroxime is a 2nd Generation cephalosporin.

Dosage
1. Adults: The dose range is 750 mg–1.5 g three times daily by intramuscular or intravenous bolus injection or rapid intravenous infusion over 30 minutes. The intravenous infusion may be given in most common infusion fluids.
2. An oral dose of 250 mg three or four times daily may be used in the treatment of infections due to sensitive organisms, e.g. urinary tract infections.
3. Children: The dose range varies from 30–100 mg/kg body weight per day in total given in three or four divided doses.

Nurse monitoring
See the section on cephalosporins.

General notes
1. The drug in injectable form should be stored in a refrigerator and protected from light.
2. After reconstitution solutions may be kept for 5 hours at room temperature or 48 hours if refrigerated.
3. To prepare injections:
   a. For intramuscular use add 1 ml of water for injection to the 250 mg vial or 3 ml to the 750 mg vial.
   b. For intravenous use each 250 mg should be diluted in 2 ml of water for injection.

CELIPROLOL (Celectol)

Presentation
Tablets—200 mg

Actions and uses
Celiprolol is a beta-blocker and the section under beta-adrenoreceptor blocking drugs should be consulted for a general account of these compounds. However, celiprolol is notably different from other beta-blockers in that it is a potent beta$_2$ partial antagonist (i.e. it **stimulates** rather than blocks the effects of sympathetic stimulation at this site) and it possesses **additional** vasodilator activity. Thus celiprolol is particularly useful in the treatment of hypertension and for patients with peripheral vascular insufficiency which is aggravated by therapy with other beta-blockers. Celiprolol is also less likely to interfere with lipid profile and indeed it may have a beneficial effect on the blood lipid pattern so improving this recognised risk factor for coronary heart disease.

Dosage
Adults: 200–400 mg once daily in the morning.

Nurse monitoring
See the section under beta-adrenoreceptor blocking drugs. Although celiprolol has pronounced beta$_2$ stimulant properties its use is contraindicated in asthma, despite an early report that it improved airways performance in a small group of asthmatics.

General note
Celiprolol tablets are stored at room temperature.

CEPHALEXIN (Ceporex, Keflex)

(See Note 3, p.362)

Presentation
Tablets—250 mg, 500 mg
Capsules—250 mg, 500 mg
Syrup—125 mg in 5 ml, 250 mg in 5 ml, 500 mg in 5 ml

Actions and uses
This drug is a member of the cephalosporin group of antibiotics and its actions and uses are described in the section dealing with the group. Cephalexin is a 1st Generation cephalosporin. It may be given orally.

Dosage

1. Adults: 1–4 g in total per day given in divided doses either 6-hourly or 12-hourly.
2. Children: 25–50 mg/kg body weight in total is given each day in divided doses either 6-hourly or 12-hourly. For severe infections up to 100 mg/kg in total daily given in four divided doses has been used.

Nurse monitoring
See the section on cephalosporins.

General notes

1. The drug may be stored at room temperature.
2. The syrup should be used within 10 days of preparation.

CEPHALOSPORINS

A group of antibiotics which includes:

Cefaclor	Ceftizoxime
Cefadroxil	Ceftriaxone
Cefamandole	Cefuroxime
Cefotaxime	Cephalexin
Cefoxitin	Cephalothin
Cefsulodin	Cephazolin
Ceftazidime	Cephradine

Actions and uses

The cephalosporin group of antibiotics has a bactericidal action, i.e. they kill organisms present in body tissues. They have a wide spectrum of activity which resembles that of ampicillin and other broad spectrum penicillins, although a few important differences exist between different cephalosporins. This has led to the classification of these drugs into three distinct categories termed 1st, 2nd and 3rd Generations.

1. 1st Generation cephalosporins are usually effective against Gram-positive microorganisms (streptococcus, staphylococcus and clostridia) and some Gram-negative microorganisms (*Neisseria meningitidis* and *Neisseria gonorrhoea*). However, enterobacteria, Proteus (with the exception of *P. mirabalis*), *Haemophilus influenzae* and the coliforms (*E. coli, Ps. aeruginosa* and Klebsiella) are generally unaffected by these drugs. Some organisms rapidly develop resistance to 1st Generation cephalosporins by producing a cephalosporin inactivating substance called beta-lactamase.
2. 2nd Generation cephalosporins have a similar spectrum to 1st Generation drugs but, in addition, they are less liable to inactivation by beta-lactamase and are therefore often effective against bacteria which have developed resistance to 1st Generation drugs. They also extend the spectrum to include activity against *Haemophilus influenzae* and enterobacteria.
3. 3rd Generation cephalosporins further extend the spectrum of the cephalosporin group by their action against *Pseudomonas aeruginosa* and they may be particularly useful for the prevention and treatment of infections due to this microorganism.

The cephalosporins, in addition to their use in the treatment of infections produced by the above, are also used for the prophylactic prevention of post-operative infection after gynaecological, abdominal, neurological and orthopaedic surgery and in patients treated with anti-cancer drugs who have a diminished (natural) immunity to infection with a host of pathogenic microorganisms.

Dosage

See individual drugs.

Nurse monitoring
1. Allergy is the most common problem with these drugs. This may be:
   a. Immediate, comprising variable reactions ranging from itch and rash to bronchospasm and anaphylactic shock.

C

b. Skin rash, fever and lymphadenopathy may develop after several days of treatment. It is important to note that patients already sensitive to penicillin have a higher risk of developing sensitivity to cephalosporins than do patients who are not allergic to penicillin.

2. It is important to note that intravenous administration of cephalosporins may produce irritation and thrombophlebitis.

3. Intramuscular injections are painful.

4. Cephaloridine (an early cephalosporin now no longer used) was particularly noted for its ability to cause renal damage, especially at higher doses. Other cephalosporins have a lesser risk of causing this problem. The risk of renal damage is especially high if other nephrotoxic drugs such as gentamicin, kanamycin, tobramycin or amikacin are given at the same time.

5. All cephalosporin drugs may accumulate if renal function is impaired and this may lead to toxicity. Reduced doses should therefore be given to patients with renal disease.

General note
See specific drugs.

CEPHALOTHIN (Keflin)
(See Note 3, p. 362)
Presentation
Injection—1 g and 4 g vials
Actions and uses
This drug is a member of the cephalosporin group of antibiotics and its actions and uses are described in the section dealing with the group. Cephalothin is a 1st Generation cephalosporin.
Dosage
1. Adults: 1 g 4 to 6-hourly to a maximum of 12 g per day by intravenous injection or infusion.
2. Children: 80–160 mg/kg body weight in total daily given in divided doses either 4 or 6-hourly.

Nurse monitoring
See the section on cephalosporins.

General notes
1. The drug may be stored at room temperature.
2. After reconstitution, solution in vials may precipitate and become cloudy. Vigorous shaking and warming in the palm of the hand are necessary to achieve resolution.
3. Reconstituted solutions may be kept for 48 hours but intravenous infusions must be given within 24 hours of preparation.
4. Reconstitution of injections:
   a. For direct intravenous administration a solution containing 1 g of cephalothin in 5 ml of diluent may be slowly injected directly into a vein over a period of 3-5 minutes.
   b. For intermittent intravenous infusion the drug may be diluted by adding 40 ml of water for injection or 5% dextrose or normal saline.
   c. For continuous intravenous infusion 4 g of cephalothin may be (after reconstitution with water) diluted in 500 ml of normal saline or 5% dextrose and given over the appropriate period.

CEPHAZOLIN (Kefzol)
(See Note 3, p. 362)
Presentation
Injection—500 mg and 1 g vials
Actions and uses
This drug is a member of the cephalosporin group of antibiotics and its actions and uses are described in the section dealing with the group. Cephazolin is a 1st Generation cephalosporin.
Dosage
The drug may be given by intramuscular and intravenous bolus injections or intravenous infusions in the following doses:
1. Adults: Dosage ranges from 500 mg 12-hourly to 1 g 6 to 8-hourly depending on the nature and severity of the infection.

2. Children: Dosage ranges from 25 mg–50 mg/kg body weight in total daily, usually given in three or four divided doses.

Nurse monitoring
See section on cephalosporins.

General notes
1. The drug may be stored at room temperature.
2. This drug should not be mixed with other antibiotics in the same syringe or infusion fluid.
3. To reconstitute vials add 2–4 ml of water for injection to each vial.
4. Intravenous infusions may be given in sodium chloride 0.9%, dextrose 5% or dextrose saline mixtures. After reconstitution 500 mg or 1 g of the drug may be diluted in 50–500 ml of any of these solutions.
5. For intravenous bolus injection the drug should be diluted after reconstitution to at least 10 ml with water for injection and it should be given over 3-5 minutes.
6. Once reconstituted, vials of injection should be used within 24 hours if kept at room temperature or 96 hours if refrigerated.

CEPHRADINE (Velosef)

(See Note 3, p. 362)
Presentation
Capsules—250 mg, 500 mg
Syrup—125 mg in 5 ml, 250 mg in 5 ml
Injection—250 mg, 500 mg and 1 g vials
Actions and uses
This drug is a member of the cephalosporin group of antibiotics and its actions and uses are described in the section dealing with the group. Cephradine is a 1st Generation cephalosporin.
Dosage
1. Adults: 2–4 g daily in total is given in four divided doses orally or by intramuscular or intravenous injection or by intravenous infusion.

2. Children: 25–50 mg/kg body weight per day in total is given in four divided doses orally. If the parenteral route is necessary the total daily dosage is higher and lies in the range of 50–100 mg/kg body weight per day in total.

Nurse monitoring
See the section on cephalosporins.

General notes
1. The drug should be stored at room temperature.
2. Syrup should be used within 7 days if kept at room temperature or 14 days if refrigerated following reconstitution.
3. Reconstitution of injections:
   a. For intramuscular injections add 1.2 ml water for injection to 250 mg of powder, 2 ml to 500 mg and 4 ml to 1 g.
   b. For intravenous injections add 5 ml water for injection to 250 mg and 500 mg vials and 10 ml water for injection to 1 g vials.
   c. For intravenous infusions the drug should be dissolved in 10 ml of water for injection prior to dilution in the appropriate infusion solution.

Cephradine may be added to isotonic (normal) sodium chloride, 5% dextrose solution or one-sixth molar sodium lactate solution. When mixed in this way it will be potent for up to 8 hours.

N.B. After adding water all vials must be shaken thoroughly for several minutes to ensure the powder is dissolved. After injections are prepared in the above manner, for intramuscular or intravenous bolus injection they should be used within 2 hours.

CHENODEOXYCHOLIC ACID (Chendol)

Presentation
Capsules—125 mg, 250 mg

Actions and uses

This drug is a naturally occurring bile acid which, after oral administration, increases the bile acid pool and thus the amount of dissolved cholesterol and phospholipid. In addition, it is likely that the output of cholesterol secreted into the bile is reduced. The net result is to prevent the precipitation of cholesterol from solution and therefore the formation of cholesterol gallstones; existing cholesterol stones will gradually redissolve, possibly obviating the need for surgical removal.

Dosage

Adults: Usually 10–15 mg/kg body weight daily in divided doses or as a single dose at bedtime. Treatment courses are determined by the size of stones, e.g. a few months for small gallstones with as long as 2 years for large stones.

Nurse monitoring

1. It is important to note that chenodeoxycholic acid therapy is not a suitable treatment for all patients with gallstones and that the nature and size of the stones are important. Those for whom treatment is unsuitable are:
   a. Patients with radio-opaque stones.
   b. Those with non-functioning gallbladders.
   c. Pregnant patients or female patients contemplating pregnancy.
   d. Patients with chronic liver disease or inflammatory bowel disease.
2. The only side-effects of treatment are diarrhoea and pruritus which commonly occur. The incidence of diarrhoea is reduced following a dosage reduction.
3. Abnormal liver function tests and liver damage have occurred during administration of this drug.

General note

Chenodeoxycholic acid capsules should be stored at room temperature in well-sealed containers.

CHLORAL HYDRATE (Noctec)

Presentation

Capsules—500 mg
Mixture—500 mg in 5 ml
Paediatric Elixir—200 mg in 5 ml

Actions and uses

Chloral hydrate is a general central nervous system depressant. It has been in clinical use for many years and has maintained its popularity as a sleep-inducing agent despite the development of many newer hypnotic drugs during this period. In particular, the drug has found widespread popularity in young and elderly patients who generally tolerate it well. The sedative action of chloral hydrate is partly due to trichloroethanol, a metabolite to which it is converted in the body.

Dosage

1. Adults: 500 mg—2 g taken on retiring.
2. Children: 30–50 mg/kg body weight as a single dose.

Nurse monitoring

1. Chloral hydrate administration may be associated with a degree of nausea and gastrointestinal upset and patients should be advised to take their dosages well diluted with water, fruit juices or beverages to minimize the irritant effect on the gut mucosa.
2. Skin rashes occasionally occur and contact of liquid chloral hydrate with skin can produce skin irritation; if this occurs the area of contact should be thoroughly washed.
3. Chloral hydrate capsules must never be bitten since they contain concentrated liquid drug which can produce severe irritation if liberated in the mouth.
4. Despite its irritant effect, chloral hydrate is generally well tolerated. In patients who suffer troublesome gastrointestinal upsets, a more palatable alternative is available (see triclofos).

General note

Chloral hydrate capsules and mixtures may be stored at room temperature. Once diluted, liquid doses must be taken immediately. Mixture and Elixir are relatively unstable and require to be freshly prepared for each prescription: these should not be kept by patients for longer than 2 weeks from time of issue.

CHLORAMBUCIL (Loukeran)

Presentation
Tablets—2 mg, 5 mg

Actions and uses
Chlorambucil is a member of the nitrogen mustard group. It damages cells by irreversibly binding important constituents which are necessary for cellular growth and reproduction. The drug has been shown in practice to be particularly active against lymphoid tissues and appears to destroy not only proliferating cells but also mature circulating lymphocytes. This makes it particularly useful in the treatment of lympho-proliferative disorders. Its main uses are as follows:

1. Lympho-proliferative disorders such as chronic lymphatic leukaemia and the lymphomas.
2. It is the drug of choice for the rare condition of Waldenstrom's microglobulinaemia.
3. It has been used in the treatment of carcinoma of the breast, lung and ovary.
4. It has an immunosuppressant action and may be used in the management of some autoimmune diseases such as rheumatoid arthritis, and systemic lupus erythematosus. It is worth noting that it is used only in severe cases of rheumatoid arthritis which have proved rapidly progressive and resistant to treatment with alternative regimes.

Dosage
1. As a cytotoxic drug:
   a. Initial dosage for adults and children is 0.1–0.2 mg/kg body weight and it is taken for up to 6 weeks at this dosage.
   b. Once remission is obtained continuous maintenance therapy is with 0.03–0.1 mg/kg body weight daily.
   It has been found that short, interrupted courses appear to be safer and are usually preferred.
2. The dosage when used as an immunosuppressive is as follows: high doses of the order 200–300 microgram/kg per day.

Nurse monitoring
1. Chlorambucil exerts a depressant effect on the bone marrow and may cause leucopenia, thrombocytopenia and anaemia. Patients may therefore suffer from severe and life-threatening infection or may develop severe haemorrhage. Patients who are given the drug for a considerable period of time may develop irreversible bone marrow damage leading to fatal aplastic anaemia.
2. Nausea and vomiting are uncommon at the usual dose levels but may occur with higher doses.
3. Skin rash, alopecia and liver damage are occasional complications.
4. As the drug affects dividing cells it reduces sperm formation and may affect the growing fetus.
5. The nurse should be constantly aware that most cytotoxic drugs are irritant to the skin and mucous surfaces, and are in general very toxic. Great care should therefore be exercised when handling these drugs, and in particular spillage or contamination of personnel or the environment must be avoided. If cytotoxic drugs are handled regularly it is theoretically possible that repeated skin contact or inhalation may produce systemic toxic effects and in nurses who have developed hypersensitivity, severe local and general hypersensitivity reactions.

General note

Tablets may be stored at room temperature.

C

CHLORAMPHENICOL
(Chloromycetin)

(See Note 3, p. 362)

Presentation

Capsules—250 mg
Suspension—125 mg in 5 ml
Injection—1 g and 1.2 g vials
Eye ointment—1 %
Eye drops—0.5%
Ear drops—10%

Actions and uses

Chloramphenicol is an antibiotic which has a bacteriostatic action, i.e. it inhibits further growth and replication of bacteria. Its mechanism of action is by inhibiting protein synthesis in cells and therefore preventing their growth. It is a highly effective antibiotic. Because of its possible severe toxicity its use is restricted to certain serious infections where it is known to be superior to other antibiotics. These are:
1. Typhoid fever
2. Meningitis due to *Haemophilus influenzae.*

Topical applications of the drug are not associated with its more serious side-effects and it is used widely for the treatment of infections of the eye and external ear.

Dosage

1. Oral:
   a. Adults: 500–750 mg four times a day.
   b. Children: 50 mg/kg daily in total usually taken in four divided doses.
2. By intramuscular or intravenous infection:
   a. Adults: up to 1 g 6-hourly,
   b. Children: 50 mg/kg daily usually divided into four or six doses. For serious infections in children, twice the above dosage may occasionally be used.
   c. Premature and newborn infants: 25 mg/kg in total per day in four divided doses.

3. Eye drops 0.5% or eye ointment 1 %: A small quantity of ointment or two eye drops in the affected eye every 1 to 3 hours until the eye has been free of visible signs of infection for 48 hours is recommended.
4. For ear drops: 1–3 drops every 3 to 4 hours is recommended.

Nurse monitoring

1. The reason that this highly effective antibiotic is now recommended for restricted use only is that it has a number of serious and potentially fatal side-effects. These are as follows:
   a. The drug may depress bone marrow function. This may be detected by serially examining the blood and usually reversion to normality will follow stoppage of treatment.
   b. An irreversible aplastic anaemia with depression of formation of all types of blood cells leaving the patient anaemic and at risk of severe haemorrhage and infection may occur independently from the above effect. Although this side-effect is more common when the drug is used in high dosage and for prolonged periods, the fact that it is irreversible and commonly fatal makes it a strong contra-indication to the general use of this drug for mild infections.
   c. A syndrome known as 'grey baby syndrome' may occur in babies. Babies' livers cannot metabolize chloramphenicol as well as adults and as a result high concentrations of chloramphenicol itself occur in the blood. This leads to circulatory collapse with shock, respiratory difficulty, cyanosis, vomiting, refusal to suckle and passage of loose green stools. If this syndrome is not recognized the child may die.

2. Other side-effects which may occur with this drug include nausea, vomiting, an unpleasant taste in the mouth, abdominal pain and diarrhoea and optic neuritis. The latter side-effect is very rare.

General note
The drug may be stored at room temperature.

CHLORDIAZEPOXIDE (Librium)

Presentation
Tablets—5 mg, 10 mg, 25 mg
Capsules—5 mg, 10 mg

Actions and uses
Chlordiazepoxide is a member of the benzodiazepine group (q.v.). Its principal use is in the treatment of anxiety but it has been found to be particularly useful in addition for the control of symptoms associated with acute withdrawal of alcohol in chronic alcoholism (delirium tremens).

Dosage
1. For treatment of anxiety:
   a. Adults receive a total of up to 30 mg daily in divided doses. Up to 100 mg may very occasionally be required.
   b. Children receive doses in the range of 5–20 mg per day in total usually given in divided doses.
   c. Use in acute alcohol withdrawal requires careful titration of dose for individual needs, under close supervision, e.g. 25–100 mg every 2-4 hours until control is achieved.

Nurse monitoring
1. For general notes see the section on benzodiazepines.
2. It is essential that the nurse notes that chlordiazepoxide injection may be given by the deep intramuscular route but should never be given intravenously.

General note
Preparations containing chlordiazepoxide may be stored at room temperature.

CHLORMETHIAZOLE (Heminevrin)

Presentation
Capsules—192 mg
Syrup—250 mg in 5 ml (as edisylate)
Injection—0.8% solution for intravenous infusion

Actions and uses
Chlormethiazole is a central nervous system depressant which has several uses in clinical practice:
1. It is a general sedative and hypnotic drug which alleviates acute restlessness and anxiety (particularly delirium tremens in alcohol withdrawal) and induces sleep.
2. It possesses anticonvulsant activity and is administered by intravenous infusion in acute convulsive states, e.g. status epilepticus, pre-eclampsia.

Dosage
1. Oral:
   a. For sedative effects: Adult dose is 1 capsule (or 5 ml syrup) three times daily.
   b. For hypnotic effects: Adult dose is 2 capsules (or 10 ml syrup) at night.
   c. For delirium tremens: Adult dose is up to 12 capsules in total daily given in 3-4 divided doses.
2. Intravenous infusion: Adults: dose range is 4–20 ml/minute of 0.8% chlormethiazole infusion depending upon indication and severity.

Nurse monitoring
1. It is important that the nurse fully understands the apparent major differences in the strengths of chlormethiazole capsules and syrup since confusion when substituting one dosage form for another can lead to overdosage or underdosage. Capsules contain 192 mg chlormethiazole

(base) while the syrup contains 250 mg chlormethiazole edisylate/5 ml. The difference in weight is due to the inactive edisylate group and is irrelevant to the clinical effect. Therefore when substituting capsules for syrup or vice versa, note that 1 capsule is equivalent to 5 ml syrup.

2. It should be noted that chlormethiazole administration is commonly associated with nasal congestion and irritation and occasionally conjunctival irritation about 15-30 minutes after a dose is administered. If these effects are severe or prevent sleep, alternative treatment may be necessary. A less common but equally important side-effect is severe headache.

3. Chlormethiazole is often used as a hypnotic in elderly subjects because it is generally well tolerated and is short-acting. However, it should be stressed that occasionally a prolonged 'hangover' effect lasting into the following day is noted which can impair mobility and awareness in elderly patients.

4. Intravenous administration may produce a fall in blood pressure and depression of respiration, particularly if given rapidly, and it may be necessary to monitor patients accordingly.

5. Irritation at the intravenous site may be noted as superficial thrombophlebitis.

6. Since chlormethiazole is a depressant of the central nervous system, concurrent use of other CNS depressant drugs (including alcohol) will produce excessive sedation.

General note

Chlormethiazole capsules and syrup may be stored at room temperature. The solution for intravenous infusion, however, should be stored in a refrigerator.

CHLOROQUINE (Nivaquine, Avloclor)

Presentation

Tablets—200 mg (as sulphate), 250 mg (as phosphate)
Syrup—50 mg in 5 ml.

Actions and uses

Chloroquine is a drug which was originally used for the treatment of malaria. Recently it has been found to be effective in a number of situations which are as follows:
1. Malaria
2. Amoebic hepatitis
3. Systemic lupus erythematosus (although it is only really useful for the control of skin lesions in this disease)
4. Rheumatoid arthritis.

Dosage

1. Malaria:
   a. Acute attacks:
      i. Adults. An initial dose of 600 mg is given followed by 300 mg 6-8 hours later and then 300 mg on each of 2 following days.
      ii. Children: Age 1-4—150 mg by mouth followed 6 hours later by 75 mg and then 75 mg daily for 2 days; Age 5-8—300 mg followed 6 hours later by 150 mg then 150 mg for 2 days.
   b. Cerebral malaria:
      i. Adults: An intramuscular or intravenous injection of 200–300 mg is given initially followed by 200 mg at intervals of 6 hours up to a total of 800 mg during the first 24 hours.
      ii. Children are treated with an initial injection of 5 mg/kg body weight intramuscularly repeated once 6 hours later if necessary.
   c. For the suppression of malaria:
      i. Adults: 300–600 mg is given weekly during exposure to risk and for 4-8 weeks thereafter.

ii. Children: Weekly doses of 5 mg/kg body weight are given for the same duration of time.
2. Hepatic amoebiasis:
   a. Adults: 300 mg of chloroquine base is given orally twice daily for 2 days and then once a day for a further 2–3 weeks.
   b. Children: The dosage is 6 mg/kg body weight twice daily for 2 days initially and then 6 mg/kg daily for 2–3 weeks.
3. Rheumatoid arthritis: Control of symptoms is achieved by treatment for 2-3 months with doses of between 75–300 mg of chloroquine base daily.
4. Discoid lupus erythematosus: The usual initial dose is 150 mg of chloroquine base twice or thrice daily reducing to a maintenance dose of 150 mg or less daily.

Nurse monitoring

1. Chloroquine is generally well tolerated when given in anti-malarial doses and toxic effects are rarely seen.
2. The higher prolonged doses given for treatment of rheumatoid arthritis and lupus erythematosus are associated with side-effects and it is in the early detection of these side-effects that the nurse's major role lies in the management of patients on these drugs. Pruritus is commonly found. Headache, and gastrointestinal upset occur less frequently. Rarely the bone marrow may be suppressed inducing blood dyscrasias such as agranulocytosis, thrombocytopenia and neutropenia. Other rare side-effects include altered skin pigmentation and muscle weakness.
3. The major problem with prolonged or high dosage treatment with chloroquine is damage to the retina which may result in permanent visual impairment. Patients should therefore be regularly assessed by measurement of visual acuity and other

---

means and the drug should, if possible, be stopped should this side-effect develop.
4. The drug should be used with great caution in patients with liver disease, psoriasis, gastrointestinal, neurological or blood disorders.

General note

Chloroquine tablets may be stored at room temperature. The syrup must be protected from light.

CHLOROTHIAZIDE (Saluric)

Presentation

Tablets—500 mg

Actions and uses

See the section on thiazide and related diuretics.

Dosage

1. Adults. The daily adult dose range is 500 mg–1 g twice daily. The duration of action of chlorothiazide is approximately 12 hours.
2. Children: Up to 1 year—125 mg; 1–7 years—250 mg; 7 years plus—500 mg. The above doses are taken as a single daily dose. Premature infants require much lower doses, e.g. 62.5 mg.

Nurse monitoring

See the section on thiazide and related diuretics.

General note

Chlorothiazide tablets may be stored at room temperature.

CHLORPHENIRAMINE (Piriton)

Presentation

Tablets—4 mg, 8 mg and 12 mg (slow release)
Syrup—2 mg in 5 ml
Injection—10 mg/ml

Actions and uses

Chlorpheniramine is an antihistamine. The actions and uses of antihistamines in general are described in the section on antihistamines. In clinical practice chlorpheniramine is used:

1. To suppress generalized minor allergic responses to allergens such as foodstuffs and drugs.
2. To suppress local allergic reactions, i.e. inflammatory skin responses to insect stings and bites, contact allergens, urticaria etc.
3. Orally for allergic conditions, e.g. hay fever and allergic rhinitis.

Dosage
1. Adults:
   a. Orally: Standard preparation: 4 mg three to four times daily. Slow release preparation: 8–12 mg twice per day.
   b. By intravenous, intramuscular or subcutaneous injection: 10–20 mg.
2. Children:
   Standard preparation (tablets or syrup): Less than 1 year—(syrup recommended) 1 mg (2.5 ml) twice per day; 1 to 5 years—(syrup recommended) 1–2 mg (2.5–5 ml) three times daily; 6 to 12 years—(tablets or syrup) 2–4 mg three times daily.

Nurse monitoring
See the section on antihistamines.

General note
The drug may be stored at room temperature.

CHLORPROMAZINE (Largactil)

Presentation
Tablets—10 mg, 25 mg, 50 mg, 100 mg
Syrup—25 mg in 5 ml
Suspension—100 mg in 5 ml
Injection—25 mg in 1 ml, 50 mg in 2 ml
Suppositories—100 mg

Actions and uses
1. Chlorpromazine is a phenothiazine drug and its actions and uses are described in the section on phenothiazine drugs.
2. The drug has a particular use in the control of intractable hiccoughs.

3. It is used in rare circumstances when the induction of hypothermia is desirable.
4. It is used in obstetric practice for the treatment of pre-eclampsia and eclampsia.

Dosage
1. Adults: The dosage varies widely with individual patients. As a rough guide the following regimes are suggested:
   a. Oral: 25 mg three times is an average dose, although in some cases total dosage may be increased up to 1 g per day if necessary.
   b. Intramuscularly: 25–50 mg is administered and repeated at 6-8 hourly intervals as required.
   c. Intravenously: The drug should be diluted with at least 10 times its own volume of normal saline and given extremely slowly. It is worth pointing out that only very rarely should this drug be given intravenously and only under strict medical supervision.
   d. Rectally: One 100 mg suppository is given and repeated at intervals of 6-8 hours if necessary. By the rectal route the onset of action is slower and the duration of effect more prolonged.
2. Children:Under the age of 5 the oral dose is 5–10 mg three times daily. Over the age of 5 one-third to one-half of the adult dosages are recommended.

Nurse monitoring
See the section on Phenothiazine drugs.

General notes
1. Preparations containing chlorpromazine may be stored at room temperature.
2. Syrup, suspension and solution for injections should be protected from light.
3. Injection solutions may develop a pink or yellow discolouration and if this is noted the solution should be discarded.

CHLORPROPAMIDE (Diabinese)

Presentation
Tablets—100 mg, 250 mg
Actions and uses
See the section on hypoglycaemic drugs, oral (1).
Dosage
50–500 mg as a single morning dose.

Nurse monitoring
See the section on hypoglycaemic drugs, oral (1).

General note
Tablets may be stored at room temperature.

CHLORTETRACYCLINE (Aureomycin)

(See Note 3, p. 362)
Presentation
Capsules—250 mg
Ointment and cream—3%
Eye ointment—1 %
Actions and uses
See the section on tetracyclines.
Dosage
The adult oral dose is 250 mg four times a day.

Nurse monitoring
See the section on tetracyclines.

General note
The drug may be stored at room temperature.

CHLORTHALIDONE (Hygroton)

Presentation
Tablets—50 mg, 100 mg
Actions and uses
See the section on thiazide and related diuretics.
Dosage
The usual adult dose range is 50–100 mg daily or on alternate days. Single daily doses are sufficient because of the very long action of chlorthalidone (48 hours or more).

Nurse monitoring
See the section on thiazide and related diuretics.

General note
Chlorthalidone tablets may be stored at room temperature.

CHOLESTYRAMINE (Questran)

Presentation
Sachets—4 g
Actions and uses
Cholestyramine is an anionic ion exchange resin with the following actions:
1. It binds bile acids present in the gut and therefore increases faecal excretion of bile acids: this in turn causes an increase in cholesterol and lipid metabolism.
2. It reduces the rate of fat absorption from the gut; it therefore has the following uses in clinical practice:
   i. To reduce plasma cholesterol in patients with hyper-cholesterolaemia.
   ii. To relieve pruritus associated with elevated plasma bile acid levels in patients with cholestatic jaundice.
   iii. To treat diarrhoea associated with vagotomy and other gastrointestinal surgery or radiotherapy which is effective because bile acids when they are bound to cholestyramine do not have the laxative effect that they would have if they were free in the gut.

Dosage
1. For the treatment of hyper-cholesterolaemia the usual dose is of the order 3-6 sachets (12–24 g) daily, taken as a single dose or in up to 4 divided doses.
2. For the treatment of pruritus—1 or 2 sachets (4–8g) daily.
3. For the treatment of diarrhoea—as for hypercholesterolaemia.
4. For the treatment of children (aged 6-12 years): The initial dose (which may be modified according to the response) is determined by the formula: Body weight in lb x adult dose.

Nurse monitoring

Cholestyramine is a particularly unpleasant preparation for patients to consume. This unpleasantness may be alleviated by encouraging patients to mix it with water, fruit juice, soup or soft fruit.

1. It is important for the nurse to note that cholestyramine may also bind and inactivate other drugs in the gastrointestinal tract and it is advisable to take any other medication 30 minutes to 1 hour before any dose of cholestyramine.
2. The drug interferes with fat absorption and therefore may reduce absorption of the fat soluble vitamins A, D and K. A description of deficiency syndromes associated with these vitamins is given under each vitamin in the text. When a vitamin deficiency is identified, parenteral vitamin supplementation may be required.
3. The most frequent side-effects associated with this treatment are gastrointestinal upsets and constipation. As the drug is not absorbed, systemic toxicity does not occur.

General note

Cholestyramine sachets may be stored at room temperature.

CHOLINE THEOPHYLLINATE (Choledyl)

Presentation

Tablets—100 mg, 200 mg
Syrup—2.5 mg in 5 ml

Actions and uses

This drug is chemically related to aminophylline whose actions and uses are described in the section on aminophylline. It is used in the management of bronchospasm associated with asthma and other conditions such as chronic bronchitis.

Dosage

1. Adults: 400–1600 mg daily in four divided doses.

2. Children: 3-6 years—62.5–125 mg three times per day; over 6 years—100 mg three to four times per day.

Nurse monitoring

The nurse monitoring aspects for aminophylline (q.v.) apply to this drug.

General notes

1. This drug may be stored at room temperature.
2. The drug should be protected from light.
3. The commercial syrup contains a high quantity of sugar and this should be taken into account when treating diabetic patients, or when treating patients who are intolerant of disaccharide.

CILAZAPRIL (Vascace)

Presentation

Tablets—0.5 mg, 1 mg, 2.5 mg, 5 mg

Actions and uses

See the section on ACE inhibitors.

Dosage

Range—2.5–5 mg as a single daily dose.

Nurse monitoring

See the section on ACE inhibitors

General note

Cilazapril tablets may be stored at room temperature.

CIMETIDINE (Tagamet, Dyspamet)

Presentation

Tablets—200 mg, 400 mg, 800 mg
Syrup—200 mg in 5 ml
Injection—200 mg in 2 ml, 400 mg in 100 ml

Actions and uses

See histamine H_2-receptor antagonists.

Dosage

Dosage for all indications is based on that used in the treatment of peptic ulceration, as follows:

1. Adults:
   a. Oral, treatment: 800 mg daily, in 2 divided doses or as a single evening dose. Occasionally patients are required to take up to 1.6 g in 4 divided doses.
   b. Oral, maintenance therapy: usually a single bed-time dose of 400 mg or 800 mg since it appears that overnight acid output is important in determining ulcer relapse rates.
   c. Injection: Intramuscular therapy can be substituted for oral treatment when necessary. Intravenous doses of 200 mg, given slowly over several minutes, repeated at intervals of 4-6 hours of 400 mg over 1 hour, or continuous intravenous infusion (50–100 mg/hour) can all be used in the actively bleeding patient.
2. Children: a dose based on 25–30 mg/day in suitably divided daily doses has been given.

Nurse monitoring
1. The nurse monitoring aspects described for histamine H_2-receptor antagonists apply.
2. It should be noted that from 1994 this drug will be available in the U.K. by purchase over-the-counter. Patients who self-medicate may require guidance on the correct use of cimetidine and, in particular, be encouraged to seek medical advice for chronic dyspepsia.

General note
Cimetidine preparations may be stored at room temperature. The syrup and injection solutions must be protected from light during storage.

CINNARIZINE (Stugeron)

Presentation
Tablets—15 mg
Capsules—75 mg

Actions and uses
Cinnarizine is an antihistamine. The actions and uses of antihistamines in general are described in the section on antihistamines. In clinical practice cinnarizine is used:
1. In the treatment of nausea and vomiting, particularly motion sickness.
2. In the treatment of vertigo and the symptoms of vertigo and nausea due to Menière's disease.
3. To improve blood flow to ischaemic tissues (due to its vasodilator action) in peripheral vascular disease.

Dosage
1. Nausea/vomiting and Menière's disease:
   a. Adults: 30 mg initially, then 15–30 mg every 8 hours.
   b. Children: Half the adult dose.
2. As a vasodilator: 75 mg every 8 hours for adults only.

Nurse monitoring
See the section on antihistamines.

General note
The drug may be stored at room temperature

CIPROFLOXACIN (Ciproxin)

(See Note 3, p. 362)
Presentation
Tablets—250 mg
Injection—100 mg in 50 ml, 200 mg in 100 ml
Actions and uses
Ciprofloxacin is the first drug in a new series of aminoquinolone antibiotics. It has some chemical similarities to nalidixic acid but its potential uses are greater. It is active against most Gram-positive and Gram-negative organisms and in particular, it has useful activity against Pseudomonas species. The major role for ciprofloxacin to date is in the following settings:
1. Urinary tract infections where resistance to standard drugs has been demonstrated.

2. Respiratory infections, particularly associated with bronchiectasis and cystic fibrosis, in which Pseudomonas is frequently implicated.
3. Skin and soft tissue infections.
4. Infections of bone and joint tissues.

Dosage
1. Urinary tract infections: oral—250 mg twice daily is sufficient since high, effective urine levels are usually achieved.
2. Respiratory infections: oral—750 mg twice daily is usually required for those less sensitive microorganisms which are frequently implicated.
3. Other infections: oral—500 mg twice daily is generally an effective intermediate dose. N.B. *Children:* see note under nurse monitoring. If treatment is however required, this is based on 7.5–15 mg/kg/day given in two divided doses.
4. Injection (Adults): 100–200 mg by intravenous injection over 30 minutes to 1 hour. The higher dose is used for infections of the respiratory with lower doses for urinary tract infections.

N.B. *Children:* see note under nurse monitoring. If treatment is however required, this is based on 5–10 mg/kg/day given in two divided doses. In patients with cystic fibrosis however, much higher doses are required e.g. up to 40 mg/kg/day orally.

Nurse monitoring
1. Ciprofloxacin is a new drug whose toxicity has yet to be clearly established. There is evidence to suspect a possible neurotoxic potential and patients with a history of convulsions must be closely monitored during treatment.
2. Serum levels of theophylline may be elevated by ciprofloxacin and an appropriate dosage reduction in theophylline should therefore be considered.
3. Crystalluria (precipitation of insoluble ciprofloxacin in the urinary tract) may occur unless patients are well hydrated. Also excessive alkalinization of the urine should be avoided, e.g. ingestion of sodium bicarbonate and other antacids.
4. The safety of ciprofloxacin in children is uncertain. Evidence from experimental animal studies indicates possible arthropathy in weight-bearing joints associated with ciprofloxacin and there is concern that growing joints may be affected adversely.
5. Commonly reported side-effects include gastrointestinal upsets (nausea, pain, diarrhoea) and dizziness and/or drowsiness. Ciprofloxacin is a contact irritant and intravenous injection may be associated with redness of the injection site and phlebitis.

General note
Ciprofloxacin tablets and injections may be stored at room temperature. The injection solution must be protected from light during storage. It is compatible with sodium chloride, glucose and fructose solutions but such dilutions should be administered within 24 hours of preparation.

CISPLATIN (Neoplatin)

Presentation
Injection—10 mg, 50 mg vials

Actions and uses
Cisplatin is a cytotoxic drug which appears to interfere with cellular reproduction. Since tumour cells reproduce at a rapid rate they are particularly sensitive to the effects of this drug. It has been used in the treatment of cancer of the testes, ovaries, bladder, head and neck, cervix, prostate, oesophagus and lung.

Dosage
1. When used as a sole anti-tumour agent the recommended dose for adults and children is 50–75 mg/m^2 body surface area as a single intravenous infusion every 3-4 weeks. An alternative regime is to give 15–20 mg/m^2 by intravenous infusion daily for 5 days every 3-4 weeks.

2. When used in combination with other cytotoxic drugs low doses may be given.
3. In practice it has been found that repeated courses are often necessary.

Nurse monitoring

1. Cisplatin is particularly toxic to the kidney and a progressive fall in renal function may occur. As this effect is dose related it must be shown by laboratory testing that renal function has returned to normal before repeat courses are given. Regular 24 hour urine collections for creatinine clearance are therefore obtained.
2. Almost all patients treated with this drug suffer from anorexia, nausea and vomiting.
3. Bone marrow suppression may occur leading to anaemia, haemorrhage due to thrombocytopenia and infection due to suppression of white cell function.
4. Other adverse effects include tinnitus, hearing loss, peripheral neuropathy, abnormal liver function and abnormal cardiac function.
5. Anaphylactic reaction characterized by facial oedema, wheezing, tachycardia and hypotension may occur within minutes of drug administration.
6. In common with all cytotoxic drugs there are potential risks to normal fetal development if treatment is given during pregnancy.

General notes

1. Cisplatin vials may be stored at room temperature.
2. They should be reconstituted with 10 ml or 50 ml of water for injection to provide a solution containing 1 mg in 1 ml.
3. The drug is diluted in 2 litres of dextrose/saline mixture and infused over a 6-8 hour period.
4. Prepared solutions should be kept at room temperature and are stable for up to 24 hours.

5. Refrigeration will produce precipitation from solution and is therefore not advised.

CLARITHROMYCIN (Klaricid)

(See Note 3, p. 362)

Presentation

Tablets—250 mg
Oral suspension—125 mg in 5 ml
Injection—500 mg vial

Actions and uses

Clarithromycin is an antibiotic of the erythromycin group which is however more active and longer acting than erythromycin and also reaches higher tissue concentrations. It is also claimed that gastrointestinal tolerance is improved with this drug. The antibacterial activity of clarithromycin is nevertheless similar to that of erythromycin and its indications are therefore similar also. In particular this drug is indicated for the treatment of lower respiratory tract infections, skin and soft tissue infections and upper respiratory infections including acute otitis media.

Dosage

1. Adults: 250–500 mg twice daily for courses of 7-14 days depending upon the nature and severity of infection.
2. Children: Up to 1 year (<8 kg)—7.5 mg/kg twice daily; 1-2 years (8-11 kg)—62.5 mg twice daily; 2-6 years (12-19 kg)—125 mg twice daily; 6-9 years (20-29 kg)—187.5 mg twice daily; older children—250 mg twice daily.

Nurse monitoring

The nurse monitoring section for erythromycin also applies to this drug with the additional comment that gastrointestinal upsets are less likely or less severe.

General notes

1. Clarithromycin preparations are stored at room temperature and protected from light.
2. To reconstitute injection, 10 ml water for injection is first added to

the vial to produce a stock solution containing 50 mg in 1 ml. This stock solution can be stored at room temperature or under refrigeration for up to 24 hours. The required volume is then transferred to 250–500 ml sodium chloride or glucose injection and administered over 4-6 hours. Prepared infusions can be stored under refrigeration only but must be used within 24 hours.

CLEMASTINE (Tavegil)

Presentation
Tablets—1 mg
Elixir—0.5 mg in 5 ml

Actions and uses
Clemastine is an antihistamine. The actions and uses of antihistamines in general are described in the section on antihistamines.
Clemastine is used in clinical practice:
1. To suppress generalized minor allergic responses to allergens such as foodstuffs and drugs.
2. To suppress local allergic reactions, i.e. inflammatory skin responses to insect stings and bites, contact allergens, urticaria etc.

Dosage
Adults: 1 mg twice daily.

Nurse monitoring
See the section on antihistamines.

General note
The drug may be stored at room temperature.

CLINDAMYCIN (Dalacin C, Dalacin T)

(See Note 3, p. 362)
Presentation
Capsules—75 mg, 150 mg
Syrup—75 mg in 5 ml
Injection—150 mg in 1 ml
Topical solution—l0 mg in 1 ml, 30 ml

Actions and uses
Clindamycin is an antibiotic with a bacteriostatic action, in that it inhibits further growth and multiplication of bacterial microorganisms in the body. It has been found to be effective against the Gram-negative bacillus Bacteroides, a major anaerobic pathogen. Also it is particularly useful for the treatment of:
1. Staphylococcal or streptococcal infections in patients who are sensitive to penicillins.
2. Staphylococcal or streptococcal infections where the organism is known to be resistant to penicillin.
3. Staphylococcal infections of bone and skin and soft tissue.
4. Prophylaxis of bacterial endo-carditis in 'at risk' dental patients.
5. Topically in the treatment of acne vulgaris when an infective component is involved.

Dosage
1. Adults:
   a. Orally: 150–300 mg 6-hourly. Prophylaxis of endocarditis: a single dose of 600 mg taken 1 hour before the dental procedure.
   b. Intramuscular injection: 600 mg–2.7 g daily in total, in two, three or four divided doses.
   c. Intravenously the dosages are identical for intramuscular injection but up to 4.8 g may be given in a life-threatening infection.
2. Children:
   a. Orally (over 1 month): 3–6 mg/kg every 6 hours and in serious infection no less than 300 mg/day regardless of age. Prophylaxis of endocarditis: a single dose of 6 mg/kg as above.
   b. Intramuscular dosage for children is 15–40 mg/kg body weight per day in total given in three or four divided doses.
   c. Intravenous dosage is identical to intramuscular dosage.
3. For treatment of acne, in adults and children: apply topical solution to the affected area twice daily for up to 12 weeks.

Nurse monitoring
1. Intramuscular injections should be made deeply into the gluteal muscles.
2. For intravenous injection: 600 mg should be diluted in 100ml or more of 5% glucose or normal saline and be given over a period of not less than 1 hour. Children's doses should be diluted appropriately.
3. Gastrointestinal upsets are the only major side-effects associated with clindamycin. If diarrhoea occurs in any patient the drug should be immediately stopped as a proportion of these patients may develop pseudomembranous enterocolitis. This serious condition arises as the result of the action of one or more endotoxins on the gut mucosa following release by the bowel organism *Clostridium difficile.*
4. The drug must be given with caution to the newborn or to patients with pre-existing kidney, liver, endocrine or metabolic disease.
5. It is important to avoid contact with the eyes or mucous membranes when applying topical solutions.

General note
All preparations containing clindamycin should be stored at room temperature. Avoid refrigeration.

CLOBAZAM (Frisium)

Presentation
Capsule—10 mg
Actions and uses
Clobazam is a member of the benzodiazepine group (q.v.) and its principal use is the treatment of anxiety.
Dosage
1. Adults: 10 mg two or three times daily.
2. Children: Children over the age of 3 should receive half the adult dose.

3. In hospitalized patients with severe anxiety states maximum doses of 60 mg per day in total have been given.

Nurse monitoring
See the section on benzodiazepines.

General notes
1. Clobazam capsules may be stored at room temperature.
2. The capsules should be protected from light.

CLOBETASOL (Dermovate)

Presentation
Ointment and cream—0.05%
Scalp application—0.05%
Actions and uses
Clobetasol is a very potent topical corticosteroid (q.v.) which is applied topically for the treatment of inflammatory skin conditions, e.g. psoriasis, eczema, dermatitis, etc.
Dosage
Cream, ointment and scalp application are applied sparingly once or twice daily to the affected area.

Nurse monitoring
Although applied topically, significant amounts of this drug may be absorbed to produce some or all of the side-effects described in the section on corticosteroids.

General note
Ointment, cream and scalp application containing clobetasol may be stored at room temperature.

CLOBETASONE (Eumovate)

Presentation
Ointment and cream—0.05%
Actions and uses
A moderately potent corticosteroid (q.v.) which is applied topically for the treatment of inflammatory skin conditions, e.g. psoriasis, eczema, dermatitis, etc.

Dosage
   Apply sparingly to the affected area
   up to four times daily.

Nurse monitoring
   Although applied topically, significant amounts of this drug may be
   absorbed to produce some or all of
   the side-effects described in the
   section on corticosteroids.

General note
   Ointment and cream containing
   clobetasone may be stored at room
   temperature.

CLODRONATE (Loron)

Presentation
   Tablets—520 mg
   Injection—300 mg in 10 ml
Actions and uses
   Clodronate is a member of the
   bisphosphonate group of drugs
   which are metabolically active in
   bone tissue. The sections on
   etidronate and pamidronate should
   be consulted for an account of the
   action of these drugs. In practice
   clodronate is used in the treatment
   of hypercalcaemia associated with
   malignant disease.
Dosage
   1. Malignant hypercalcaemia:
      a. Acute intravenous therapy: By
         slow infusion in a daily dose of
         300 mg until serum calcium has
         normalized, usually for periods
         of 7-10 days. Single high dose
         therapy has been attempted.
      b. Maintenance of serum calcium
         using oral therapy: The dose
         range is one to two tablets
         (1040 mg to 2080 mg) daily.

Nurse monitoring
   1. The nurse monitoring section for
      etidronate also applies to this
      drug
   2. Intravenous infusions are
      prepared in 500 ml sodium
      chloride 0.9% and administered
      over 2-4 hours.

General note
   Clodronate preparations are stored
   at room temperature.

CLOFIBRATE (Atromid-S)

Presentation
   Capsules—500 mg
Actions and uses
   Clofibrate has a number of complex
   and as yet not clearly defined
   actions on body metabolism. Its
   overall effect is to reduce blood
   cholesterol. It may be used to
   reduce the cholesterol level in the
   blood of patients who have a familial
   predisposition to high blood
   cholesterol and who tend to develop
   ischaemic heart disease early in life.
Dosage
   The recommended dose for adults
   and children is 20–30 mg/kg body
   weight given in two or three divided
   doses.

Nurse monitoring
   1. This drug may produce side-
      effects of nausea, abdominal
      pain and diarrhoea.
   2. One of the mechanisms by which
      clofibrate reduces blood
      cholesterol is to raise the level of
      cholesterol in the bile and
      prolonged use may be
      associated with the development
      of gall stones.
   3. If patients have liver disease
      associated with impaired liver
      function they should not receive
      this drug.

General note
   Clofibrate capsules may be stored at
   room temperature.

CLOMIPHENE (Clomid)

Presentation
   Tablets—50 mg
Actions and uses
   In the normal female during each
   menstrual cycle the growth of a
   follicle, ovulation and the development of the endometrium is stimulated by two hormones from the

pituitary known as luteinizing hormone (LH) and follicle stimulating hormone (FSH). Late in the menstrual cycle, sufficient oestrogen is produced during the menstrual process for these pituitary hormones to be inhibited and by this process a regular cycle of menstruation is produced. Clomiphene blocks the inhibitory action of oestrogens on the pituitary and therefore stimulates further production of the pituitary hormones. This action is useful in the treatment of infertility when it has been shown that ovulation is not taking place, as the stimulation of pituitary hormones may induce ovulation.

Dosage
50 mg daily for 5 days with subsequent courses for up to six cycles until pregnancy occurs.

Nurse monitoring
1. Because of its mechanism of action clomiphene is likely to lead to the stimulation of the development of more than one ovum and multiple pregnancies may occur. This risk is usually explained to patients prior to commencing treatment.
2. As clomiphene stimulates the ovaries and produces ovarian enlargement its administration is contraindicated should the patient be known to have an ovarian cyst.
3. Common side-effects include hot flushes and abdominal pain and distension.
4. Less common side-effects include blurring of vision, ocular damage, fatigue, dizziness, headache, nausea, vomiting, breast tenderness, heavy periods, urinary frequency and very rarely loss of hair.
5. Abnormalities in liver function have occurred when patients receive this drug.

General notes
1. The drug may be stored at room temperature.

2. Tablets should be protected from moisture, light and excessive heat.

CLOMIPRAMINE (Anafranil)

Presentation
Capsules—10 mg, 25 mg, 50 mg
Syrup—25 mg in 5 ml
Injection—25 mg in 2 ml
Tablets—75 mg, slow release
Actions and uses
Clomipramine is a tricyclic antidepressant drug. Its actions and uses are described in the section on tricyclic antidepressants.
Dosage
For the treatment of depression the following regimes may be used:
1. By the oral route: 30–50 mg per day may be taken in three divided doses. Alternatively the entire daily dose may be taken on retiring or as a single dose using 75 mg slow release tablets.
2. Where injections are necessary, e.g. for the treatment of uncooperative patients or at the beginning of therapy when a more rapid effect is required: 25 mg by intramuscular injection may be given up to six times daily.

Nurse monitoring
See the section on tricyclic antidepressant drugs.

General notes
1. Preparations containing clomipramine must be stored at room temperature.
2. Solutions for injection and syrup must be protected from light.

CLONAZEPAM (Rivotril)

Presentation
Tablets—0.5 mg, 2 mg
Injection—1 mg in 1 ml
Actions and uses
Clonazepam is a benzodiazepine drug (q.v.) which has a marked anticonvulsant action. It is used in all forms of epilepsy particularly of the

petit mal variety. It may be given prophylactically by the oral route to prevent epilepsy and by slow intravenous injection for the treatment of status epilepticus.

Dosage

1. Oral prophylactic doses are as follows:
   a. Adults: 4–8 mg orally daily in three or four divided doses.
   b. Children: Up to 1 year—0.5–1 mg; 1-5 years—1–3 mg; 5-12 years—3–6 mg. The above doses are total dosages and should be administered in three or four divided doses daily.
2. For the treatment of status epilepticus: A slow intravenous injection is administered over a period of 30 seconds. More rapid injections produce hypotension and apnoea. Recommended doses are 1 mg for adults and 0.5 mg for infants and children.

Nurse monitoring

1. See the section on benzodiazepines for general nurse monitoring points on this drug.
2. A particular adverse effect with this drug is increased salivation and bronchial hypersecretion. This produces 'drooling' and may prove troublesome in patients with obstructive airways disease.
3. In common with anticonvulsant drug therapy in general, clonazepam should never be abruptly withdrawn but should instead be replaced with an alternative medication after gradual reduction in dose.

General notes

1. Preparations containing clonazepam may be stored at room temperature.
2. The injection should be protected from light.
3. The injection consists of a dry powder in a vial with 1 ml of solvent. For reconstitution the solvent is water for injection. It should be added immediately before use. If necessary the

injection can be diluted in an intravenous infusion containing sodium chloride or dextrose.
4. Any injection which is not used must be immediately discarded.
5. Intravenous infusions must be used within 12 hours.

CLONIDINE (Catapres, Dixarit)

Presentation

Tablets—0.025, 0.1 and 0.3 mg (or 25, 100 and 300 microgram)
Capsules—0.25mg sustained-release
Injection—0.15 mg in 1 ml

Actions and uses

1. Clonidine reduces the blood pressure in two ways:
   a. It reduces the sympathetic nerve activity stimulated by centres in the brain.
   b. If affects the peripheral blood vessels altering their response to vasoconstrictor substances.
2. Small doses of clonidine have been found to be effective in the prophylaxis of migraine.
3. The drug has also been used to treat menopausal vascular flushes. Again very small doses are used (see below).

Dosage

1. In the treatment of hypertension the recommended adult dosage is as follows:
   a. 0.15–0.3 mg may be given by slow intravenous injection. The effects last for several hours and may be repeated up to a maximum dosage of 0.75 mg in 24 hours.
   b. The initial oral dose is 50–100 microgram three times daily increasing as required to a maintenance range of between 0.3 and 1.2 mg three times per day. Alternatively, 0.25 mg sustained-release capsule in the morning and a further one or two capsules at night.
2. For the prophylaxis of migraine and the treatment of menopausal vascular flushes a dose range of 50–150 microgram per day is recommended.

Nurse monitoring
1. There is no doubt that the most important fact to remember about this drug is that if it is stopped suddenly serious rebound hypertension may occur within 24 hours. Therefore the drug should never be stopped suddenly unless the patient is under constant medical supervision.
2. Clonidine may worsen symptoms of depression and therefore is relatively contraindicated in depressed patients.
3. Recognised side-effects include bradycardia, headache, sleep disturbances, nausea, constipation and impotence in males. Facial pallor has also been noted.
4. Dry mouth, sedation and postural hypotension commonly occur during the early stages of treatment.
5. Rarely a Raynaud's type phenomenon with cyanosis, pallor and paraesthesia of the extremities may develop rapidly at the commencement of treatment .

General note
Clonidine tablets and injection may be stored at room temperature. For ease of administration the injection solution can be diluted with 5% dextrose and 0.9% sodium chloride injection.

CLOPENTHIXOL (Clopixol)

Presentation
Tablets—10 mg, 25 mg
Injection—200 mg in 1 ml ampoules as decanoate, 2g in 10 ml vials as decanoate

Actions and uses
Clopenthixol is a member of a group of neuroleptic drugs which are used for their tranquillizing or calming effect in patients with severe behavioural disorders. It therefore shares many of the actions and uses described for phenothiazines.

Dosage
Adults
1. By the oral route, initially 20–30 mg daily in divided doses with maintenance dosages in the range 20–50 mg daily. Up to 150 mg daily may be required to control severe cases.
2. Clopenthixol decanoate injection produces a long-acting (depot) effect and doses of 200–400 mg by the intramuscular route may be administered at 2-4 week intervals.

Nurse monitoring
See the section on phenothiazines

General note
Clopenthixol tablets and injections should be stored at room temperature.

CLOTRIMAZOLE (Canesten)

Presentation
Cream—1 %
Powder—1 %
Topical spray—1 %
Pessaries—100 mg, 200 mg and 500 mg

Actions and uses
This drug has a broad spectrum of action against many fungi and also exhibits activity against trichomonas, staphylococcus, streptococcus and bacteroides. It has a wide range of uses including:
1. All fungal skin infections due to dermatophytes, yeasts, moulds and other fungi including trichophyton species, candida, ringworm (tinea) infections, athletes foot, paronychia, pityriasis versicolor, erythrasma, intertrigo, fungal nappy rash, candida vulvitis and balanitis. It should be noted that the drug is not recommended as a sole treatment for pure trichomoniasis.

Dosage
1. Cream, powder or spray: To be thinly and evenly applied to the affected area two or three times daily and rubbed in gently.

Treatment should be continued for at least 1 month or for at least 2 weeks after the disappearance of all signs of infection.

2. Pessaries: Two tablets should be inserted daily preferably at night for three consecutive days. Alternatively one pessary may be inserted daily for 6 days or a single 500 mg pessary inserted once.

Nurse monitoring

Rarely patients may experience local mild burning or irritation immediately after applying the preparation.

General note

Preparations may be stored at room temperature.

CLOXACILLIN (Orbenin)

(See Note 3, p. 362)

Presentation

Capsules—250 mg, 500 mg
Syrup—125 mg in 5 ml
Injection—vials containing 250 mg and 500 mg

Actions and uses

Cloxacillin is a member of the penicillin group of antibiotics and has actions and uses similar to those described for benzylpenicillin (q.v.). In practice, however, it has a distinct advantage over benzylpenicillin in that it is often effective against infections due to *Staphylococcus aureus* which are resistant to benzylpenicillin. The drug is well absorbed after oral administration.

Dosage

1. Adults:
   a. Orally: 500 mg four times a day
   b. Intravenous and intramuscular: 250–500 mg 4 to 6-hourly.
   c. Intra-articular and intrapleural: 500 mg is given once daily.
2. Children: Less than 2 years one-quarter of the adult dose; over 2 years—one-half of the adult dose.

Nurse monitoring

See the section on benzylpenicillin.

General notes

1. Preparations containing cloxacillin may be stored at room temperature.
2. Once reconstituted injection solutions must be used immediately.
3. Once reconstituted the syrup should be used within 7 days.
4. Injections are prepared as follows:
   a. For intramuscular injection the vials should be diluted with 1.5–2 ml of water for injection.
   b. For intravenous injection: 1 g should be dissolved in 20 ml of water for injection and given either directly over 3-4 minutes or added to 0.9% sodium chloride, 5% dextrose or dextrose/saline mixtures and infused over 4-6 hours.
   c. For intra-articular or intrapleural injection: The vials should be diluted with 5–10 ml water for injection.

CO-AMOXICLAV (Augmentin)

(See Note 3, p. 362)

Co-amoxiclav or Augmentin is a combination of amoxycillin and clavulanic acid

Presentation

Tablets—each tablet contains amoxycillin 250 mg and clavulanic acid 125 mg (375 mg); amoxycillin 500 mg and clavulanic acid 125 mg (625 mg)
Suspensions—Amoxycillin 250 mg and clavulanic acid 62 mg in 5 ml; amoxycillin 125 mg and clavulanic acid 31 mg in 5 ml
Injection—Amoxycillin 500 mg and clavulanic acid 100 mg; amoxycillin 1 g and clavulanic acid 200 mg

Actions and uses

The actions and uses of amoxycillin are described in the section on amoxycillin. The addition of clavulanic acid broadens the spectrum of activity of amoxycillin since this substance prevents the breakdown and therefore inactivation of amoxycillin by the enzyme penicillinase (beta-lactase). This enzyme is produced by a number of bacteria and effectively renders them penicillin-resistant. Some bacteria therefore resistant to amoxycillin alone may be effectively treated by co-amoxiclav. In practice this may prove particularly important in the treatment of urinary tract pathogens such as *E. coli* and skin and soft tissue infection due to staphylococcus.

Dosage

Doses may be calculated on the basis of the amoxycillin content and full prescribing instructions are given under amoxycillin.

Nurse monitoring

1. The nurse monitoring aspects already discussed for amoxycillin apply to this drug.
2. The addition of clavulanic acid appears to increase the incidence of diarrhoea due to amoxycillin.
3. Cholestatic jaundice is reported to occur in association with co-amoxiclav but not amoxycillin or clavulanic acid alone. Liver function tests should be monitored if prolonged therapy is required.

General note

Co-amoxiclav tablets, suspension and injections may be stored at room temperature.

CODEINE PHOSPHATE

Presentation

Tablets—15 mg, 30 mg and 60 mg
Linctus—15 mg in 5 ml
Syrup—25 mg in 5 ml

Actions and uses

Codeine phosphate is a member of the narcotic group of analgesics. It has, however, a very mild analgesic action. It has the following uses:

1. As a mild analgesic, usually in combination with aspirin in codeine compound tablets (Codis).

2. It may be used for the treatment of diarrhoea when it has a constipating effect.
3. It may be used as a cough suppressant.

Dosage

1. For mild analgesia: In combination with aspirin, adults should receive two codeine compound tablets 4-6 hourly.
2. For constipating action:
   a. Adults should receive 15–60 mg three or four times a day.
   b. Children: Less than 1 year old: It is not recommended that such children receive this drug; 1-7 years—1.25–2.5 ml of the linctus (15 mg in 5 ml) three or four times a day.
3. As a cough suppressant: 2.5–10 ml of syrup or 5–10 ml of linctus three to four times daily.

Nurse monitoring

The drug has none of the severe problems associated with narcotic analgesics (q.v.), but if used as a mild analgesic constipation may be a problem.

General note

The drug may be stored at room temperature.

COLCHICINE

Presentation

Tablets—250 microgram, 500 microgram

Actions and uses

Colchicine interferes with the uptake of uric acid crystals by white cells in gouty joints. The result of this is that inflammation is rapidly reduced and symptoms of pain are relieved. Its main use is in the treatment of acute gout but it is occasionally used as an alternative to the non-steroidal anti-inflammatory analgesics to prevent attacks of gout, especially during the introduction of allopurinol therapy.

Dosage

1. Adults: A single course is used in acute gout. Initially 1 mg is given followed by subsequent doses of

500 microgram every 2 hours until relief of pain is obtained or vomiting or diarrhoea occur or a total dose of 10 mg has been reached. Courses should not be repeated within 3 days.
2. For prophylaxis, a dose of 500 microgram twice daily may be used.

Nurse monitoring
1. Although colchicine is a very effective drug its use is limited by the frequent occurrence of side-effects such as nausea, abdominal pain and diarrhoea. Indeed these side-effects may necessitate withdrawal of treatment.
2. High dosage may cause skin rashes, renal damage and alopecia has followed prolonged use.
3. It is recommended that colchicine be used with caution in elderly patients with heart disease and in patients with kidney or gastrointestinal disease.
4. It is worth noting that fatalities have occurred after overdosage of colchicine with doses as low as 7 mg and therefore any patient accidentally or purposefully ingesting excess doses of this drug must be referred to a hospital urgently for treatment.

General note
Colchicine tablets may be stored at room temperature. They should be protected from light.

CONTRACEPTIVES, ORAL

Oestrogen + Progestogen
Ethinyloestradiol + Norethisterone
(Trade names: Binovum, Brevinor, Loestrin 20, Loestrin 30, Neocon 1/35, Norimin, Ovysmen, Synphase, Trinovum)
Ethinyloestradiol + Ethynodiol
(Trade names: Conova 30)
Ethinyloestradiol + Levonorgestrel
(Trade names: Eugynon 30, Eugynon 50, Logynon, Microgynon 30, Ovran, Ovran 30, Ovranette, Trinordiol)

Ethinyloestradiol + Desogestrel
(Trade names: Marvelon, Mercilon)
Ethinyloestradiol + Gestodene
(Trade names: Femodene, Minulet, Triadene)
Mestranol + Norethisterone
(Trade names: Norinyl-1, Ortho-Novin 1/50)
Progestogen-only
Norethisterone
(Trade names: Micronor, Noriday)
Ethynodiol*
(Trade name: Femulen)
Levonorgestrel
(Trade names: Microval, Neogest, Norgeston)
* Converted in the body to Norethisterone

Actions and Uses
Oral contraceptives act by a number of mechanisms:
1. They act on an area of the brain called the hypothalamus which normally releases substances which in turn cause another area of the brain called the pituitary to release substances known as gonadotrophins. These gonadotrophins stimulate ovulation. Oral contraceptives halt this action.
2. Oral contraceptives affect the endometrium (the lining of the uterus) making the implantation of an ovum less likely and therefore reducing the chances of successful pregnancy.
3. The cervical mucus is made more viscous and therefore spermatozoa have greater difficulty in reaching the uterus and fertilizing the ovum.
Oral contraceptives may be made up of two main types of hormones:
1. Oestrogens which principally inhibit ovulation.
2. Progestogens which also inhibit ovulation but have in addition an effect on the cervical mucus.
For the most part combinations of both oestrogens and progestogens are used as they are thought to be more reliable. Recently it has been found that the dose of oestrogen required for successful contraception is lower than was previously thought necessary. These two hormones

may be combined for the purposes of contraception in two different ways:

1. The combination of both drugs may be started on the 5th day after the start of menstruation and continued for 20 days. No further drugs are taken until the 5th day of the next episode of bleeding.
2. Oestrogen only may be given for 15-21 days with progestogen being added to the last 5-10 days of the 21 day course.

It is important in addition to note that some contraceptive pills are now being produced which contain progestogens only.

Dosage

1. For combination tablets: One tablet is taken daily for 21 days starting on the 5th day of menstruation. To assist patients who have difficulty remembering when to stop and start treatment, many contraceptives come in packs of 28 days, 7 of these being dummy tablets.
2. Progestogen-only tablets are taken every day without break during the cycle.

Nurse monitoring

The taking of the contraceptive pill has, because of considerable publicity given to it in the national press, created many anxieties in women's minds. In addition various situations arise in which women may wonder whether it is appropriate either to commence or continue such treatment. Nurses may find themselves being asked about such situations and therefore the nurse monitoring section on these drugs will be based on the type of question which the nurse may have to answer.

1. Are there any women who should not take the pill? It is recommended that the pill be avoided in certain groups of patients and these are as follows:
   a. Patients with cardiovascular disease including hypertension, previous stroke, angina pectoris, myocardial infarction or venous thrombosis.
   b. Patients with liver disease (some authorities believe that the contraceptive pill may be given to patients with liver disease if their liver function tests are normal).
   c. Any patient who has or has in the past had breast cancer or cancer of gynaecological origin.
   d. It is felt that patients who have or have had hypertension, facial nerve palsy or migraine may be at risk of cerebral thrombosis and therefore they should be discouraged from using the contraceptive pill.
2. How soon after having a baby can I start the pill? It is advisable to wait for the first period to occur prior to commencing the contraceptive pill. It is important, however, to ensure that alternative precautions are taken as even if a patient is breast feeding, there is a risk of pregnancy.
3. Can I breast feed when taking the pill? There is very little risk to the suckling infant from the low doses of oestrogen and progestrogen in the contraceptive pill and therefore it is not contraindicated from the point of view of the infant. However, there may be a reduction in milk production after recommencing the pill and this may lead to failure of breast feeding.
4. What must I do if I forget a dose?
   a. If a combined preparation is being taken, the dose may be taken up to 12 hours after the usual time safely.
   After 12 hours there is a definite risk and if 3 days or more have elapsed then the course should be completed, missing out the tablets which have been omitted, but alternative precautions to avoid pregnancy must be used.
   b. With the progestogen-only pills, missing a dose by even 3 hours or more may be important and additional precautions are advised until at least 14

consecutive days treatment have again been taken.

5. If I stop the pill to become pregnant how long should I wait before attempting to become pregnant? It is best to wait until at least one true period has occurred after stopping the pill. This allows calculation of dates and assessment of maturity and development of the fetus to be performed more accurately.

6. Will the pill damage my baby if I do become pregnant? Although there is a theoretical risk that the baby might be damaged, in practice there is no evidence that any damage occurs.

7. How long can I take the pill for? Provided no severe side-effects occur, and regular checks are made at visits to a general practitioner or family planning clinic, the pill may be continued for as long as the patient desires. More specific advice on this point should be sought from the patient's own general practitioner or family planning clinic.

8. What do I do if I require an operation? A combined preparation should be stopped 6 weeks prior to operation. Progestogen-only pills may be continued. If surgery is necessary at short notice the doctor or surgeon involved should be informed that the patient is on the pill.

9. Will my periods be regular when I take the pill? It is important to point out that the bleeding which occurs is not actually a period but episodes of bleeding will tend to occur regularly if the combined preparations are used. A beneficial effect is that bleeding may become lighter and pain encountered with periods may be abolished. If progestogen-only pills are used, irregularities in the menstrual cycle and therefore irregular bleeding may occur in the early months of treatment and occasionally periods may be missed altogether.

10. Can other drugs I take interfere with the pill? A number of drugs including antibiotics (particularly Rifampicin), Ergotamine, barbiturates, anticonvulsants, Aminocaproic Acid, tranquillizers, corticosteroids, antihistamines, Phenylbutazone and Oxyphenbutazone have been thought to have a theoretical risk of reducing the effectiveness of oral contraceptives. The evidence is more firm for barbiturates, anticonvulsants and Rifampicin. Alternative means of contraception should be used if these drugs are taken in short courses and if they are to be taken for more prolonged courses this problem should be discussed further with the patient's medical practitioner.

11. Side-effects with the contraceptive pill are common and these may be divided into two major groups:
    a. Those arising just after the commencement of the contraceptive pill for the first time. These are largely due to the oestrogen and include nausea, vomiting, breast discomfort, fluid retention, depression, headache, lethargy, abdominal discomfort, vaginal discharge, cervical erosions and a syndrome of general irritability.
    b. Actual side-effects include depression, altered sexual drive, jaundice, salt and water retention, hypertension, altered glucose tolerance, thrombophlebitis and thromboembolism.

12. The results of many biochemical tests may be altered in patients taking the pill and in order to avert unnecessary worry for the patient and unnecessary use of health service resources, nurses may play an important role in encouraging patients always to tell medical staff at consultation that they are using the oral contraceptive.

CORTICOSTEROIDS

The following corticosteroids are in current clinical use:
Alclomethasone
Beclomethasone
Betamethasone
Budesonide
Clobetasol
Clobetasone
Cortisone
Dexamethasone
Difluocortolone
Fluclorolone
Fludrocortisone
Fluocinolone
Fluocinonide
Fluocortolone
Flurandrenolone
Halcinonide
Hydrocortisone
Methylprednisolone
Prednisolone
Prednisone
Triamcinolone

Actions and uses

Corticosteroids are a group of mainly synthetic substances which are derived from a hormone, hydrocortisone, which is produced in the body by the cortex of the adrenal glands. All these drugs have two major effects which are described as glucocorticoid and mineralocorticoid. The glucocorticoid activity is responsible for the anti-inflammatory action of corticosteroids which makes the drug useful in a wide range of diseases including rheumatoid disease, connective tissue disease, inflammatory bowel disease, allergic conditions, asthma and inflammatory skin conditions such as eczema, dermatitis and psoriasis. The mineralocorticoid activity has little usefulness clinically and is responsible for a number of side-effects including salt and water retention. Corticosteroids are used both systemically and topically in the form of tablets, injections, ointments, creams, eye drops, enemas and suppositories.

Dosage

For dosage and route of administration see individual drugs.

Nurse monitoring

1. Corticosteroids produce many side-effects, especially if given in high dose or for prolonged periods of time. By far the most important side-effect is suppression of the ability of the adrenal gland of the body to produce hydrocortisone. This means that any patient who is either on steroids or has recently been on prolonged or high doses of steroids will be unable to produce steroids in response to any stress such as infection or injury. As a consequence they may demonstrate more severe reactions to such stresses and on occasion this may result in a fatal outcome. The nurse's primary role in the management of patients on corticosteroids, therefore, is to bear in mind that any patient who is on, or who has recently been on corticosteroids will, if they suffer injury or infection or require an operation, need to have their dosage at least doubled during such stress periods. In addition, any patient who has been on prolonged courses of corticosteroids should never have their drug stopped suddenly for any reason.
2. Patients who have been on steroids for a long period develop what is known as 'Cushingoid' symptoms. These include a moon face, obesity, purple striae and acne.
3. The electrolyte disturbances associated with corticosteroid treatment include:
   a. Salt and water retention with hypertension
   b. Hypokalaemia with resultant muscle weakness
   c. Altered glucose metabolism with the possible precipitation of diabetes
   d. Altered calcium/phosphorus balance producing osteoporosis and a tendency towards bone fracture.
4. Depression and psychosis are occasionally associated with steroid treatment.

5. Gastric upset and occasionally peptic ulceration may be associated with steroid treatment.
6. Wound healing may be delayed significantly. This is especially important in patients who have to undergo an operation while on steroid treatment.
7. Corneal ulceration and cataract formation may occur.
8. There is an increased risk of infection by bacteria, viruses and fungi, such as oral candidiasis, when patients are treated with steroids.
9. It is important to note that the above effects can occur with prolonged or high dosage of steroids administered by any route including topical application to the skin.
10. It is also extremely important to note that corticosteroids should not be given to patients who have active infection such as chickenpox, poliomyelitis, tuberculosis and infection due to herpes virus.

CORTISONE (Cortelan, Cortistab, Cortisyl)

Presentation
Tablets—5 mg, 25 mg
Injection—25 mg in 1 ml

Actions and uses
Cortisone is a corticosteroid drug and has actions and uses as described in the section on corticosteroids. It is converted in the body to the active component hydrocortisone. As this conversion varies greatly between patients it is usually preferable to administer hydrocortisone itself as this enables medical staff to more accurately predict the active amount of drug being received.

Dosage
Dosages vary widely depending on the type of illness, severity of the disease, and the route of administration. It is therefore impossible to outline dosage regimes in this text.

Nurse monitoring
See the section on corticosteroids.

General note
Tablets containing cortisone may be stored at room temperature.

CO-TRIMOXAZOLE (Septrin, Bactrim)

(See Note 3, p. 362)
Co-trimoxazole is a combination of a sulphonamide (sulphamethoxazole) and trimethoprim.

Presentation
Tablets—
400 mg sulphamethoxazole + 80 mg trimethoprim
800 mg sulphamethoxazole + 160 mg trimethoprim
100 mg sulphamethoxazole + 20 mg trimethoprim (Paediatric)
Suspension—
400 mg sulphamethoxasole + 80 mg trimethoprim in 5 ml
200 mg sulphamethoxazole + 40 mg trimethoprim in 5 ml (Paediatric)
Injection—
800 mg sulphamethoxazole + 160 mg trimethoprim in 3 ml (intramuscular)
400 mg sulphamethoxazole + 80 mg trimethoprim in 5 ml (for intravenous infusion)

Actions and uses
Sulphonamide drugs and trimethoprim when used alone are bacteriostatic, i.e. they prevent further growth and division of bacteria. It has been found that the combined use of these two substances is preferable for two reasons:
1. The combination of the two substances is bactericidal in action, i.e. bacteria present are killed rather than simply inhibited from further growth and division.
2. The combination of the two different mechanisms of action makes it more difficult for bacteria to develop resistance to the drug.
The organisms against which cotrimoxazole is effective include Haemophilus, Proteus, Escherichia,

Neisseria, Salmonella, Shigella, *Streptococcus pyogenes* and staphylococcus. It should be noted that infections with Pseudomonas organisms are usually not success-fully treated with this compound. In clinical practice the drug is widely used in treatment of chest and urinary tract infections and for the prophylaxis of urinary tract infec-tions.

Co-trimoxazole, in very high dosage has a special use in the treatment of pneumocystic lung infection in patients with compromised immunity e.g. AIDS. See Note 7.

Dosage

1. Oral:
   a. Adults should receive 800 mg of sulphamethoxazole and 160 mg of trimethoprim twice daily.
   b. Children should receive the following doses: Less than 1 year—20 mg of sulphamethoxazole and 4 mg of trimethoprim per kg twice daily; 1-7 years—one-quarter of the adult dose; over 7 years—one-half of the adult dose.
2. Parenteral administration:
   a. Adults should receive 1 ampoule (3 ml) twice daily.
   b. Children over 6 should receive half the adult dose. It is not recommended that the intra-muscular preparation be used in younger children due to the inadequacy of muscle mass in which to inject the preparation.
3. By the intravenous route adults should receive 2 ampoules (10 ml) twice daily. Each ampoule (5 ml) should be diluted to 125 ml immediately prior to infusion. A number of solutions may be used for dilution including 5 and 10% dextrose, 5% laevulose, 0.9% sodium chloride, dextran 40, dextran 70, Ringer's' solution and sodium chloride 0.18% and dextrose injection.
4. The intravenous doses for children are as follows: 6 weeks to 6 months of age—1.25 ml diluted appropriately twice per day; 6 months to 6 years—2.5 ml diluted appropriately twice daily; 6 years

to 12 years—5 ml diluted appropriately twice per day; over 12 years—adult doses are recommended.

N.B. Reduced doses are used for patients with renal disease.

Nurse monitoring

1. The nurse monitoring notes on sulphonamides (q.v.) and trimethoprim (q.v.) are applicable to this drug.
2. It is worth noting that the risk of macrocytic (megaloblastic) anaemia with this drug is only really important with prolonged full dose therapy and can be prevented by giving folinic acid, although if macrocytic anaemia develops it is preferable to use an alternative antibiotic.

General notes

1. Oral preparations may be stored at room temperature.
2. As noted above intravenous infusion ampoules should be diluted immediately before use and if not used immediately should be disposed of.
3. No other substances should be added to intravenous infusions of co-trimoxazole.
4. Intravenous infusions should be administered slowly with each dose being given over approxi-mately $1-1\frac{1}{2}$ hours.

CYANOCOBALAMIN—VITAMIN B_{12} (Cytamen, Cytacon)

Presentation

Tablets—50 microgram per tablet
Injection—250 microgram in 1 ml, 1000 microgram in 1 ml
Oral liquid—35 microgram in 5 ml

Actions and uses

Cyanocobalamin (Vitamin B_{12}) is indicated for the treatment of megaloblastic anaemia where this has been shown to be due to a deficiency of Vitamin B_{12} by the appropriate laboratory test. Deficiency of Vitamin B_{12} occurs either where there is a deficiency in the gut of a substance (intrinsic factor) normally produced by the stomach which is essential for the absorption of Vitamin B_{12}, this condition being known as pernicious anaemia, or it may be due to other forms of malabsorption. More rarely Vitamin B_{12} deficiency may be seen in people who have a strict vegan diet.

Dosage
1. Parenterally:
   a. For the treatment of pernicious anaemia: Initially 250–1000 microgram intramuscularly on alternate days for 2 weeks and then 1000 microgram monthly
   b. For the prophylaxis of megalo-blastic anaemia due to gastrectomy, malabsorption syndrome or strict veganism: 250–1000 microgram monthly.
2. Orally:
   a. Adult: 300 microgram per day
   b. Children: 35–70 microgram 2-3 times per day.

Nurse monitoring
1. Sensitization to Vitamin B_{12} is extremely rare. It may present as an itching rash and very exceptionally as anaphylactic shock.
2. Cyanocobalamin contains cyanide. This is contraindicated for use in patients suffering from either tobacco amblyopia or Leber's optic atrophy (optic atrophy and optic neuritis).
3. Hydroxycobalamin is in general to be preferred to cyanocobalamin as it has a longer duration of action.

General note
Ampoules should be protected from light.

CYCLIZINE (Valoid)

Presentation
Tablets—50 mg
Injection—50 mg in 1 ml

Actions and uses
Cyclizine is an antihistamine. The actions and uses of antihistamines in general are described in the section on antihistamines. Cyclizine is used in clinical practice:

1. In the treatment of nausea and vomiting, particularly motion sickness.

Dosage
1. Adults: Orally, intramuscularly or intravenously: 50 mg three times daily.
2. Children: (1-10 years): Up to 25 mg orally three times per day.

Nurse monitoring
See the section on antihistamines.

General note
The drug may be stored at room temperature.

CYCLOPENTHIAZIDE (Navidrex)

Presentation
Tablets—0.5 mg

Actions and uses
See the section on thiazide and related diuretics.

Dosage
The daily adult range is 0.25–1 mg usually as a single daily dose. The duration of action is 12 hours plus.

Nurse monitoring
See the section on thiazide and related diuretics.

General note
Cyclopenthiazide tablets may be stored at room temperature.

CYCLOPHOSPHAMIDE (Endoxana)

Presentation
Tablets—10 mg, 50 mg
Injection—100 mg, 200 mg, 500 mg, 1 g

Actions and uses
Cyclophosphamide is a member of the nitrogen mustard group. It is converted by the liver to a number of highly reactive metabolites. These metabolites interfere with the enzyme systems essential for cell growth and therefore diminish tumour growth. It has a wide range of uses which are as follows:

1. It is widely used to good effect in Hodgkin's disease, lympho-sarcoma, multiple myeloma, reticulum cell sarcoma, chronic lymphocytic leukaemia and ovarian carcinoma.
2. It has also been used in the treatment of carcinoma of the breast and lung.
3. It is used in a number of non-malignant diseases including rheumatoid arthritis, systemic lupus erythematosus, nephrotic syndrome and other autoimmune diseases.

Dosage

1. As a cytotoxic drug: This depends on the tumour type, the state of the patient and other factors including coincident administration of other cytotoxic drugs. Various regimes are used and include:
   a. 2–6 mg/kg body weight daily by single intravenous injection
   b. 2–6 mg/kg body weight in divided oral doses
   c. 10–15 mg/kg as single intravenous doses at weekly intervals
   d. 60–80 mg/kg as single intravenous injections at 3-4 weekly intervals.
2. For an immunosuppressant effect, daily oral doses of 1.5–3 mg/kg are used.

N.B. All above doses are for adults.

Nurse monitoring

1. Cyclophosphamide may be given orally or intravenously but it is unsuitable for intramuscular use.
2. It is essential that all patients receiving this drug should maintain an adequate fluid intake as this has been shown to reduce the incidence of haemorrhagic cystitis which results from an irritant effect on the bladder surface due to metabolites.
3. Bone marrow suppression is a common side-effect of this drug. The white cells are more commonly affected than platelets and therefore infection in patients on this drug may be particularly severe and life threatening.

4. Gastrointestinal toxicity is common with this drug and may present as anorexia, nausea and vomiting.
5. Alopecia is a common side-effect and the risk increases as higher doses of the drug are used. As alopecia is a particularly distressing side-effect, patients require a good deal of psycho-logical support and should be constantly encouraged by the fact that their hair will return after cessation of treatment, and indeed in some patients the hair will reappear while they are still receiving the drug.
6. Uncommon side-effects include liver toxicity, cardiac damage, skin and nail pigment-ation, dizziness, diarrhoea, thyroid dysfunction and the syndrome of inappropriate secretion of antidiuretic hormone. Jaundice, colitis, mucosal ulceration, interstitial pulmonary fibrosis and side-effects on the clotting mechanism are also seen.
7. Cyclophosphamide enhances the effect of oral anti-diabetic drugs and should therefore be used with caution in diabetics. Any diabetic receiving this drug should be carefully monitored as change in hypoglycaemic therapy may be necessary.
8. The nurse should be constantly aware that most cytotoxic drugs are irritant to the skin and mucous surfaces, and are in general very toxic. Great care should therefore be exercised when handling these drugs, and in particular spillage or contamination of personnel or the environment must be avoided. If cytotoxic drugs are handled regularly it is theoretically possible that repeated skin contact or inhalation may produce systemic toxic effects and in nurses who have developed hypersensitivity, severe local and general hypersensitivity reactions.

General notes

1. It is important to note that solutions prepared using water for injection should be used within 2 hours.
2. The drug is usually injected directly into the vein over a period of about 2 minutes or added to the drip tubing of a running 0.9% sodium chloride or 5% dextrose infusion.
3. Cyclophosphamide tablets and vials for injection may be stored at room temperature.

CYCLOSPORIN (Sandimmun)

Presentation

Injection—50 mg in 1 ml, 150 mg in 5 ml
Oral solution—100 mg in 1 ml

Actions and uses

The drug cyclosporin is an immunosuppressant which is used for organ transplantation (involving skin, heart, kidney, pancreas, cornea, bone marrow, etc.) to reduce the likelihood of rejection and graft-versus-host disease. It acts on human t-lymphocytes which undergo a complex change during the development of the normal immune response. Cyclosporin is also used in the control of a variety of autoimmune diseases (e.g. psoriasis) as a steroid sparing agent and alternative to other first line immunosuppressants.

Dosage

1. These vary considerably depending upon the nature of the organs transplanted, and the manufacturer's literature should be consulted.
2. A typical dose in psoriasis and other autoimmune diseases is 2.5–5 mg/kg daily in 2 divided doses.

Nurse monitoring

1. Intravenous infusions should be administered in glass, not PVC, containers.
2. Cyclosporin produces a series of side-effects which are dose-related, i.e. will diminish when dosage is reduced, including; increased growth of body hair (hirsutism), tremor, kidney and liver impairment, gingival hypertrophy and gastrointestinal upsets.
3. Close monitoring of liver and kidney function and of blood level of the drug itself should be carried out.
4. Intravenous infusion may be associated with hypersensitivity reactions, usually to an inactive constituent of the preparation rather than to the drug itself.
5. Cyclosporin given in combination with other drugs which carry a known risk of producing renal damage will increase the possibility of kidney dysfunction.
6. Concurrent administration of many other drugs has been shown to increase blood levels of cyclosporin and hence the incidence of side-effects. These include the antiarrhythmics, erythromycin, doxycycline, various antifungals, calcium antagonists, colchicine, danazol, oral contraceptives and hormone replacement therapy.
7. In contrast to the above, drugs which may reduce cyclosporin levels and so increase the risk of tissue rejection include the barbiturates, other anticonvulsants, and rifampicin.

General notes

1. Cyclosporin oral solution must not be refrigerated since precipitation of the drug will occur.
2. Once opened, the oral solution should be discarded if unused after 2 months.

CYPROHEPTADINE (Periactin)

Presentation

Tablets—4 mg
Syrup—2 mg in 5 ml

Actions and uses

Cyproheptadine is an antihistamine. The actions and uses of antihistamines in general are discussed in the section on antihistamines. In clinical practice cyproheptadine is used:

1. To suppress local allergic reactions, i.e. inflammatory skin responses to insect stings and bites, contact allergens, urticaria etc.
2. To stimulate the appetite in patients who have problems with eating sufficiently, such as anorexia nervosa sufferers.
3. To counteract the effects of the chemical released in the rare syndrome known as carcinoid syndrome which is characterized by diarrhoea, flushing and skin rash.

Dosage
Adults: 4 mg three times daily.

Nurse monitoring
See the section on antihistamines.

General note
The drug may be stored at room temperature.

CYPROTERONE ACETATE
(Androcur, Cyprostat, Dianette)

Presentation
Tablets—50 mg
Capsules—100 mg

Actions and uses
Cyproterone acetate has as anti-androgenic action. The actions of androgens are described in the section on androgens. In clinical practice the drug is used for the following conditions:

1. It may be used to treat hirsutism in the female.
2. It can also be given to treat symptoms of sexual precocity and sexual deviation in the male.
3. It reduces sebum secretion and is administered cyclically in combination with ethinyloestradiol (Dianette) in female acne unresponsive to oral antibiotic therapy.
4. It is used in the treatment of symptomatic metastatic cancer of the prostate which is an androgen-dependent tumour.

Dosage
1. For hirsutism in females: 50 mg daily for short courses during each menstrual cycle, usually combined with oestrogenic treatment.
2. For deviant sexual behaviour in males: 50 mg twice daily.
3. In female acne: a low dose (2 mg) in combination with ethinyloestradiol is taken from day 1 to day 21 of the menstrual cycle and repeated after a 7 day interval.
4. Prostatic cancer: 300 mg daily in 2-3 divided doses.

Nurse monitoring
1. When administered to male patients:
   a. A reduction in sperm count and therefore fertility usually occurs.
   b. Gynaecomastia (breast enlargement) and tenderness of the breast may occur.
2. When administered to females: Galactorrhoea and breast enlargement may occur.
3. The Dianette combination with ethinyloestradiol is contraceptive and may be used as such in patients with acne who also require an oral contraceptive.
4. Common symptoms during the first few weeks of treatment include tiredness, fatigue and lassitude. These symptoms usually disappear after 3 months of treatment.
5. Weight gain is a common problem with prolonged administration of this drug.
6. This drug should not be given to patients with adrenal dysfunction or diabetes mellitus.
7. Other contraindications to treatment include a history of thrombosis or embolism and a history of depression.
8. With long-term treatment hypochromic anaemia may occur.

General note
The drug may be stored at room temperature.

C

CYTARABINE (Alexan, Cytosar) (Also described as Cytosine Arabinoside and Ara-C)

Presentation
Injections—100 mg and 500 mg in vials with 5 ml ampoules containing solvent or as ready-mixed solutions. Also 1 g in 10 ml ready-mixed solution.

Actions and uses
Cytarabine is a cytotoxic drug which is thought to act by inhibiting an enzyme essential in the synthesis of DNA which in turn is an essential step in the growth and division of any cell. It has two major uses:

1. Its use as a cytotoxic drug has been confined to the treatment of leukaemias, especially acute myeloid leukaemia in adults.
2. As it also exerts an anti-viral action it has been used in the treatment of infections due to herpes virus.

Dosage
Cytarabine is given by intravenous infusion and intravenous, subcutaneous and intrathecal injections. It is often given in combination with a variety of other cytotoxic agents.

1. For remission in acute myeloid leukaemia:
   a. 2–4 mg/kg body weight daily may be given by rapid intravenous injection.
   b. 0.5–1 mg/kg daily may be given by continuous injection. Courses of up to 10 days of either of the above are usually given.
   c. An alternative regime is to administer 3–5 mg/kg on 5 consecutive days with further 5 day courses repeated after periods of up to 10 days until an effect is achieved.
   d. A further alternative is to administer very short courses of extremely high dosages, e.g. of the order 2 g per square metre of body surface by intravenous infusion.
2. For maintenance treatment: 1 mg/kg has been given by subcutaneous injection once or twice weekly.

3. In the treatment of leukaemic meningitis intrathecal doses of up to 50 mg have been given on two to three occasions.
4. In the treatment of infection due to herpes virus 100 mg/m^2 body surface area has been given by intravenous injection daily. An alternative regime is 2–4 mg/kg body weight daily.
5. For the treatment of encephalitis intrathecal doses of 10 mg/m^2 body surface area have been given.

Nurse monitoring

1. When patients are receiving this drug nausea, vomiting, diarrhoea, and oral ulceration frequently occur.
2. A most important side-effect of this drug is suppression of bone marrow with resultant increased risk of haemorrhage, anaemia and infection.
3. More rarely skin rashes, pain in the abdomen, chest and joints and neurotoxic and nephrotoxic side-effects have been reported.
4. Patients with impaired liver function are at an increased risk of suffering toxic effects.
5. As animal studies on this drug have demonstrated adverse effects on fetal development it is completely contraindicated in pregnancy and any woman receiving the drug should be encouraged to take adequate contraceptive measures.
6. The nurse should be constantly aware that most cytotoxic drugs are irritant to the skin and mucous surfaces, and are in general very toxic. Great care should therefore be exercised when handling these drugs, and in particular spillage or contamination of personnel or the environment must be avoided. If cytotoxic drugs are handled regularly it is theoretically possible that repeated skin contact or inhalation may produce systemic toxic effects and in nurses who have developed hypersensitivity, severe local and general hypersensitivity reactions.

General notes

1. The injection should be stored in a refrigerator.
2. Reconstituted solutions may be retained for up to 48 hours at room temperature.
3. Any solution in which a slight haze has developed must be immediately discarded.
4. Solutions are prepared by adding the accompanying 5 ml diluent to provide an injection containing 20 mg/ml.
5. Note that intrathecal injections must be prepared by using water for injection as the solvent provided contains benzyl alcohol and may be irritant if injected into the CSF.
6. Intravenous infusions are given in 0.9% sodium chloride or 5% dextrose solution.

D

DACARBAZINE (DTIC)

Presentation
Injection—100 mg, 200 mg.

Actions and uses
Dacarbazine is a cytotoxic drug. The precise method of action remains to be discovered. Its most important use is in the treatment of malignant melanoma. It is also used in the treatment of sarcoma and Hodgkin's disease and to a lesser extent in tumours of the colon, ovary, breast, lungs and testis.

Dosage
1. 2–4.5 mg/kg body weight daily may be given by intravenous injection for 10 days, repeated at intervals of 4 weeks.
2. An alternative regime is to give 250 mg/m² daily intravenously for 5 days and repeat at intervals of 3 weeks.
3. Intravenous injections should be given over a period of about 1 minute.

Nurse monitoring
1. Bone marrow depression producing anaemia, haemorrhage due to thrombocytopenia and infection due to suppression of white cell production may occur in a severe degree.
2. Frequent and distressing side-effects include anorexia, nausea and vomiting.
3. Other less common adverse effects include diarrhoea, muscle pain, tiredness, alopecia, facial flushing, paraesthesia and altered liver function.
4. It is extremely important for the nurse to note that dacarbazine is a very irritant drug and contact with the skin or eyes must be avoided.
5. The nurse should be constantly aware that most cytotoxic drugs are irritant to the skin and mucous surfaces, and are in general very toxic. Great care should therefore be exercised when handling these drugs, and in particular spillage or contamination of personnel or the environment must be avoided. If cytotoxic drugs are handled regularly it is theoretically possible that repeated skin contact or inhalation may produce systemic toxic effects and in nurses who have developed hypersensitivity, severe local and general hypersensitivity reactions.

General notes
1. Dacarbazine injection must be stored in a refrigerator and protected from light.
2. Solutions are prepared by adding 9.9 ml to each 100 mg vial or 19.7 ml to each 200 mg vial using water for injection.
3. Prepared solutions are stable for 72 hours under refrigeration.

DANAZOL (Danol)

Presentation
Capsules—100 mg and 200 mg

Actions and uses
This drug inhibits the production of the hormones normally secreted by the pituitary which stimulate function of the ovaries and endometrium of the ovaries during the menstrual

cycle. It is used most commonly in clinical practice for the treatment of endometriosis but it has also been used for the treatment of gynaecomastia, fibrocystic mastitis, precocious puberty and pubertal breast hypertrophy.

Dosage

It is important to note that the therapeutic effect of danazol is controlled by careful dosage adjustment, according to individual response.

1. For the treatment of endometriosis the usual adult dose range is between 200 and 800 mg daily.
2. For the treatment of precocious puberty in children: 100–400 mg may be given daily according to the child's age and weight.

Nurse monitoring

1. The drug's androgenic properties can produce side-effects of acne, oily skin, fluid retention, hirsutism, deepening voice and clitoral hypertrophy.
2. Other side-effects include flushing, reduction in breast size, skin rash, anxiety, dizziness, vertigo, headache, nausea and loss of hair.
3. Due to the risk of fluid retention, the drug should be used with great caution in patients with heart disease, kidney disease or epilepsy.
4. If patients have impaired liver function, the dosage required will usually be reduced.

General note

The drug may be stored at room temperature.

DAUNORUBICIN (Cerubidin, Rubidomycin)

Presentation

Injection—20 mg

Actions and uses

This drug is an anthracycline antibiotic and although it has a similar action to doxorubicin (q.v.) it has a different spectrum of clinical use in that it is of great value in the treatment of acute leukaemia but has little place in the treatment of solid tumours for which doxorubicin is frequently used.

Dosage

The drug is given by intravenous injection. The usual dosage is 0.5–3 mg/kg body weight. The intervals between injection vary widely according to the treatment schedule being used. The total number of injections required varies considerably between patients.

Nurse monitoring

The nurse monitoring notes on daunorubicin are identical to those for doxorubicin (q.v.).

General notes

1. Daunorubicin injection should be stored in a cool place and protected from light. It is normally recommended that it be kept under refrigeration.
2. The injection is prepared by dissolving the required dose in 10–20 ml of sodium chloride 0.9% and it is then injected into the tube of a fast running intravenous infusion of normal saline.
3. Any unused solution should be immediately discarded.

DEBRISOQUINE (Declinax)

Presentation

Tablets–10 mg

Actions and uses

See the section on guanethidine.

Dosage

The initial adult dosage is usually 10 mg once or twice a day. This is built up gradually to a maximum of 60 mg per day in total. In cases of severe hypertension the starting dose may be 20 mg once or twice daily building up to 120 mg per day in total and doses as high as 300 mg have been used.

Nurse monitoring

See the section on guanethidine.

General note
Debrisoquine tablets may be stored at room temperature.

DEGLYCYRRHIZINISED LIQUORICE (Caved-S)

Presentation
Tablets—380 mg (also includes antacids)

Actions and uses
Deglycyrrhizinised liquorice is known to have a healing action on peptic ulcers. The mechanism of this healing action is unknown. It has been used to treat both gastric and duodenal ulcers and is usually given in courses of up to 6 weeks in duration.

Dosage
1. Gastric ulcer: 2 tablets three times daily.
2. Duodenal ulcer: 2 tablets three to six times daily.

Nurse monitoring
Mild diarrhoea occasionally occurs in patients receiving this drug.

General notes
Nil.

DEMECLOCYCLINE (Ledermycin)

(See Note 3, p. 362)
Note: Previously referred to as Demethylchlortetracycline

Presentation
Tablets—300 mg
Capsules—150 mg
Syrup—75 mg in 5 ml
Oral drops—60 mg in 1 ml

Actions and uses
1. The actions and uses of demeclocycline as an antibacterial are identical to those described for tetracyclines in general (q.v.).
2. The drug has a peculiar effect on the kidney in that it blocks the action of antidiuretic hormone (ADH, Vasopressin) on the renal tubules. This hormone is important in maintaining plasma volume by stimulating reabsorption of free water by the kidney and under certain rare circumstances an excess of ADH may be produced leading to dilutional hyponatraemia. This syndrome of inappropriate ADH secretion (SIADH) can be treated by administration of demeclocycline in the doses described below.

Dosage
1. For the treatment of infection:
   a. Adults: 150 mg four times a day or 300 mg twice a day.
   b. Children: less than 1 year— 30 mg/day in total given in two divided doses; 1-5 years— 60–120 mg/day in total given in four divided doses; 5-9 years—120–240 mg/day in total given in two or three divided doses; 9-15 years— 270–600 mg in total per day given in four divided doses.
2. For the treatment of inappropriate ADH secretion (SIADH), 600–1200 mg per day in total is given in divided doses.

Nurse monitoring
1. The general nurse monitoring notes on tetracyclines (q.v.) are applicable to demeclocycline.
2. It is important to note that the incidence of photosensitivity reactions is particularly high with this drug.
3. It is absolutely essential to remember that the drug in syrup should not be diluted for ease of administration.

General note
The drug may be stored at room temperature.

DESIPRAMINE (Pertofran)

Presentation
Tablets—25 mg

Actions and uses
Desipramine is a tricyclic antidepressant drug. Its actions and uses are described in the section on tricyclic antidepressants.

Dosage
For the treatment of depression 25 mg three or four times per day orally

is usually given. This may be increased to a maximum total daily dose of 200 mg if required.

Nurse monitoring
See the section on tricyclic antidepressant drugs.

General note
Desipramine tablets may be stored at room temperature.

DESMOPRESSIN (DDAVP)

Presentation
Nasal drops—100 microgram/ml
Intranasal spray—10 microgram/metred 0.1 ml dose
Injection—4 microgram in 1 ml
Tablets—100 microgram, 200 microgram

Actions and uses
Desmopressin is a chemical derivative of vasopressin, the posterior pituitary antidiuretic hormone (ADH). It has a much longer action than ADH and does not possess the marked vasoconstrictor effect of the natural hormone and is therefore a more convenient and safer alternative in the treatment of diabetes insipidus.

Very high doses of desmopressin have been given by intravenous injection as a means of stimulating clotting Factor VIII synthesis in deficiency states (haemophilia and von Willebrand's Disease). This use is highly specialized and only carried out under the haematologist's supervision.

Dosage
This is highly variable in the individual and is adjusted in order to produce sufficient diuresis each day so that water overload is prevented.
1. Intravenous: used only for initial therapy and postoperatively—1–4 microgram daily for adults and as little as one-tenth of the upper limit for children.
2. Intranasal: for maintenance therapy a dose range of 5–20 microgram, once or twice daily, is common.
3. Oral: 100–200 microgram three times daily.

Nurse monitoring
1. The wide variation of dosage between individuals and in the same subject during long-term maintenance must be stressed. The poor oral bioavailability of this drug is reflected in the major differences between oral and intranasal dosage. It is therefore important to monitor urine output during therapy.
2. The method of administration of the intranasal forms of desmopressin vary and require careful patient education in order to achieve optimum control. The nurse has therefore an important task in confirming patient compliance.
3. Although desmopressin lacks the potent vasoconstrictor action of ADH and is much less likely to produce constriction of the coronary arteries or hypertension, patients with cardiovascular disease should nevertheless be carefully monitored.
4. Following pituitary surgery for diabetes insipidus, desmopressin may only be required for the relatively short-term.

General note
Desmopressin nasal solutions and injection must be stored in the refrigerator.

DEXAMETHASONE (Oradexon, Decadron)

Presentation
Tablets—0.5 mg, 0.75 mg, 2 mg
Injection—5 mg in 1 ml, 8 mg in 2 ml, 100 mg in 5 ml

Actions and uses
See the section on corticosteroids.

Dosage
Doses vary considerably with the nature and severity of the illness being treated and it is not therefore appropriate to quote specific instances.

D

Nurse monitoring
See the section on corticosteroids.

General notes
1. Preparations containing dexamethasone may be stored at room temperature but should be protected from light.
2. Intravenous infusions are prepared by adding dexamethasone injection to saline or dextrose solution. They must be discarded if unused after 24 hours.

DEXTROMORAMIDE (Palfium)

Presentation
Tablets—5 mg and 10 mg
Injection—5 mg in 1 ml, 10 mg in 1 ml
Suppositories—10 mg

Actions and uses
Dextromoramide is a narcotic analgesic and its general actions and uses are described in the section on narcotic analgesics.

Dosage
For adults:
1. Orally or by subcutaneous or intramuscular injection: 5 mg repeated 4-6 hourly according to the patient's response.
2. Rectally: a 10 mg suppository should be administered 4-6 hourly according to patient response.

Nurse monitoring
1. See the section on narcotic analgesic drugs.
2. Dextromoramide may also be administered sublingually in which case its onset of action is rapid and first pass metabolism by the liver during absorption is avoided. This is a particularly useful route if rapid onset short-term analgesia is required e.g. to assist with a painful procedure such as a dressing change, bathing or other movement which evokes severe pain.

General notes
1. The drug should be stored in a locked (controlled drug) cupboard.
2. The drug should be stored at room temperature.

DEXTROPROPOXYPHENE (Doloxene, Depronal SA, Distalgesic)

Presentation
Capsules—65 mg
N.B. Dextropropoxyphene is also included in a few preparations with salicylate or paracetamol. Distalgesic is the best example of this: this combination of dextropropoxyphene and paracetamol is now officially called co-proxamol.

Actions and uses
Dextropropoxyphene is a derivative of the narcotic analgesic group of drugs. It has a much milder analgesic effect than other members of the group and it is used for the treatment of mild or moderately painful conditions such as headache or musculoskeletal pain.

Dosage
Adults: two tablets 4-6 hourly when required for pain. If slow release capsules of the pure drug are used, the dosage is 150 mg 8 to 12-hourly.

Nurse monitoring
1. The incidence of problems with addiction due to prolonged use of dextropropoxyphene is not as great as with other stronger members of the narcotic analgesic group of drugs but it is worth noting that some degree of dependence may occur in some cases.
2. The drug is not subject to the legal requirements of 'controlled drugs' such as morphine.
3. Dextropropoxyphene enhances the effect of warfarin and may lead to an increased bleeding tendency in patients receiving this drug. Warfarin dosage should be carefully monitored

when dextropropoxyphene is
introduced.
4. The drug is associated with few
side-effects. However, a major
problem which should probably
severely restrict the general use
of dextropropoxyphene is that if
it is taken in overdose it can
cause profound respiratory
depression. This has led to a
number of fatalities.

General note
The drug may be stored at room
temperature.

DIAMORPHINE (Heroin)

Presentation
Injection—Diamorphine is available
in a variety of strengths from 5 mg to
500 mg.
Actions and uses
Diamorphine is a narcotic analgesic
and its general actions and uses are
described in the section on narcotic
analgesics. It is in fact the most
potent analgesic available when
administered by injection being
converted to an active metabolite
(6-methylmorphine) which rapidly
achieves very high concentrations in
the CNS. When taken orally,
however, diamorphine is virtually
completely metabolized to morphine
by the liver during first pass and it
has no advantages over morphine
by this route. Diamorphine is the
drug of first choice when parenteral
analgesia is indicated in severe,
often chronic severe, pain.
Dosage
Dosage varies widely depending on
the condition under treatment and
the individual's response to the drug,
Initial doses (given as a guideline
only) would be 5–10 mg by
subcutaneous, intramuscular or
intravenous routes, repeated
4-hourly as required according to the
patient's response and increased
appropriately as tolerance develops.
In the control of pain associated with
advanced cancer, for example, daily
doses of 1 g or more may eventually
be required.

Nurse monitoring
1. See the section on narcotic
analgesics.
2. Parenteral diamorphine,
commonly administered by
continuous subcutaneous
infusion, is often preferred for
patients with chronic severe pain
when the oral route is no longer
available. When transferring
from oral morphine a suggested
dose of diamorphine by injection
of one-third the oral morphine
dosage is suggested.
3. The solubility of diamorphine is
exceedingly high so that even
very large doses can be
dissolved in a fraction of 1 ml so
facilitating subcutaneous bolus
administration.

General notes
1. The drug should be stored in a
locked (controlled drug) cupboard.
2. The drug should be stored at
room temperature.

DIAZEPAM (Diazemuls, Stesolid, Valium)

Presentation
Tablets—2 mg, 5 mg, 10 mg
Capsules—2 mg, 5 mg
Syrup—2 mg in 5 ml
Injection—10 mg in 2 ml, 20 mg in
4 ml
Rectal solution—5 mg and 10 mg
Suppositories—5 mg and 10 mg
Actions and uses
Diazepam is a member of the
benzodiazepine group (q.v) and of
this group it has perhaps the widest
application:
1. It may be taken orally during the
day for the treatment of anxiety.
2. In large doses it may be taken as
an hypnotic.
3. It may be administered intravenously or intramuscularly for the
control of acute muscle spasm in
such conditions as tetanus or
status epilepticus
4. It may be given orally for the relief
of muscle spasm associated with
chronic neurological abnormalities

such as cerebral palsy and disseminated sclerosis

5. It may be given intravenously for sedation immediately prior to minor surgical, dental and investigative procedures.

6. It may be administered by the rectal route as an alternative to the oral or injectable routes. Suppositories are often useful prophylaxis if used during febrile illness in patients with a history of febrile convulsions, and rectal solution is an alternative to injections in the control of convulsions.

Dosage

1. For the treatment of anxiety: 6–30 mg may be given daily either by the oral or intramuscular route.

2. For the treatment of insomnia: A single dose ranging from 5–30 mg may be taken on retiring.

3. In tetanus: 0.1–0.3 mg/kg body weight by intravenous injection of 1-4 hours.

4. In status epilepticus: An initial dose of 0.15–0.25 mg/kg body weight may be given by the intravascular or intravenous route. A second dose may be given 30 minutes to 1 hour later. Occasionally continuous intravenous infusions of 3–10 mg/kg body weight for 24 hours may be required.

5. For the control of muscle spasm associated with chronic neurological disorders: Dosages are adjusted on an individual basis to try to obtain the best relief from spasm without inducing excess sedation.

6. When given intravenously for sedation prior to dental, surgical or investigative procedures doses of between 5 and 15 mg are given. It must be emphasized that the intravenous administration of diazepam in such circumstances is not entirely safe and facilities for resuscitation must always be available as respiratory arrest may occur.

7. By the rectal route: 5 mg or 10 mg as suppository or rectal solution.

Nurse monitoring

1. For general notes see the section on benzodiazepines.

2. During intravenous injection (where 5 mg/minute is a reasonable infusion rate) the patient becomes drowsy and develops slurred speech. This is generally an indication that the optimum dose has been administered. Patients who have received intravenous diazepam should remain under observation for at least an hour after the procedure has been completed as they may be quite markedly sedated.

3. As emphasized above, there is always the danger of respiratory arrest with intravenous administration of diazepam.

4. The injection solution is irritant and may cause redness around the injection site and thrombophlebitis for a period after administration. It should be noted that for this reason the intravenous use of 'Diazemuls' which contains diazepam in a fat emulsion is preferred. The fat emulsion provides a protective coating along the vein tract and hence reduces the irritant effect.

General notes

1. Preparations containing diazepam may be stored at room temperature.

2. The injection solution should never be mixed with other drugs in the same syringe.

3. If at all possible injection solution should be administered undiluted. However, when intravenous infusion is necessary, it may be added to normal saline or 5% dextrose. When such infusions are prepared they should be used within 6 hours and if some solution remains it should be discarded and replaced with a fresh solution.

DIAZOXIDE (Eudemine)

Presentation
Tablets—50 mg
Injection—300 mg in 20 ml

Actions and uses
1. Diazoxide is a potent vasodilator drug, its effect being mainly on the arterioles. When given intravenously it produces a rapid fall in blood pressure and it has been widely used in the treatment of hypertensive crises. It has tended to be replaced by other drugs which allow more effective control of blood pressure.
2. As an oral hyperglycaemic agent, diazoxide should be titrated to the desired hyperglycaemic effect. Total daily dosages range from 400–1000 mg.

Dosage
The drug is only effective intravenously and as it is rapidly inactivated it must be given rapidly, i.e. in less than 30 seconds. Patients should be lying flat during administration. The duration of action is usually 4-6 hours. It may be given as required up to four times in 24 hours.

Nurse monitoring
1. As mentioned above the drug effect is so rapid and profound that patients should be supine during administration. Even so hypotension not rapidly reversible is not uncommon.
2. Pain may commonly be felt at the injection site.
3. Repeated dosage may produce the following effects:
   a. Hyperglycaemia: Thus the urine should be tested for glucose. Treatment with oral hypoglycaemic drugs may be necessary.
   b. Salt and water retention: Thus a careful check for symptoms of heart failure must be made.
   c. Hyperuricaemia: Actual joint pain is rarely noted.
4. There have been reports that when the drug is used in hypertensive crises in labouring patients, delivery may be delayed unless oxytocin is concurrently administered.
5. Long-term dosage is usually not recommended because of the following effects: Hyperglycaemia, salt and water retention, hypertrichosis, skin rash, leucopenia, thrombocytopenia, extrapyramidial effects, hyperuricaemia.

General notes
1. Diazoxide injection may be stored at room temperature. It must be given undiluted and never mixed with other drugs.
2. Tablets may be stored at room temperature.

DICHLORALPHENAZONE (Welldorm)

Presentation
Tablets—414 mg chloral hydrate equivalent

Elixir—143 mg chloral hydrate equivalent in 5 ml

Actions and uses
Dichloralphenazone is an hypnotic drug which is taken to induce sleep. It is converted in the body to the active substance chloral hydrate.

Dosage
1. Adults: 2-4 tablets taken on retiring.
2. Children: 30—50 mg/kg as chloral hydrate, up to 1 g in total.

Nurse monitoring
1. Patients receiving this drug commonly suffer what is known as a hangover effect. Symptoms are of tiredness and drowsiness the day after administration of the drug and headache is a common feature. There is no way of dealing with this problem other than to change to a shorter acting hypnotic.
2. Dichloralphenazone can affect patients' requirements for anticoagulants such as warfarin and patients should be closely

observed and have their clotting times frequently checked. During commencement of the drug warfarin dosage may require to be increased to maintain its effect and when the drug is stopped the dose may require to be decreased to avoid the possibility of bleeding.

3. Other side-effects which occur with this drug include skin rashes, nausea and vomiting.
4. In patients with the rare disease of acute intermittent porphyria this drug may precipitate acute symptoms and is therefore contraindicated

General notes
1. Preparations containing dichloralphenazone may be stored at room temperature.
2. The elixir should be stored in well sealed bottles and away from direct sunlight.
3. If necessary it may be diluted with syrup for ease of administration.

DICHLORPHENAMIDE (Daranide)

Presentation
Tablets—50 mg

Actions and uses
Dichlorphenamide is a carbonic anhydrase inhibitor with a similar mechanism of action to acetazolamide (q.v.). It is used for the treatment of glaucoma.

Dosage
Adults: Initially up to 200 mg 12-hourly with maintenance dosage in the range of 25–50 mg one to three times a day.

Nurse monitoring
The nurse monitoring aspects of acetazolamide (q.v.) apply to this drug.

General note
The drug may be stored at room temperature.

DICLOFENAC (Voltarol)

Presentation
Tablets—25 mg, 50 mg
Tablets, slow release—75 mg, 100 mg
Suppositories—100 mg
Injection—75 mg in 3 ml

Actions and uses
See the section on non-steroidal anti-inflammatory analgesic drugs.

Dosage
The adult oral dose range is 25–100 mg three times a day or 75 mg (once or twice) or 100 mg once daily as slow release tablets. 100 mg may be administered at night by the rectal route and 75 mg by intramuscular injection once or twice daily.

Nurse monitoring
See the section on non-steroidal anti-inflammatory analgesic drugs.

General note
Diclofenac preparations may be stored at room temperature.

DICYCLOMINE (Merbentyl)

Presentation
Tablets—10 mg
Syrup—10 mg in 5 ml

Actions and uses
Dicyclomine is an anticholinergic drug. It has a specific antispasmodic action on the smooth muscle of the gastrointestinal tract. It is therefore used for the following conditions: irritable colon, spastic constipation, infant colic, spasm associated with colitis, diverticulitis, Crohn's disease, gastritis, peptic ulcer and cholecystitis.

Dosage
1. Adults: 10–20 mg three times daily taken before or after meals.
2. Children:
   a. Infants (less than 2 years): 5–10 mg 15 minutes before feeding. The total daily dose in this age group should not exceed 40 mg.
   b. Older children may receive dosages as necessary up to the equivalent of the adult dose.

D

Nurse monitoring
Dicyclomine has identical side-effects to those described under hyoscine-N-butylbromide (Buscopan). In addition dizziness, nausea, vomiting, anorexia, headache, constipation, fatigue, sedation and skin rash may occur.

General note
Dicyclomine preparations may be stored at room temperature. Syrup should however be protected from light by storing in amber glass bottles. For ease of administration, if required, the syrup may be diluted immediately before use with an equal quantity of water.

DIETHYLCARBAMAZINE (Banocide)

Presentation
Tablets—50 mg
Actions and uses
This antihelminthic drug is used in the treatment of filarial infection due to *W. bancrofti, B. malayi, Onchocerciasis volvulus and loa loa*. It may also be used for the prophylaxis of bancrofti in malarian filariasis and loaiases.
Dosage
1. Treatment of disease for adults and children: An initial dose of 1 mg/kg body weight, gradually increased over 3 days to 6 mg/kg body weight daily in three divided doses is recommended. Duration of treatment should be 3 weeks.
2. For prophylaxis of bancrofti, malarian filariasis: 50 mg monthly.
3. For prophylaxis of loaiases: 4 mg/kg for 3 successive days each month.

Nurse monitoring
1. Allergic reactions caused by destruction of the organisms are common and take the form of generalized itching and conjunctival congestion. These may be reduced by increasing the dosage slowly as recommended above and by the concurrent administration of antihistamines or corticosteroids.
2. Anorexia, nausea, vomiting, dizziness and mild drowsiness may occur with this drug.

General note
The drug may be stored at room temperature.

DIETHYLPROPION (Tenuate, Apisate)

Presentation
Tablets—75 mg (slow release)
Actions and uses
Anorexogenic drugs abolish hunger by a direct action on the central nervous system. They are thought to have a supplementary effect in that they increase the ability to perform mental and physical work without the need for increased food intake.

Dosage
Adults only: One 75 mg slow release tablet taken mid-morning.

Nurse monitoring
1. As this drug is related to the amphetamine group, there is a definite risk of physical and psychological dependence and addiction developing. Diethylpropion is therefore classified as a controlled drug and it is recommended that patients are treated for short (6-8 week) courses only and that the drug is immediately discontinued if they fail to lose weight.
2. Again, because of its relationship to the amphetamine group of drugs, this drug should not be given to patients who suffer from cardiovascular disease such as angina or hypertension.
3. The drug should never be given to patients who are undergoing treatment or have recently been given treatment with monoamine oxidase inhibitors (q.v.).
4. Side-effects may be divided into three groups:

a. Neurological: insomnia, nervousness, depression and anxiety.
b. Gastrointestinal: nausea, vomiting and constipation.
c. Cardiovascular: tachycardia, hypertension and headache.
5. Rare side-effects include dry mouth and allergic skin rashes
6. If an excess dose is taken psychosis may be produced. This rapidly resolves after discontinuation of the drug.

General note

The drug may be stored at room temperature. It is subject to storage restrictions which apply to 'controlled drugs'.

DIFLUCORTOLONE (Nerisone)

Presentation

Cream—0.1 %
Ointment and oily cream—0.1%, 0.3%

Actions and uses

This potent corticosteroid (q.v.) is used topically in the treatment of inflammatory skin conditions such as psoriasis, eczema and dermatitis.

Dosage

Cream, oily cream and ointment are applied one to three times daily to affected areas.

Nurse monitoring

Although applied topically, significant amounts of this drug may be absorbed through the skin producing some or all of the side-effects described in the section on corticosteroids.

General notes

1. The ointment, cream and oily cream should be stored under cool, dry conditions.
2. These products have a shelf life of 5 years from the date of manufacture.

DIFLUNISAL (Dolobid)

Presentation

Tablets—250 mg, 500 mg

Actions and uses

1. See the section on aspirin.
2. Diflunisal is a long-acting aspirin-like drug which is less irritant to the stomach and therefore may produce fewer gastrointestinal problems than aspirin.

Dosage

1. Adults. The average adult dose is 250–500 mg twice daily. Occasionally higher doses are required.
2. Children: It is not recommended that children receive this form of aspirin.

Nurse monitoring

1. See the section on aspirin for general nurse monitoring points on this drug.
2. It is important to note that there is an increased incidence of severe skin rashes with diflunisal as compared to other salicylate drugs.

General note

Diflunisal tablets may be stored at room temperature.

DIGOXIN (Lanoxin)

Presentation

Tablets—0.0625 mg, 0.125 mg, 0.25 mg
Injection—0.5 mg in 2 ml
Elixir—0.05 mg in 1 ml

Actions and uses

1. 'Inotropic' effect: Digoxin increases the force of contraction of heart muscle, thus improving its pumping action. This makes it useful in the treatment of heart failure.
2. 'Chronotropic' effect: The rate at which impulses pass down the atrioventricular (A-V) nodal conducting pathway of the heart is slowed, allowing in turn more efficient pumping of blood through

the heart. Thus the drug is useful in the treatment of atrial tachyarrhythmias, such as atrial fibrillation.

Dosage

1. 'Loading' dose: After administration the drug is slowly distributed throughout a number of body tissues and the therapeutic plasma concentration is only slowly achieved. Therefore, if rapid control is necessary this can be overcome using a high initial or 'loading' dose. The amount given, and the route of administration depend on a number of factors.

   a. Amount given: This depends mainly on the age, weight and renal function of the patient, and also to a certain extent on how rapidly the drug's effect is required. Thus a patient under 60 with normal renal function who has heart failure because of a supraventricular tachycardia might be given 0.5 mg intravenously followed by 0.25 mg three times a day until an adequate clinical effect is obtained. On the other hand, an older patient with atrial fibrillation in mild heart failure might only be given 0.25 mg once or twice a day orally until a clinical response is obtained. In the majority of cases, a loading dose is unlikely to be required in which case a single daily maintenance dose can be used from the outset.

   b. Route of administration: This depends on the required rapidity of onset. As mentioned above, in cases of heart failure due to supraventricular tachycardia, intravenous administration may be preferred, whereas oral treatment would be the choice with less urgent cases. Intramuscular digoxin may be given in emergency situations where absence of adequate monitoring facilities makes intravenous administration impossible, but the absorption of this drug from the muscle is erratic and unpredictable and this route should be avoided as far as possible.

2. Maintenance dose: This varies according to the age, weight and renal function of the patient. Two ways of approaching the problem of calculating the required dosage are as follows:

   a. The use of a 'nomogram', where dosage is calculated according to age, weight and renal function.

   b. By monitoring the clinical effects (i.e. pulse rate) and the appearance of side-effects, and tailoring the dose to suit individual patient needs.

Plasma levels of digoxin can be measured. These are particularly useful for testing patient compliance, and for detecting excessive dosage but the levels obtained do not reflect accurately the clinical effect of the drug. Suggested dosages (given as a guideline only):

1. Intravenous administration in adults: 0.5 mg diluted in 50 ml of saline and given over 30 minutes

2. Oral loading dose: 0.25 mg three times a day for three doses.

3. Maintenance dosage: 0.25 mg once a day in the age groups 12-70 years old and 0.0625 mg once a day over the age of 70.

4. Children's dosage: Less than 1 year—loading dose 0.02 mg/kg three times a day (oral), maintenance 0.01 mg/kg daily; 1-5 years—loading 0.2 mg three times a day (oral), maintenance 0.01 mg/kg daily; 6-12 years—loading 0.375 mg three times a day (oral), maintenance 0.25 mg per day.

Nurse monitoring

1. The nurse's role in patients on digoxin therapy is a particularly important one for two reasons:

   a. Non-cardiac side-effects (see below) are most likely to be observed by the nurse and therefore warning may be given and the dose changed before life-threatening complications arise.

b. The nurse has an active role to play in the day-to-day manipulation of drug dosage, as it is generally accepted that digoxin should be withheld at least until medical staff are consulted, if the pulse rate is less than 55 per minute.
2. Non-cardiac side-effects include anorexia, nausea, vomiting, diarrhoea, yellow vision, gynaecomastia.
3. Cardiac side-effects include bradycardia, paroxysmal atrial tachycardia and ventricular arrhythmias of any kind.

General notes
1. The drug should be stored in a dry place at room temperature.
2. The drug should be protected from light.

DIHYDROCODEINE (DF 118)

Presentation
Tablets—30 mg
Elixir—l0 mg in 5 ml
Injection—50 mg in 1 ml

Actions and uses
Dihydrocodeine is a narcotic analgesic drug. Its general actions and uses are described in the section on narcotic analgesics. The oral form is used for the treatment of mild painful conditions which would not usually be considered appropriate for treatment with other more powerful drugs of the narcotic analgesic group.

Dosage
Adults:
1. Orally: 30 mg every 4 to 6 hours.
2. By intramuscular or deep subcutaneous injection: 50 mg 4 to 6-hourly as required.

Nurse monitoring
See the section on narcotic analgesic drugs.

General notes
1. It is important to note that although oral preparations are not subject to legal requirements of 'controlled drugs' dihydrocodeine injection is a controlled drug and should be stored in a locked (controlled drug) cupboard.
2. The drug should be stored at room temperature.

DIHYDROTACHYSTEROL (Tachyrol, AT 10)

Presentation
Tablets—200 microgram (Tachyrol)
Oral solution—250 microgram/ml (AT 10)

Actions and uses
The actions and uses of dihydrotachysterol are identical to those described for vitamin D (q.v.), of which this drug is a very potent metabolite.

Dosage
For the treatment of resistant rickets and hypoparathyroidism: 750–1250 microgram per day initially depending on the age of the patient and the severity of the disorder. The dosage should subsequently be adjusted according to individual needs.

Nurse monitoring
See the section on vitamin D.

General note
The drug may be stored at room temperature.

DILTIAZEM (Adizem, Britiazem, Tildiem)

Presentation
Tablets—60 mg
Capsules (delayed release)—90 mg, 120 mg, 180 mg
Tablets (slow release)—90 mg, 120 mg
Capsules (very slow release)—300 mg

Actions and uses

Diltiazem blocks the movement of calcium into cardiac muscle and vascular smooth muscle cells, an action which explains its description as a 'calcium channel blocker' or calcium antagonist and which results in reduced muscle activity or tone. Thus cardiac muscle cells become less excitable, with consequent reduction in heart work and atrioventricular nodal (A-V) conduction. At higher doses, peripheral vasodilatation occurs with reduction in vascular resistance and a fall, therefore, in blood pressure.

As a result of the above, diltiazem is used in the treatment of angina pectoris and hypertension.

Dosage

The total adult daily dose varies from 180 mg to 480 mg which, depending upon the nature of the preparation prescribed, may be taken once, twice or three times in the day.

Nurse monitoring

1. The introduction over the years of a bewildering series of diltiazem preparations has created major confusion among patients and doctors alike. This is exemplified by the description of 'standard', 'slow' and even 'slower' release products, above. In fact, it should not be assumed that all preparations which are labelled 'slow' or 'sustained release' are equivalent. To avoid confusion, therefore, it is strongly recommended that diltiazem be prescribed as a recognised branded product so that patients will receive consistency in terms of bioavailability and activity. Nurses may find themselves in the position whereby they must rationalize therapy and reassure patients accordingly.
2. Diltiazem depresses cardiac function and care should be exercised when it is prescribed with other cardiac depressant drugs (e.g. beta-blockers). Note that digoxin also depresses A-V nodal conduction. Patients with mild bradycardia or a prolonged P-R interval on ECG should be carefully monitored.
3. The heart rate should be carefully monitored in elderly patients and those with kidney and/or liver impairment.
4. Diltiazem should not be used in patients with A-V block, sick sinus syndrome or severe bradycardia.
5. The peripheral vasodilator effect of diltiazem may manifest as flushing.

General notes

1. Diltiazem tablets and capsules may be stored at room temperature.
2. Note that slow release tablets, if scored, can be halved only. Otherwise slow or modified release products must not be crushed or dissolved for ease of administration. If in doubt, seek advice from the Pharmacy.

DIMENHYDRINATE (Dramamine)

Presentation

Tablets—50 mg

Actions and uses

Dimenhydrinate is an antihistamine. The actions and uses of antihistamines in general are discussed in the section on antihistamines. Dimenhydrinate is used in clinical practice:

1. For the treatment of nausea and vomiting, particularly motion sickness.
2. For the treatment of vertigo and the symptoms of vertigo and nausea due to Menière's disease.

Dosage

1. Adults: Orally: 50–100 mg 4-hourly.
2. Children: Orally: 1-6 years—12.5–25 mg two or three times daily; 7-12 years—25–50 mg two to three times daily.

Nurse monitoring

See the section on antihistamines.

General note

The drug may be stored at room temperature.

DIPHENOXYLATE (Lomotil)

Presentation

Tablets—2.5 mg
Liquid—2.5 mg in 5 ml
Diphenoxylate is combined with a small quantity of atropine and occasionally also with neomycin.

Actions and uses

This drug is chemically related to morphine-like compounds, all of which tend to produce constipation by a direct action on the motility of the gut. It is frequently combined with atropine because atropine also affects gut movement and the two drugs have an additive effect. It is occasionally also combined with neomycin because neomycin was in the past used to treat episodes of diarrhoea thought to be due to bacterial infection.

Dosage

1. Adults. Initially 10 mg followed by 5 mg every 6 hours until control of symptoms is achieved.
2. Children: 1-3 years—2.5 mg daily; 4-8 years—2.5 mg three times daily; 9-12 years—2.5 mg four times daily; 12-16 years—5 mg three times daily. All until control of symptoms is achieved.

Nurse monitoring

1. Perhaps the most important point for the nurse to note about this drug is that although it is used for a frequently trivial and self-limiting disorder, it has potentially serious side-effects and may be fatal in overdosage. It should only, therefore, be used in the short-term and patients must be continually encouraged to use it only as directed.
2. Diphenoxylate may produce nausea, vomiting, sedation, dizziness, skin rash, restlessness and depression.
3. The inclusion of atropine in the preparation may give rise to

side-effects including dry mouth, tachycardia and urinary retention, the latter being particularly frequent in children.

4. If this drug is taken in overdose, particularly in young children, it has a marked depressive function on the respiratory system and the central nervous system which may lead to fatality. Overdoses, therefore, should be referred immediately to hospital.
5. The drug should not be given to children under the age of 1 year.
6. The drug should not be given to patients who also are in receipt of sedative drugs such as barbiturates and tranquillizers
7. Patients should be advised that the combination of this drug and alcohol may cause excessive sedation.
8. The drug should not be given to patients receiving monoamine oxidase inhibiting drugs (q.v.)
9. The drug should not be given to patients with jaundice.

General note

Preparations containing diphenoxylate may be stored at room temperature.

DIPHENYLPYRALINE (Histryl)

Presentation

Capsules, slow release-2.5 mg, 5 mg

Actions and uses

Diphenylpyraline is an antihistamine. The actions and uses of antihistamines in general are described in the section on antihistamines. Diphenylpyraline is used in clinical practice:

1. To suppress generalised minor allergic responses to allergens such as foodstuffs and drugs.
2. To suppress local allergic reactions, i.e. inflammatory skin responses to insect stings and bites, contact allergens, urticaria etc.

3. As a nasal decongestant, e.g. in the treatment of allergic rhinitis and hay fever.
Dosage
1. Adults: 5-10 mg of the slow release preparation twice daily.
2. Children:
Over 7 years-2.5 mg of the slow release preparation twice daily.

Nurse monitoring
See the section on antihistamines.

General note
The drug may be stored at room temperature.

DIPIPANONE (Diconal)

N.B. Diconal tablets contain dipipanone 10 mg in combination with cyclizine 30 mg.
Actions and uses
Dipipanone is a narcotic analgesic drug and its actions and uses are described in the section on narcotic analgesics. It is produced in combination with cyclizine for the latter drug's anti-emetic effect.
Dosage
Adults: 1-3 tablets 6-hourly as required.

Nurse monitoring
See the section on narcotic analgesic drugs

General notes
1. This drug is subject to the legal requirements of 'controlled drugs' and should be kept in a locked (controlled drug) cupboard.
2. The drug should be stored at room temperature.

DIPYRIDAMOLE (Persantin)

Presentation
Tablets—25 mg, 100 mg
Injection—10 mg in 2 ml

Actions and uses
1. The drug reduces the blood pressure by dilating peripheral blood vessels and thus reduces the work done by the heart.
2. It dilates coronary vessels increasing blood flow and oxygen supply to the heart. The combination of these two actions makes the drug potentially useful for the treatment of angina. It is not effective in relieving the pain of an acute attack but is more useful when administered on a regular basis for the prevention of attacks of angina, usually when control of symptoms has been found to be difficult or impossible with established anti-anginal drugs (i.e. beta-blockers, nitrates, nifedipine, perhexiline).
3. It also affects blood clotting by reducing platelet aggregation.
Dosage
1. For the prophylaxis of angina:
Oral: 50 mg three times a day.
Intravenous: 10–20 mg three times a day.
2. To decrease platelet aggregation:
Oral: 100 mg three to four times a day increasing to 800 mg if necessary.

Nurse monitoring
1. After an intravenous dose a bitter taste in the mouth, facial flushing and hypotension may occur.
2. With oral therapy, hypotension manifest by dizziness and fainting may occur. Other side-effects such as skin rash, gastric upset, and diarrhoea are rare.

General note
Dipyridamole tablets and injection solution can be stored at room temperature.

DISOPYRAMIDE (Rythmodan)

Presentation
Capsules—100 mg, 150 mg
Tablets—250 mg, slow release
Injection—50 mg in 5 ml

Actions and uses

Disopyramide has a number of effects on the heart muscle and the conducting tissues of the heart, which make it useful in the treatment of the supraventricular and ventricular tachyarrhythmias. These effects are:

1. Prolongation of the refractory period of cardiac muscle
2. Decrease in excitability of cardiac muscle
3. Decrease in conduction velocity.

Dosage

1. Intravenous:
   a. Initial dose: 2 mg/kg body weight given over 5 minutes (to a maximum of 150 mg irrespective of body weight).
   b. Maintenance infusion: 0.4 mg/kg/hour (to a maximum of 800 mg in 24 hours).
2. Oral dose range for adults is 300–800 mg/day divided into four equal doses.
3. Alternatively, an oral dose of 250–375 mg twice daily may be given using slow release tablets.

Nurse monitoring

1. Disopyramide has anti-cholinergic side-effects such as dry mouth, blurred vision, and urinary retention, the latter being especially important in elderly men, particularly those with prostatism.
2. Nausea, diarrhoea and dizziness may also occur.
3. Occasionally heart failure may be precipitated.
4. Serious rhythm disturbances may occur in patients with hypokalaemia or heart block.
5. Too rapid intravenous injection may cause profuse sweating.

General note

Disopyramide capsules, tablets and injections may be stored at room temperature. When given by intravenous infusion the injection solution may be added to sodium chloride, dextrose, compound sodium chloride or Ringer's injection solution.

DOBUTAMINE (Dobutrex)

Presentation

Injection—250 mg vials

Actions and uses

Dobutamine indirectly stimulates heart muscle and leads to an increase in its force of contraction, thus improving cardiac output. It is used intravenously by infusion to try to increase cardiac output in patients who are suffering from cardiogenic shock, the commonest cause of this being a massive heart attack, with subsequent severe impairment of the heart's ability to pump blood and therefore maintain blood pressure.

Dosage

For adults: 2.5–10 microgram/kg/minute. Doses up to 40 microgram/kg/minute have been used if lower dosages fail to produce a reasonable effect.

Nurse monitoring

See the section on dopamine.

General notes

1. Dobutamine injection as dry powder in vials may be stored at room temperature.
2. The injection solution is reconstituted by adding water for injection or 5% dextrose injection to the vial.
3. Reconstituted solution may be stored in a refrigerator for up to 48 hours or at room temperature for 6 hours.
4. This solution is further diluted by addition to solutions of sodium chloride, dextrose, dextrose/saline, laevulose or compound sodium lactate injection.
5. Infusion solutions must be used within 24 hours of preparation; they may develop a slight pink discolouration which does not necessarily indicate an alteration in potency.

DOCUSATE SODIUM (Dioctyl Medo)

Presentation

Tablets—100 mg
Syrup—12.5 mg in 5 ml, 50 mg in 5 ml

Actions and uses

The actions of laxatives are discussed in the section on laxatives. Docusate sodium falls into the third group, i.e. it is a wetting agent which softens hard, impacted stools. It is used in the treatment of constipation.

Dosage

1. Adults: Up to 600 mg per day in three divided doses.
2. Children:
   a. Infants: up to 30 mg per day in three divided doses.
   b. Older children: up to 60 mg per day in three divided doses.
3. The syrup may be given by the rectal route as an enema:
   a. Adults: 15–40 ml
   b. Children: 7.5–15 ml
   c. Infants: 5–10 ml
      Above doses as syrup 12.5 mg in 5 ml.

Nurse monitoring

There are no specific problems with this drug.

General notes

1. Preparations containing docusate sodium may be stored at room temperature.
2. For an optimum effect, doses should be taken with plenty of fluid.

DOMPERIDONE (Motilium)

Presentation

Tablets—10 mg
Suspension—5 mg in 5 ml
Suppositories—30 mg

Actions and uses

Domperidone has similar actions and uses to those of metoclopramide, though it does not produce the adverse effects on the CNS which are associated with metoclopramide. Its major use is as an anti-emetic.

Dosage

1. Adults: 10–20 mg every 4-8 hours by the oral route, or 60 mg rectally every 4-8 hours.
2. Children: 0.2–0.4 mg/kg body weight every 4-8 hours, or 4 mg/kg body weight daily by the rectal route given as 3-4 doses.

Nurse monitoring

1. While it is generally considered that this drug produces few, if any, side-effects, patients should be carefully assessed for the occurrence of adverse effects similar to those described for metoclopramide.
2. Children are usually very sensitive to metoclopramide-produced CNS effects and treatment in children should be restricted to the control of nausea and vomiting associated with anti-cancer therapy.

General note

Preparations containing domperidone are stored at room temperature.

DOPAMINE (Intropin)

Presentation

Injection—200 mg in 5 ml

Actions and uses

Dopamine is inactive orally but when given intravenously it directly stimulates the heart's action increasing its force of contraction. It also increases the blood flow through the kidneys, by dilating renal blood vessels. Urine output may be increased. This effect may be reversed at higher dosage. It is used in the treatment of cardiogenic shock (see the section on dobutamine, its actions and uses).

Dosages

Adult intravenous dosage is initially 2–5 microgram/kg/minute increasing by 1–4 microgram/kg/minute every 15-30 minutes until an adequate effect is achieved. Doses of up to 50 microgram/kg/minute have been used but 9 microgram/kg/minute is the average maintenance dose needed.

Nurse monitoring

This drug is rarely used outside intensive or coronary care units. The major problem with administration is an increase in the heart rate which may progress to fatal cardiac tachyarrhythmia. Cardiac monitoring is therefore obligatory. Both dopamine and dobutamine are less likely to produce this effect than isoprenaline which is an alternative treatment for cardiogenic shock. High dosages of dopamine may produce peripheral vasoconstriction, hypertension, cardiac conduction defects, and reduced renal blood flow.

General note

Dopamine injection solution may be stored at room temperature. An infusion solution is prepared by adding the injection to solutions of sodium chloride, dextrose, laevulose, dextrose/saline and compound sodium lactate injection.

DORNASE ALFA (Pulmozyme, rhDNase)

Presentation

Nebulizer solution—2,500 unit (2.5 mg) per ampoule.

Actions and uses

Impaired lung function is a major problem in patients with cystic fibrosis and demands frequent and vigorous physiotherapy. Viscous purulent secretions which are retained within their airways contain high concentrations of an extracellular DNA, released during the breakdown of white blood cells which have migrated to the area. Dornase alfa is a form of a naturally occurring enzyme (DNase or deoxyribonuclease) which biochemically degrades extracellular DNA so reducing the viscoelasticity of

sputum and increasing its clearance. When used in conjunction with physiotherapy, which is greatly facilitated by the drug, significant symptomatic benefit and an improved quality of life can be achieved.

Dosage

Contents of one ampoule, 2,500 unit, administered by jet nebulizer once daily or twice daily for adult patients.

Nurse monitoring

1. The use of this drug must be continuous since benefits rapidly subside when treatment is interrupted. The cost of therapy is very substantial and good compliance is important to reduce unnecessary waste.
2. Dornase alfa does not obviate the need for other treatments in cystic fibrosis including regular physiotherapy (which is nevertheless improved by it).
3. The drug is delivered via a compressed air jet (not ultrasonic) nebulizer system. Suitable devices include the Hudson T Up-draft II/Pulmoaide, Airlife Misty Pulmo-Aide, and Acor II Pulmo-aide.
4. Apart from local irritation manifest as pharyngitis, laryngitis and hoarseness, the drug is otherwise well tolerated.

General notes

1. Store in a refrigerator and protect from light.
2. Brief (less than 24 hour) exposure to room temperature does not adversely affect the solution.
3. Do not mix with other drugs in the same nebulizer.

DOTHIEPIN (Prothiaden)

Presentation

Capsules—25 mg
Tablets—75 mg

Actions and uses

Dothiepin is a tricyclic antidepressant drug. Its actions and uses are described in the section dealing with these drugs.

Dosage

For the treatment of depression 75–150 mg may be given daily orally in three divided doses or alternatively the total daily dose may be taken in the evening on retiring.

Nurse monitoring

1. For general notes on nurse monitoring see the section on tricyclic antidepressant drugs.
2. It is worth noting that dothiepin produces a lesser incidence of the troublesome anticholinergic side-effects described in the section on tricyclic antidepressant drugs, and may therefore be particularly suitable for use in elderly patients.

General note

Dothiepin capsules and tablets may be stored at room temperature.

DOXAPRAM (Dopram)

Presentation

Injection—100 mg in 5 ml
Intravenous infusion—1 g in 500 ml dextrose 5%

Actions and uses

This drug has a direct stimulant action on centres in the brain associated with respiration. It is, therefore, used to stimulate respiration in:

1. Acute respiratory failure associated with overdosage of drugs which depress breathing such as barbiturates and opiates.
2. Depressed respiration produced by anaesthesia in the postoperative recovery period.

Dosage

Doxapram is administered by intravenous injection or infusion:

1. For the treatment of acute respiratory failure due to overdosage of drugs:
   0.5–4 mg/minute by infusion.
2. To aid recovery from anaesthesia: hourly injections of 1–1.5 mg/kg are given.

Nurse monitoring

1. The drug is contraindicated for use in patients who suffer from severe hypertension, coronary artery disease, thyrotoxicosis, status asthmaticus and cerebrovascular accident. It should be used with great care in patients who are either epileptic or are on monoamine oxidase inhibiting drugs.
2. Side-effects include raised blood pressure and a fast pulse rate.
3. In postoperative conditions restlessness, muscle twitching, sweating, confusion, nausea and vomiting may be produced.

General notes

1. Solutions for intravenous injection and infusion are stored at room temperature, and should never be refrigerated.
2. Doxapram is unstable when added to infusion fluids containing alkaline substances such as aminophyline, frusemide and barbiturates.

DOXEPIN (Sinequan)

Presentation

Capsules—10 mg, 25 mg, 50 mg, 75 mg

Actions and uses

Doxepin is a tricyclic antidepressant drug. Its actions and uses are described in the section on these drugs.

Dosage

10–100 mg three times daily.

Nurse monitoring

1. For general notes see the section on tricyclic antidepressant drugs.
2. Doxepin induces fewer of the troublesome anticholinergic side-effects described in the section on tricyclic antidepressant drugs and may therefore be particularly useful for treating elderly patients.

General note
Doxepin capsules may be stored at room temperature.

DOXORUBICIN (Adriamycin)

Presentation
Injection—10 mg vials, 50 mg vials

Actions and uses
Doxorubicin is an anthracycline antibiotic which is used in clinical practice for its cytotoxic effect. It inhibits the division of cells, particularly those of rapidly multiplying malignant tumours. It is often used in combination with other cytotoxic drugs to treat a wide range of neoplastic diseases including acute leukaemias, lymphomas, soft tissue and bone malignancies in childhood and solid tumours (in particular breast and lung carcinoma).

Dosage
The drug is given by intravenous injection over 2-3 minutes to the drip tubing of a running infusion. The dosage is usually calculated on a body surface area basis. When used alone 60–75mg/m² is the recommended dose to be given at intervals of 3 weeks. When used in combination with other cytotoxic drugs, 30–40 mg/m² at intervals of 3 weeks is recommended.
Occasionally a dose regime of 1.2–2.4 mg/kg body weight is used.

Nurse monitoring
1. The drug is extremely caustic and must be given into a fast running infusion to prevent severe local effects. It is therefore important to ensure that an infusion is working correctly prior to administration of the drug.
2. An important side-effect peculiar to this type of antibiotic is its cardiotoxicity. Initially tachycardia and electrocardiogram changes are seen but this can progress to gross cardiomyopathy resulting in cardiac failure and death.
3. Bone marrow suppression produces anaemia, leucopenia and thrombocytopenia with a resultant increased risk of severe infection and haemorrhage.
4. Gastrointestinal side-effects such as oral ulceration, nausea, vomiting and diarrhoea may occur.
5. The drug must be used at a reduced dose level in patients with impaired renal function.
6. The drug usually produces a red discolouration of the urine. It is important that the patient be warned of this side-effect in advance and be reassured that the red discolouration is of no significance.
7. The nurse should be constantly aware that most cytotoxic drugs are irritant to the skin and mucous surfaces, and are in general very toxic. Great care should therefore be exercised when handling these drugs, and in particular spillage or contamination of personnel or the environment must be avoided. If cytotoxic drugs are handled regularly it is theoretically possible that repeated skin contact or inhalation may produce systemic toxic effects and in nurses who have developed hypersensitivity, severe local and general reactions.

General notes
1. Doxorubicin dry powder in vials may be stored at room temperature.
2. The solution is prepared by adding 5 ml of water for injection or sodium chloride 0.9% injection to the 10 mg vial. 25 ml of these solvents may be added to the 50 mg vial.
3. Solutions thus prepared are injected into the drip tubing of a running sodium chloride 0.9%, dextrose 5% or dextrose saline infusion.

DOXYCYCLINE (Vibramycin)

(See Note 3, p. 362)

Presentation

Capsules—50 mg, 100 mg
Syrup—50 mg in 5 ml

Actions and uses

See the section on
tetracyclines.

Dosage

1. Adults: 100–200 mg once or
   twice daily.
2. Children: Tetracyclines
   should be avoided in children.
   If essential however,
   4 mg/kg initially, then 2 mg/kg
   body weight in total
   per day given as one or two
   doses.

Nurse monitoring

The general nurse
monitoring notes for tetracyclines
(q.v.) apply to doxycycline
with two important
exceptions:

1. Doxycycline is less likely
   to cause deterioration of renal
   function in patients with
   renal impairment.
2. Food and milk are less
   likely to affect its absorption
   and therefore the timing
   of administration in
   relation to meals is less
   important with this
   drug.

General notes

1. The drug should be stored at
   room temperature.
2. Once prepared the syrup
   should be used within
   14 days.

DYDROGESTERONE (Duphaston)

Presentation

Tablets—10 mg

Actions and uses

1. The actions and uses of
   progestational hormones in
   general are described in the
   section dealing with these
   drugs.

2. In clinical practice duphaston is
   recommended for the treatment
   of:
   a. Endometriosis
   b. Threatened abortion
   c. Habitual abortion
   d. Irregular menstrual cycles
   e. Functional uterine bleeding
   f. Infertility
   g. Premenstrual tension

Dosage

1. For the treatment of
   endometriosis: 10 mg two to
   three times per day from day
   5-25 of the cycle.
2. For the treatment of threatened
   abortion: 40 mg initially and
   then 10 mg 8-hourly until
   symptoms remit. Persistence
   of symptoms or return of
   symptoms during treatment
   are indications to double the
   dose. The effective dose must
   be maintained for a week after
   the symptoms have ceased and
   should be gradually decreased
   thereafter.
3. For the treatment of habitual
   abortion, infertility or irregular
   cycles: 10 mg twice daily from
   day 11-25 of the cycle.
4. For the treatment of
   dysmenorrhoea: 10 mg twice
   daily from day 5-25 of the
   cycle.
5. For the treatment of functional
   bleeding:
   a. To arrest bleeding: 10 mg
      twice daily together with an
      oestrogen for 5-7 days.
   b. To prevent bleeding:
      10 mg twice daily together
      with an oestrogen from
      day 11-25 of the cycle.
6. For the treatment of
   amenorrhoea: 10 mg twice
   daily in combination with an
   oestrogen from day 11-25 of the
   cycle.
7. For the treatment of
   premenstrual tension: 10 mg
   twice daily from day 12-26 of the
   cycle.

Nurse monitoring
1. The nurse monitoring aspects of progestational hormones in general are described in the hormones (2) section.
2. No contraindications are known to the administration of this drug.
3. Side-effects are rare and the only one of note is that breakthrough bleeding may occur in a few patients.

General note
The drug may be stored at room temperature.

E

ECONAZOLE (Ecostatin, Pevaryl)

Presentation

Cream and lotion—1 %
Pessaries—150 mg

Actions and uses

Econazole is effective in the
treatment of fungal infection due to
Candida albicans and its main use in
clinical practice is for the treatment
of vaginal and vulval candidiasis
(thrush).

Dosage

1. Pessaries: one pessary should be
   inserted at bedtime for three
   consecutive nights.
2. Cream: The cream should be
   applied twice daily, in the
   morning and the evening, to the
   ano-genital area.

Nurse monitoring

1. It is important that patients
   should be advised that should
   menstruation commence the
   course of treatment may be
   continued.
2. The nurse may play an important role in emphasizing to the
   patient that despite disappearance of symptoms full courses of
   treatment should be taken.
3. Occasional local irritation may be
   produced giving symptoms of
   burning, stinging or itching.

General note

The drug may be stored at room
temperature.

EDROPHONIUM CHLORIDE (Tensilon)

Presentation

Ampoules containing 10 mg
edrophonium chloride in 1 ml

Actions and uses

Edrophonium has the same
mechanism of action as
neostigmine (q.v.). It has a very
short duration of action and its
major clinical use arises when
clinicians are faced with a patient
who has myasthenia gravis and
who is already on an anticholinergic
drug, but who has developed an
increase in weakness. This may
be due to under- or overdosage with
the anticholinergic drug and
administration of edrophonium will
produce a rapid, short-lived
improvement in muscle power if
inadequate dosage is the cause of
weakness, but it will not have this
effect if the patient has already
received too much anticholinergic
drug. It may also be used to confirm
the diagnosis of myasthenia gravis
as its administration to a patient with
myasthenia gravis produces a rapid
and short-lived improvement in
muscle power.

Dosage

1. In adults with myasthenia gravis
   to differentiate the cause of an
   increase in weakness: 10 mg is
   given intravenously 2 hours after
   the last dose of their treatment. If
   therapy has been inadequate
   there is a rapid, transient increase
   in muscle strength. If the patient
   has been over-treated there is a
   transient increase in muscle
   weakness.

2. As a diagnostic test for myasthenia gravis: 2 mg is given intravenously initially. If no reaction occurs within 30 seconds a further 8 mg is administered.

Nurse monitoring
This drug has a very short duration of action and therefore only high dosage or prolonged administration may lead to problems. It has the potential to produce the same problems described under the nurse monitoring section of neostigmine (q.v.).

General note
The ampoule solution should be protected from light.

ENALAPRIL (Innovace)

Presentation
Tablets—2.5 mg, 5 mg, 10 mg, 20 mg
Actions and uses
See section on ACE inhibitors.
Dosage
Range: 10–40 mg as a single daily dose.

Nurse monitoring
See section on ACE inhibitors

General note
Enalapril tablets may be stored at room temperature.

ENOXACIN (Comprecin)

Presentation
Tablets—200 mg
Actions and uses
Enoxacin is an aminoquinolone antibiotic chemically related to nalidixic acid, ciprofloxacin and ofloxacin. Its spectrum of activity is similar to these other drugs and as a result enoxacin is used in the treatment of infections of the genitourinary tract, skin and soft tissue, and shigellosis.

Dosage
Adults: Dosage varies according to the condition which is treated. Simple urinary tract infections are very sensitive and respond to a dose of 200 mg twice daily for 3 days. A single 400-mg dose is usually adequate in the treatment of uncomplicated gonorrhoea. Skin and soft tissue infections, on the other hand, require higher prolonged dosage, e.g. 400 mg twice daily for 1-2 weeks. For treatment of shigellosis, the dose is 400 mg twice daily for 5 days. Lower doses may be used in the elderly in whom higher blood levels are often produced.

Nurse monitoring
1. In common with other broad spectrum antibiotics, disturbances of gastrointestinal function are possible.
2. A few patients may develop allergy to enoxacin. This usually presents as skin rashes but in more severe cases breathlessness, tachycardia, angioedema, and even anaphylaxis may occur.
3. Central nervous system side-effects include restlessness, agitation, hallucinations and confusion. Seizures have been reported in a few cases and treatment in epileptics should be avoided.
4. Since enoxacin has been shown to impair development of joint tissue in immature animals it should be avoided in infants and young children if possible.

General note
Enoxacin tablets are stored at room temperature.

EPIRUBICIN (Pharmorubicin)

Presentation
Injection—10 mg, 20 mg, 50 mg
Actions and uses
Epirubicin is an anthracycline antibiotic which is used in clinical practice for its cytotoxic effect. It has

the actions and uses described for the related agent doxorubicin but there is some evidence to suggest that it is better tolerated than is doxorubicin and has better overall safety.

Dosage

As a single agent, usually in the range 75–90 mg/m² body surface area given once and repeated in cycles of 21 days. In combination with other cytotoxic agents a dose of 50 mg/m² is commonly used.

Nurse monitoring

The nurse monitoring aspects of doxorubicin apply also for this drug.

General note

Epirubicin vials may be stored at room temperature and exposure to direct sunlight should be avoided; reconstituted solutions retain their chemical stability for up to 48 hours if stored in a refrigerator.

EPOETIN (Eprex, Recormon)

Presentation

Injection—1000, 2000, 4000, 5000 and 10,000 international unit vials

Actions and uses

Epoetin is recombinant alpha or beta human erythropoietin i.e. forms of a natural hormone which is produced by genetic biotechnology. Erythropoietin is a protein normally present in low concentrations in plasma which is largely produced as a result of the action of a renal enzyme (erythrogenin) on a plasma protein or preformed and released directly by the kidney. It acts on the bone marrow to stimulate production of erythrocytes and so maintains circulating haemglobin levels which adequately oxygenate the tissues of the body.

Anaemia as a result of erythropoietin deficiency occurs in chronic renal failure and is associated with significant morbidity, despite the fact that a small proportion (10-15%) of the protein is normally produced by the liver. Replacement therapy is therefore indicated for patients with anaemia of chronic renal failure sufficiently severe to require renal dialysis, and other patients with severe symptoms of anaemia though not yet receiving dialysis. Alpha and beta forms are equally active and indeed are interchangeable.

Dosage

1. Erythropoietin is usually administered by subcutaneous injection but may also be given by the intravenous route over 2 minutes.
2. Dialysis patients: Initially 20–50 units/kg body weight 3 times weekly increased according to response in increments of 20–25 units/kg at intervals of 4 weeks up to a maximum of 600 units/kg weekly. Once Hb 10–12 g/dl (10–12 g/100 ml) is reached maintenance doses as low as 20–50 units twice weekly can be used.
3. Severe symptomatic anaemia in patients not yet requiring dialysis: As above by subcutaneous injection.

Nurse monitoring

1. An influenza-like syndrome is reported in some patients as a result of hypersensitivity, especially when intravenous injections are administered too quickly.
2. A dose-dependent rise in blood pressure can occur and may be hazardous for patients with existing hypertension, if poorly controlled. Hypertensive encephalopathy and tonic-clonic convulsions have been reported. Blood pressure must be carefully monitored in all patients.
3. There may also be a dose-related rise in blood platelets during the early treatment stage and shunt thrombosis in patients who are prone to complications with arteriovenous shunts may arise.
4. Other side-effects include hyperkalaemia, raised creatinine, urea and phosphate; skin reactions and palpebral oedema. Myocardial infarction and anaphylaxis are rare but severe

untoward events attributed to
erythropoietin.
5. Note that no more than 1 ml
should be administered at any
one subcutaneous site.

General notes
1. Both alpha and beta epoetin
preparations must be stored in a
refrigerator and protected from
light.
2. Alpha epoetin is ready mixed and
unpreserved. No more than one
dose should therefore be
administered from each vial.
3. Beta epoetin is diluted and used
immediately. Do not mix with any
other drug.

ERGOMETRINE MALEATE

Presentation
Tablets—250 microgram and 500
microgram
Injection—500 microgram in 1 ml
Actions and uses
This drug produces powerful
rhythmic contractions of the uterus
by direct action on the uterine
muscle. In clinical practice it is
administered in the management of
third stage labour to assist in the
delivery of the placenta and the
cessation of bleeding, thereby
reducing the risk of post partum
haemorrhage.
Dosage
1. Orally: 500 microgram to 1 mg up
to a maximum of 3 mg.
2. By subcutaneous, intramuscular
or intravenous injection: up to
1.5 mg.

Nurse monitoring
1. Nausea and vomiting may
occasionally be produced.
2. This drug should be used with
caution in patients who are
suffering from toxaemia of
pregnancy.

General notes
1. The tablets may be stored at room
temperature.

2. Injection solution should be
protected from light and preferably
stored in a refrigerator.

ERGOTAMINE (Migril, Cafergot)

N.B. These preparations contain
ergotamine in combination with
caffeine.
Presentation
Tablets—1 mg and 2 mg
Inhaler—0.36 mg in each metered
dose
Suppositories—2 mg
Actions and uses
Migraine classically causes severe,
throbbing, unilateral headache. It is
caused by alteration in the cerebral
blood vessels and ergotamine in
clinical practice is found to be
effective in the treatment of this
condition as it reverses the changes
in cerebral vasculature.
Dosage
1. Orally: 1 or 2 mg repeated every
30 minutes until relief is obtained
to a maximum of 6 mg in 1 day
and 12 mg in any 1 week.
2. Rectally: 2 mg at the onset of an
attack, repeated half-hourly to a
total of 6 mg per day or 12 mg per
week.
3. Inhalation: One dose repeated
after 5 minutes if required to a
total of six doses per day or 15
doses per week.

Nurse monitoring
1. If it is to be effective in the acute
attack it should be administered
as soon as possible after the
onset of either the premonitory
symptoms if they occur, or the
headache.
2. This drug causes generalized
vasoconstriction which may
produce, in minor cases,
coldness of the skin and limbs
and in extreme cases gangrene.
3. Other side-effects include
nausea, vomiting, diarrhoea,
dizziness, ocular disturbance,
muscular weakness, confusion,
anxiety, drowsiness and
convulsion.

4. The drug should be used with great care in patients who suffer from heart diseases as it may produce angina, alter the blood pressure and alter the rhythm of the heart.
5. The nurse may play an important role in reminding patients that they must never exceed the maximum advised doses.

General note

The drug may be stored at room temperature.

ERYTHROMYCIN (Erythrocin, Erymax, Ilotycin, Ilosone)

(See Note 3, p. 362)

Presentation

Tablets—250 mg, 500 mg
Capsules—250 mg
Syrup—100 mg in 5 ml, 125 mg in 5 ml, 250 mg in 5 ml, 500 mg in 5 ml
Injection—100 mg in 5 ml (intramuscular)
—300 mg and 1 g vials (intravenous)

Actions and uses

Erythromycin is an antibiotic with a bacteriostatic action. This means that it inhibits growth and multiplication of bacterial cells in the body but does not kill them. It is effective principally against staphylococci and streptococci. Unfortunately resistance to erythromycin can develop if treatment persists longer than 1 week. It is a useful alternative to penicillin for the treatment of staphylococcal and streptococcal infections, when the infections have been proven to be resistant to penicillin or when the patient is allergic to penicillin. It is also used in the treatment of rarer infections due to myco-plasma, rickettsia, chlamydia and in the treatment of Legionnaire's disease.

Dosage

1. Adults:
   a. Orally: 250–500 mg four times a day.
   b. Intramuscularly: 100 mg 4-8 hourly.
   c. Intravenously: 300 mg 6-hourly or 600 mg 8-hourly. These intravenous doses may be doubled in the case of severe infection.
2. Children: Less than 1 year—12 mg/kg orally four times day; 1-7 years—125-250 mg orally four times a day; over 7 years—adult doses may be given.

Intramuscular injections should be avoided in children as they usually have insufficient muscle mass to tolerate the injection. Intravenous doses in children are identical to the above oral doses.

Nurse monitoring

1. Mild and occasionally severe gastrointestinal upsets with nausea and vomiting, and diarrhoea may occur. This may be reduced by ensuring that the tablets are taken with meals.
2. The estolate form of erythromycin (Ilosone) has been associated with liver injury which usually manifests as fever, pain and obstructive jaundice. This occurs only very rarely but it is recommended that the dosage of erythromycin estolate be reduced in patients with previously diagnosed liver disease.
3. Erythromycin for intravenous administration and infusion must be in a final concentration of not more than 1 %, i.e. 10 mg per ml. It is usually diluted in 0.9% sodium chloride or 5% dextrose.
4. In recent years it has become apparent that erythromycin is a potent inhibitor of the liver's capacity to produce drug-metabolizing enzymes (i.e. the hepatic microsomal enzyme system). This has resulted in the marked potentiation of certain common drugs which are normally extensively metabolized by the liver during absorption and passage into the systemic circulation: these include theophylline, warfarin, and phenytoin. Extreme caution is therefore warranted when

E

erythromycin is prescribed for
any patient regularly taking drugs
of this type since sudden and
severe toxicity might develop.

General notes
1. The drug may be stored at room
temperature.
2. Intravenous erythromycin is
prepared by adding water for
injection to the vial before addition
to infusion fluid.
3. As noted above the maximum
concentration of an intravenous
injection should be 10 mg per ml.

ESMOLOL (Breviblock)

Presentation
Injection—100 mg in 10 ml, 2.5 g in
10 ml
Actions and uses
Esmolol is a beta-blocker and the
section under beta-adrenoreceptor
blocking drugs should be consulted
for a general account of these compounds. However esmolol is notably
different from other beta-blockers, so
far, in that it has an ultra-short action
and is administered only by continuous infusion. Esmolol is used peri-
operatively for short-term prevention
and treatment of supraventricular
arrhythmias (atrial fibrillation, atrial
flutter and sinus tachycardia) and
hypertension in at risk patients.
Because of its very rapid and total
inactivation in the circulation, it is
administered by continuous
intravenous infusion when control is
readily titrated against drip rate.
Dosage
Esmolol is administered under
specialist supervision when the
infusion rate is determined by the
individual's response. The usual
dose rate is in the range 50–200
microgram/kg/minute.

Nurse monitoring
See under the section on beta-
adrenoreceptor blocking drugs.
The dosing rate of esmolol is
carefully adjusted throughout by
patient response so that excessive
beta-blockade should not occur.

General notes
1. Esmolol injection is stored at room
temperature and protected from
light.
2. Ampoules containing 100 mg in
10 ml are for use undiluted. The
2.5 g vial must be first diluted (5 g
to 500 ml) to provide a final
concentration of 10 mg in 1 ml.
Sodium chloride and glucose
injections or mixtures of these are
used for dilution. Hartmann's
lactated Ringer's solution can
also be used but not sodium
bicarbonate injection.

ESTRAMUSTINE (Estracyt)

Presentation
Capsules—140 mg
Actions and uses
This drug is a combination of an
oestrogenic substance (oestradiol)
and a cytotoxic agent (mustine). It
readily concentrates in prostatic
tissue and is used for the treatment
of cancer of the prostate, particularly
when unresponsive to conventional
oestrogenic treatment.
Dosage
The daily dose may vary from 140
mg to 1400 mg and it is usually
divided to be taken with meals. An
average dose is of the order of
560 mg.

Nurse monitoring
1. Relatively common side-effects
include nausea, vomiting and
diarrhoea.
2. Thrombocytopenia with resultant
increased risk of haemorrhage
may occur with this drug.
3. Other side-effects noted have
been altered liver function,
gynaecomastia and increased
risk of myocardial infarction.
4. This drug should be avoided in
patients with active peptic ulcer
disease and those with severe
liver or cardiac disease.
5. It should be used with great
caution in patients who already
have existing impairment of bone
marrow function.

6. The nurse should be constantly aware that most cytotoxic drugs are irritant to the skin and mucous surfaces, and are in general very toxic. Great care should therefore be exercised when handling these drugs, and in particular spillage or contamination of personnel or the environment must be avoided. If cytotoxic drugs are handled regularly it is theoretically possible that repeated skin contact or inhalation may produce systemic toxic effects and in nurses who have developed hypersensitivity, severe local and general hypersensitivity reactions.

General note
Capsules of estramustine should be stored in a refrigerator.

ETHACRYNIC ACID (Edecrin)

Presentation
Tablets—50 mg
Injection—50 mg as dry powder
Actions and uses
Ethacrynic acid is a 'loop' diuretic and has a similar mode of action and spectrum of use to frusemide (q.v.). Ethacrynic acid has a longer duration of action than frusemide of 6-8 hours.
Dosage
1. Adults:
   a. The oral adult dose range is 50–150 mg per day. Dosages of up to 400 mg may occasionally be required for the treatment of refractory oedema. Where the total daily dose exceeds 100 mg, divided dosage regimes should be used.
   b. The usual intravenous dose is 50 mg or 0.5–1 mg/kg up to a maximum of 100 mg.
2. Children: Oral therapy only should be used. Dosages are as follows: Up to 1 year— 2.5 mg/kg; 1-7 years—2.5 mg/kg; 7 years plus— 50 mg taken as a single dose.

Nurse monitoring
1. The nurse monitoring notes for thiazide diuretics (q.v.) are applicable to ethacrynic acid.
2. Ethacrynic acid is a very irritant drug and should never be given by the intramuscular or subcutaneous routes.
3. Ethacrynic acid is commonly associated with hearing dysfunction including persisting deafness. For this reason it is very rarely used as a first line 'loop' diuretic and if it is used, large single doses should never be given as they produce an increased incidence of this effect.

General notes
1. Ethacrynic acid tablets and powder for injection may be stored at room temperature.
2. To make up solutions for injection 50 ml sodium chloride 0.9% or dextrose 5% injections are added to the vial containing powder (occasionally dextrose solutions may produce a cloudy appearance and such solutions must be discarded.)
3. The injection is given slowly (over several minutes) either directly or via the drip tube of a running infusion.
4. Unused solution must be discarded after 24 hours.

ETHAMBUTOL (Myambutol)

Presentation
Tablets—100 mg, 400 mg
N.B. Ethambutol is often used in combination with isoniazid in the preparation 'Mynah'.
Actions and uses
Ethambutol is an antibacterial drug which is of use only for the treatment of tuberculosis caused by the organism *Mycobacterium tuberculosis*. Its action may be either bacteriostatic (inhibiting growth and replication of the organism) or bacteriocidal (killing the organism), depending on the concentration achieved in the tissues. If used on its

E

own for the treatment of tuberculosis it will be, in a large number of cases, ineffective as the organism gradually develops resistance to it and therefore it is usually used in combination with other antituberculous drugs (q.v.).

Dosage

1. For initial treatment and for prophylaxis against tuberculosis: A single daily oral dose of 25 mg/kg is recommended.
2. For maintenance treatment a single oral dose of 15 mg/kg body weight is recommended.

Nurse monitoring

1. Patients undergoing treatment for tuberculosis receive their drugs for considerable periods of time. The nurse may play an important role in reminding patients that their drug therapy must be taken regularly for as long as recommended by medical staff, whether or not they themselves feel that they have recovered.
2. Ethambutol is generally well tolerated by most patients. Rare side-effects include:
   a. An optic neuritis with visual disturbance including colour blindness to green and red
   b. Gastrointestinal upset
   c. Skin rash
   d. Jaundice
   e. Peripheral neuritis
   f. Raised serum urate level (which may give rise to joint pain due to gout).
3. It is recommended that the drug be used with great caution in patients with impaired renal function, gout or reduced visual acuity. In the latter group, regular testing of visual acuity should be performed if it is decided that it is necessary to commence such a patient on ethambutol.

General note

The drug may be stored at room temperature.

ETHINYLOESTRADIOL

Presentation

Tablets—1, 10, 50, 100 microgram and 1 mg

Actions and uses

This drug is an oestrogenic substance. In clinical practice it is used for the treatment of:
1. Menopausal symptoms.
2. The suppression of lactation.
3. The treatment of malignant disease of prostate and breast.
4. The treatment of primary amenorrhoea.
5. It is used in conjunction with a progestational agent as an oral contraceptive.

Dosage

1. For the treatment of menopausal symptoms: 10–50 microgram thrice daily is given initially and subsequent maintenance doses range from 10–20 microgram per day.
2. For the suppression of lactation: 100 microgram is given twice daily for 3 days, reducing to 50 microgram twice daily for 6 days.
3. For the treatment of malignant disease of prostate and breast: Between 1 and 3 mg is given daily.
4. For the treatment of primary amenorrhoea: 10–50 microgram is given thrice daily for 14 consecutive days every 4 weeks.

Nurse monitoring

See the section on oestrogenic hormones in hormones (1).

General note

The drug may be stored at room temperature.

ETHOSUXIMIDE (Zarontin, Emeside)

Presentation

Capsules—250 mg
Syrup—250 mg in 5ml

Actions and uses

1. The actions and uses of anticonvulsant drugs in general are discussed in the section on these drugs.
2. Ethosuximide is particularly useful for the treatment of petit mal epilepsy.

Dosage

N.B. Individual dosage requirements vary greatly. The following doses are given as a guide only.

1. Adults: The usual maintenance dose range is 1–1.5 g daily.
2. Children: An initial dose of 250 mg is recommended in children less than 6 years and 500 mg in children older than 6 years. The dose should thereafter be gradually increased until an optimum response is achieved.

Nurse monitoring

1. See nurse monitoring aspects in the section on anticonvulsant drugs in general.
2. Gastrointestinal upset including nausea, vomiting and anorexia commonly occur with this drug.
3. Neurological effects are fairly common and include drowsiness, lethargy, euphoria, dizziness, headache and behavioural disorders such as restlessness, agitation, anxiety and aggression.
4. Skin rashes and disorders of the blood may rarely occur.

General note

The drug may be stored at room temperature.

ETIDRONATE (Didronel)

Presentation

Tablets—200 mg, 400 mg (combined with calcium in Didronel PMO)
Injection—300 mg in 6 ml

Actions and uses

Etidronate is classed as a bisphosphonate or diphosphonate, a group of drugs which alter the metabolic activity of bone. Bone is metabolically very active being constantly destroyed and re-built in a process known as remodelling which maintains fresh bone throughout life. In some circumstances however the breakdown of bone (which is influenced by the activity of a cell called the osteoclast) is relatively greater than new bone synthesis (which is influenced by a cell called the osteoblast). Etidronate inhibits osteoclast activity and so redresses this balance.

Etidronate by its action inhibits the release of calcium from bone and is used therefore when this occurs excessively. Indications include the treatment of hypercalcaemia of malignancy, Paget's disease and to arrest osteoporosis after the menopause. The latter is the indication for Didronel PMO: it should be noted that in women, oestrogen produced by the ovary is important in stimulating bone synthesis. This is gradually lost once the menopause arrives as ovarian failure develops.

Dosage

1. Adults:
   a. Paget's disease—usually 5 mg/kg for up to 6 months.
   b. Malignant hypercalcaemia 7.5 mg/kg by slow intravenous infusion on 3 consecutive days. Course may be repeated after 1 week.
   c. Osteoporosis—400 mg is taken orally for 14 days then stopped. Calcium tablets are then taken daily throughout a cycle of 90 days (3 months approximately). The cycle may then be repeated.

Nurse monitoring

1. The absorption of etidronate and indeed other bisphosphonates is very poor and reduced even further by the presence of food in the gut. It should therefore be taken at a time when the least amount of food is present i.e. at the mid-point between meals.
2. Antacids also impair absorption and should not be taken at or around the same time.

3. Mild gastrointestinal disturbances are occasionally reported with oral therapy but are much more likely after intravenous administration. Intravenous therapy may also cause diarrhoea and the appearance of an unpleasant metallic taste. Etidronate should be used with caution in enterocolitis.
4. Etidronate should not be used in the presence of severe renal impairment and kidney function should be monitored during treatment.
5. A few patients with Paget's disease may complain of a transient increase or 'flare' in bone pain at Pagetoid sites.

General notes
1. Etidronate tablets may be stored at room temperature. Solution for injection too is stored at room temperature and must not be refrigerated.
2. Each dose of intravenous etidronate should be diluted in at least 250 ml sodium chloride 0.9% injection and administered over a period of no less than 2 hours.

ETODOLAC (Lodine)

Presentation
Tablets—200 mg
Capsules—200 mg

Actions and uses
See section on non-steroidal anti-inflammatory drugs.

Dosage
Adults: Usually 200 mg twice daily though occasionally 400–600 mg may be taken as a single daily dose.

Nurse monitoring
1. See the section on non-steroidal anti-inflammatory drugs.
2. Etodolac is a relatively new drug and early impressions are that it produces a low incidence of gastrointestinal upset.

Nevertheless it is important that patients treated with this drug should be carefully monitored for adverse effects.

General note
Etodolac tablets and capsules may be stored at room temperature.

F

FAMCICLOVIR (Famvir)

Presentation
Tablets—250 mg

Actions and uses
After absorption this drug is converted in the body to its active principle, penciclovir. Its actions and uses are identical to those of acyclovir but its absorption and hence bioavailability is far greater so that adequate blood levels are achieved with less frequent oral dosing. Currently, famciclovir is licensed only for the treatment of *Herpes zoster* (shingles) infection but it is likely that its uses will eventually include prophylaxis of herpes virus infections in the immune-compromised.

Dosage
Adults only: 250 mg 8-hourly, reduced to 12-hourly in patients with moderate renal impairment (creatinine clearance 30–60 ml/minute) or once daily in severe renal impairment.

Nurse monitoring
1. The nurse monitoring section under acyclovir applies to this drug also.
2. Famciclovir is generally well tolerated though a proportion of patients have complained of nausea and headache.

General note
Famciclovir tablets are stored at room temperature

FAMOTIDINE (Pepcid PM)

Presentation
Tablets—20 mg, 40 mg

Actions and uses
See histamine H_2-receptor antagonists.

Dosage
1. Treatment of peptic ulcer: 40 mg at bedtime for up to 8 weeks.
2. Prevention of relapse: usually a single bedtime dose of 20 mg which is taken continuously.

Nurse monitoring
The nurse monitoring aspects described for histamine H_2-receptor antagonists apply.

General note
Famotidine tablets may be stored at room temperature.

FENBUFEN (Lederfren)

Presentation
Capsules—300 mg
Tablets—300 mg

Actions and uses
See the section on non-steroidal anti-inflammatory analgesic drugs.

Dosage
The usual adult dose is 600 mg at night and 300 mg in the morning.

Nurse monitoring
See the section on non-steroidal anti-inflammatory analgesic drugs.

General note
Fenbufen capsules and tablets may be stored at room temperature.

FENFLURAMINE (Ponderax)

Presentation
Capsules—60 mg sustained release

Actions and uses

Anorexogenic drugs abolish hunger by a direct action on the central nervous system. They are thought to have a supplementary effect in that they increase the ability to perform mental and physical work without the need for increased food intake.

Dosage

Adults: 60–120 mg as a single daily dose, i.e. 1-2 slow release capsules.

Nurse monitoring

1. Perhaps the most important point to note about fenfluramine is that although it, like other anorexogenic drugs, is a member of the amphetamine group, it does not produce the neurological effects of drugs of this group and it, therefore, does not produce dependence or addiction and is unlikely to be abused in this way.

2. The drug is contraindicated for the treatment of patients who have recently received or are at present receiving treatment with monoamine oxidase inhibiting drugs (q.v.)

3. Patients should be warned that the mild sedative effect of this drug will be markedly increased if alcohol is taken.

4. The mild sedative effect on its own may occasionally impair driving skills and again patients should be warned of this potential effect.

5. The drug is not recommended for the treatment of patients who have a history of depressive illness.

6. Side-effects which include sedation, dizziness, diarrhoea, nausea and headache may be minimized by initiating treatment with low doses and subsequently increasing doses gradually.

General note

The drug may be stored at room temperature.

FENOPROFEN (Fenopron, Progesic)

Presentation

Tablets—200 mg, 300 mg, 600 mg

Actions and uses

See the section on non-steroidal anti-inflammatory analgesic drugs.

Dosage

The usual adult dose is 200–600 mg three or four times per day.

Nurse monitoring

See the section on non-steroidal anti-inflammatory analgesic drugs.

General note

Fenoprofen tables may be stored at room temperature.

FENOTEROL (Berotec)

Presentation

Inhaler—200 microgram/dose of metered aerosol
Nebulizer solution—0.5%

Actions and uses

This drug has a highly selective action on receptors in bronchial muscle causing relaxation of muscle tone. It is used, therefore, for the treatment of reversible airways obstruction (bronchospasm) in asthma and other conditions such as bronchitis and emphysema.

Dosage

By inhalation:
1. One or two inhalations (metered doses) three times a day using the pressurized inhaler.
2. 0.1–0.5 ml of nebulizer solution may be inhaled up to four times a day for the control of acute, severe, symptoms.

It should be noted that this drug has a long duration of action.

Nurse monitoring

1. Rarely this drug may cause palpitation, tachycardia, head-ache and fine muscle tremor.
2. The drug should be used with care in patients suffering from heart disease, hypertension or hyperthyroidism.

3. The drug should be used with great care if patients are receiving monoamine oxidase inhibitors or tricyclic antidepressants.

General notes

1. The pressurized aerosol should be stored at room temperature.
2. The container should never be punctured or incinerated at the end of use.

FERROUS FUMARATE

Presentation

Name	Also Contains
Ferrocap	Vitamin B
Ferrocap-F 350	Folic Acid
Fersaday	
Fersamal	
Folex 350	Folic Acid
Pregaday	Folic Acid

Actions and uses
See the section on irons (oral).

Dosage
300 mg of ferrous fumarate contains 100 mg of elemental iron.

1. For the treatment of iron deficiency anaemia:
   a. Adults: 300 mg of ferrous fumarate twice daily.
   b. Children: Less than 1 year—100–150 mg of ferrous fumarate per day; 1-7 years—200–300 mg per day; over 7 years—300–450 mg per day. Children over 12 years should receive the adult dose.
2. For the prevention of iron deficiency anaemia during pregnancy: 300 mg of ferrous fumarate once per day.

Nurse monitoring
See the section on irons (oral).

General note
Most iron tablets may be stored safely at room temperature.

FERROUS GLUCONATE

Presentation
Tablets—300 mg.

Actions and uses
See the section on irons (oral).

Dosage
900 mg of ferrous gluconate contains 100 mg of elemental iron.

1. For the treatment of iron deficiency anaemia:
   a. Adults: 900–1800 mg of ferrous gluconate per day.
   b. Children: Less than 1 year—225–450 mg of ferrous gluconate per day; 1-7 years—450–700 mg of ferrous gluconate per day; 7-12 years—750–900 mg of ferrous gluconate per day; over 12—Adult doses apply.
2. For the prevention of iron deficiency anaemia in pregnancy: 900 mg of ferrous gluconate per day.

Nurse monitoring
See the section on irons (oral)

General note
Most iron tablets may be stored safely at room temperature.

FERROUS SUCCINATE (Ferromyn)

Presentation
Elixir—106 mg in 5 ml

Actions and uses
See the section on irons (oral).

Dosage
106 mg of ferrous succinate contains 37 mg elemental iron.
For the treatment of iron deficiency anaemia:

1. Adults. 106 mg of ferrous succinate three times a day.
2. Children: Less than 2 years—21 mg (1 ml) of ferrous succinate twice daily; 2-5 years—53 mg (2.5 ml) of ferrous succinate three times daily; 5-10 years—106 mg of ferrous succinate twice daily; over 10—Adult doses apply.

Nurse monitoring
See the section on irons (oral).

General note
Most iron tablets may be stored
safely at room temperature.

FERROUS SULPHATE

Presentation
Proprietary preparations containing
ferrous sulphate are:

Name	Also Contains
Fefol	Folic Acid
Fefol Vit	Folic Acid+Vitamins B and C
Fefol Z	Folic Acid + Zinc
Feospan	
Ferrograd C	Vitamin C
Ferrograd Folic	Folic Acid
Ferro-Gradumet	
Fesovit Z	Vitamin B and C + Zinc
Folicin	Folic Acid + Minerals
Slow Fe	
Slow-Fe Folic	Folic Acid

Actions and uses
The actions and uses of ferrous
sulphate are identical to those
described for iron (q.v.).

Dosage
200 mg of ferrous sulphate dried
contains 60 mg of elemental iron;
300 mg of ferrous sulphate contains
60 mg of ferrous iron. The
appropriate daily dosage is therefore
as follows:
1. For the treatment of iron
   deficiency anaemia:
   a. Adults: Ferrous sulphate 300
      mg two or three times a day.
      Ferrous sulphate dried: 200 mg
      two to three times a day
   b. Children: Less than 1 year—
      100–150 mg of ferrous sulphate
      per day; 1-7 years—200–300
      mg per day; over 7 years—
      300–450 mg per day. Children
      over 12 years should receive
      the adult dose.
2. For the prevention of iron
   deficiency anaemia during
   pregnancy: 300 mg two or three
   times per day of ferrous sulphate
   is advised.

Nurse monitoring
See the section on irons (oral).

General note
Most iron tablets may be stored
safely at room temperature.

FINASTERIDE (Proscar)

Presentation
Tablets—5 mg
Actions and uses
Growth of the prostate gland and
hence prostatic hypertrophy is
dependent upon the conversion of
testosterone to its more active
metabolite dihydrotestosterone within
the gland itself by the action of an
enzyme, *5-alpha reductase.*
Finasteride is a potent inhibitor of
5-alpha reductase; it consequently
prevents the formation of the active
metabolite without interfering with
testosterone directly and as a result
reduces the gland size in benign
prostatic hypertrophy.
Dosage
A single daily dose of 5 mg is taken
for a prolonged period of up to 6
months before being re-assessed. If a
positive response is obtained continuous treatment thereafter is indicated.

Nurse monitoring
1. Patients who do not respond to
   the above dosage are unlikely to
   respond to increasingly higher
   doses and treatment should be
   abandoned if initially unsuccessful.
2. This drug may affect male sexual
   function. Impotence, decreased
   libido and reduced volume of
   ejaculate are reported in up to
   5% of patients.
3. Finasteride is otherwise well
   tolerated and does not appear to
   interact with other drugs.
4. The drug is of no benefit in the
   treatment of prostatic cancer
   which should be excluded at the
   outset and re-assessed during
   treatment.
5. Nurses should avoid handling
   broken or crushed tablets
   from which theoretically
   transcutaneous absorption can
   occur. This may present
   problems in pregnant subjects or
   those of child-bearing age.

General note

Tablets are stored at room temperature and protected from light.

FLAVOXATE (Urispas)

Presentation

Tablets—100 mg, 200 mg

Actions and uses

This drug has anticholinergic actions which in clinical practice make it useful for the treatment of disorders associated with spasm of the smooth muscle of the lower urinary tract. It is used in the treatment of dysuria, urgency, nocturia and painful spasm of the bladder due to catheterization or cystoscopy.

Dosage

100–200 mg three times a day in adults.

Nurse monitoring

1. Due to its anticholinergic action the drug produces dry mouth and blurred vision and should not be used in patients who suffer from glaucoma.
2. The drug is contraindicated in patients who have gastrointestinal obstruction.
3. Common side-effects experienced by the patient include nausea, headache and fatigue.

General note

The drug should be stored at room temperature.

FLUCLOROLONE (Topilar)

Presentation

Cream and ointment—0.025%

Actions and uses

This potent corticosteroid (q.v.) is used topically in the treatment of inflammatory skin conditions such as psoriasis, eczema and dermatitis.

Dosage

Cream and ointment are applied sparingly once or twice per day.

Nurse monitoring

Although used topically, sufficient may be absorbed through the skin for this drug to produce some or all of the side-effects described in the section on corticosteroids.

General notes

1. Fluclorolone ointment and cream may be stored at room temperature but excessively warm storage areas should be avoided.
2. Dilution with other creams may alter the stability of the drug and are therefore contraindicated; however, white soft paraffin may be used if necessary.

FLUCLOXACILLIN (Floxapen)

(See Note 3, p. 362)

Presentation

Capsules—250 mg, 500 mg
Syrup—125 mg in 5 ml
Injection—Vials containing 250 mg and 500 mg

Actions and uses

Flucloxacillin is a member of the penicillin group of antibiotics and has the same actions and uses as those described for benzylpenicillin (q.v.). It has a number of important advantages over benzylpenicillin and these are as follows:

1. It is very well absorbed from the gut and therefore is indicated when oral treatment is desired.
2. It is often highly effective against organisms especially of the staphylococcal group which are likely to be resistant to benzylpenicillin.

Dosage

1. Adults:
   a. Orally: 250–500 mg four times a day.
   b. Intramuscular or intravenous: 250–500 mg four times a day.
   c. Intrapleural and intra-articular: 250–500 mg per day.
2. Children: Less than 2 years—one-quarter of the adult dose. Over 2 years—one-half of the adult dose.

> **Nurse monitoring**
> See the section on benzylpenicillin

General notes
1. Preparations containing flucloxacillin may be stored at room temperature.
2. Once reconstituted injection solutions must be used immediately
3. Once reconstituted the syrup should be used within 7 days.
4. Injections are prepared as follows:
   a. For intramuscular injection: The vials should be diluted with 1.5–2 ml of water for injection.
   b. For intravenous injection: 1 g should be dissolved in 20 ml of water for injection and given either directly over 3-4 minutes or added to 0.9% sodium chloride, 5% dextrose or dextrose/saline mixtures and infused over 4-6 hours.
   c. For intra-articular or intrapleural injection: The vials should be diluted with 5–10 ml of water for injection.

FLUCYTOSINE (Alcobon)

Presentation
Tablets—500 mg
Intravenous infusion—2.5 g in 250 ml

Actions and uses
This drug is effective in the treatment of certain systemic fungal infections. It acts by inhibiting the production of a crucial component necessary for fungal growth and development. It is indicated for the treatment of systemic infections with *Cryptococcus neoformans, Candida albicans* and other candida species, *Torulopsis glabrata, hansenula, chromomycosis* and other rare fungal diseases.

Dosage
The total daily dose in adults and children is 200 mg/kg body weight divided into four doses. It should be administered via the giving set provided, which contains a special filter. It may be administered directly

into a vein, through a central venous catheter or by intraperitoneal infusion. The duration of each section of the infusion should be of the order of 20-40 minutes. It should be noted that recommendations are produced by the manufacturers giving recommendations of total daily dosage related to creatinine clearance (an indication of renal function). It should be noted that the total daily dose by either oral or intravenous route is identical.

> **Nurse monitoring**
> 1. The drug should never be given to patients with severe renal failure unless blood levels of the drug can be monitored.
> 2. Disease of the bone marrow is a relative contraindication to the use of this drug.
> 3. Nausea, vomiting, diarrhoea, skin rash, thrombocytopenia and bone marrow suppression may occur.
> 4. Tests of liver function may be altered by administration of this drug.

General notes
1. Infusions are supplied ready for use by direct request to the manufacturers.
2. Storage conditions for both tablets and infusion are critical. The tablets should be stored in a well-closed container, protected against moisture and light. The infusion should be stored between 15 and 20°C. Deviation outside this range in either direction will lead to degeneration and render the infusion useless.

FLUDROCORTISONE (Florinef)

Presentation
Tablets—0.1 mg, 1 mg

Actions and uses
Fludrocortisone is a corticosteroid drug which has primarily mineralo-corticoid actions. It is therefore not used for the indications described under corticosteroid drugs (q.v.). Its

only use in clinical practice is in the treatment of disorders associated with deficiency of adrenal gland function such as Addison's disease.

Dosage
For replacement of mineralocorticoid function in Addison's disease 0.1 mg daily or on alternative days is given. Adequacy of dosage is monitored by checking the urea and electrolytes and blood pressure of the patient under treatment.

Nurse monitoring
1. Fludrocortisone has mainly mineralocorticoid actions. A deficiency of replacement treatment will be manifest by weakness, nausea, vomiting, hypotension and in extreme cases shock and excessive dosage will be manifest by hypertension and hyperkalaemia. Both an excess and deficiency of fludrocortisone are highly dangerous situations and constitute a medical emergency requiring immediate further assessment in hospital.
2. It is worth noting that very few patients require more than 0.1 mg per day for replacement treatment in diseases such as Addison's disease. If these patients are accidentally given 1 mg per day they may become severely ill and die. The only indication for using 1 mg tablets is in very rare circumstances where suppression of adrenal gland over-activity is required.

General note
Fludrocortisone tablets may be stored at room temperature.

FLUMAZENIL (Anexate)

Presentation
Injection—500 micrograms in 5 ml
Actions and uses
Flumazenil is a specific antagonist of drugs of the benzodiazepine group (q.v.) i.e. it blocks the sedative effects of such drugs on the central nervous system. In practice,

Flumazenil is used to reverse anaesthesia or marked over-sedation produced by the benzodiazepine, permitting a rapid return of consciousness, spontaneous respiration and mobility. Its major roles are in anaesthesia, intensive care units, and following acute major benzodiazepine overdosage.

Dosage
Adults: Initially, a 200-microgram dose is administered by slow intravenous injection, with further doses at 1-2 minute intervals until recovery is achieved or a maximum total dose of 1–2 mg has been given. In practice, total doses exceeding 300–600 micrograms are rarely required.

Nurse monitoring
1. It is important to note that withdrawal symptoms may be precipitated in patients who have habitually taken drugs of the benzodiazepine group and who are, as a result, dependent on them. This may not always be known, and careful monitoring of the patient is essential. Note that flumazenil has been investigated under carefully controlled conditions as an aid to weaning benzodiazepine-addicted subjects off their drug. It is stressed that such use should not be attempted except under specialist supervision.
2. When used in an anaesthetized patient, prior reversal of any administered neuromuscular blocking drug is necessary since recovery may not otherwise be apparent.
3. The action of flumazenil is very short-lived (2-3 hours only) and sedation may rapidly and unexpectedly become re-established unless repeated dosages are given. Patients treated with flumazenil may therefore require prolonged monitoring, particularly if long-acting benzodiazepines have been taken. This may be

especially important if a benzodiazepine has been administered for short-term sedation in an out-patient department (e.g. prior to endoscopy) with a view to the patient returning home immediately afterwards.

4. Flumazenil may interfere with the action of other central nervous system depressants (although it is relatively specific for the benzodiazepines), including antidepressants, anticonvulsants, and neuroleptics.

5. Administration has been associated with nausea, vomiting, anxiety, agitation, raised blood pressure and heart rate, and seizures. Such effects may in fact be related to benzodiazepine withdrawal symptoms described in 1 above.

General note

Flumazenil injection may be stored at room temperature

FLUNITRAZEPAM (Rohypnol)

Presentation

Tablets—1 mg

Actions and uses

Flunitrazepam is a benzodiazepine and the section on these drugs should be consulted for a brief general account. It has a marked sedative effect and is taken as a hypnotic, to induce sleep. Of particular interest is the short action of this drug in the body which tends to produce a normal length sleep of up to 8 hours without the hang-over effect which occasionally extends into the following day with other hypnotics.

Dosage

Adults: 0.5 mg to 1 mg taken on retiring. Elderly patients should receive the lower dosage.

Nurse monitoring

See the section on benzodiazepines.

General note

Tablets containing flunitrazepam may be stored at room temperature.

FLUOCINOLONE (Synandone, Synalar)

Presentation

Ointment and cream—0.01, 0.025%, 0.2%
Gel—0.025%
Lotion—0.025%

Actions and uses

This potent corticosteroid (q.v.) is used topically for the treatment of inflammatory skin conditions such as psoriasis, eczema and dermatitis.

Dosage

Cream or ointment is applied sparingly to the affected area four times daily.

Nurse monitoring

Although applied topically, significant absorption through the skin may occur and produce some or all of the side-effects described in the section on corticosteroids.

General notes

1. Preparations containing fluocinolone should be stored in a cool, dry place.

2. The stability of the drug may be markedly altered by dilution with other ointments, creams or lotions.

FLUOCINONIDE (Metosyn)

Presentation

Cream and ointment—0.05%

Actions and uses

This potent corticosteroid (q.v.) is used topically for the treatment of inflammatory skin conditions such as psoriasis, eczema and dermatitis.

Dosage

Cream or ointment is applied sparingly to the affected area one to four times daily.

Nurse monitoring

Although fluocinonide is applied topically, sufficient absorption may occur through the skin to produce some or all of the effects described in the section on corticosteroids.

General notes

1. The cream may be stored at room temperature but warm areas, such as around a radiator should be avoided.
2. If absolutely necessary the ointment may be diluted with white soft paraffin but other creams and ointments should not be mixed with fluocinonide.

FLUOCORTOLONE (Ultradil)

Presentation

Ointment and cream—a mixture of the privalate and hexanoate esters containing 0.1% and 0.25% of each.

Actions and uses

This moderately potent corticosteroid (q.v.) is used topically for the treatment of inflammatory skin conditions such as psoriasis, eczema and dermatitis.

Dosage

Ointment or cream is applied sparingly to the affected area one to three times daily.

Nurse monitoring

Although applied topically, significant amounts of this drug may be absorbed through the skin to produce some or all of the side-effects described in the section on corticosteroids.

General notes

1. Fluocortolone ointment and cream should be stored in a cool, dry place.
2. These preparations may be used for up to 5 years from the date of manufacture.

FLUOROURACIL (5-Fluorouracil, 5-FU, Efudix)

Presentation

Injection—250 mg in 10 ml
Capsules—250 mg
Cream—5%

Actions and uses

Fluorouracil is a cytostatic drug which inhibits cell division by interfering with cellular DNA and to some extent, RNA, synthesis. Its action is that of an antimetabolite since it prevents incorporation of pyrimidine bases into the nucleic acid structure. Fluorouracil is used systemically in the palliative treatment of a variety of inoperable solid tumours including those of the breast, gastrointestinal tract, liver, pancreas, endometrium and bladder. The drug is also applied topically to treat premalignant and malignant superficial lesions and in the treatment of some warts.

Dosage

Fluorouracil is usually administered systemically as part of a wider chemotherapeutic regime.
Doses of the order 12–15 mg/kg body weight are administered by intravenous bolus injection or by continuous intravenous infusion. Oral therapy is used for long-term maintenance treatment usually in doses of 15 mg/kg given on a series of 5-7 consecutive days initially, then at intervals of 1 week as a single dose.
Topical cream is applied sparingly once or twice daily to the lesion.

Nurse monitoring

1. It is important to realize that this drug is cytotoxic and nurses applying topical therapy should wear protective gloves and wash hands thoroughly on completion.
2. Fluorouracil is a potent skin sensitizer and an allergic contact dermatitis may develop following skin contact. In any event this drug is cytotoxic and contact should be avoided or, if it occurs, the area should be washed rapidly and thoroughly.

3. Diarrhoea, nausea and vomiting commonly occur during treatment and leucopenia usually follows completion of a course of therapy.
4. Treatment must be discontinued if white cell counts fall below 3500/mm^3, platelets below 100 000/mm^3, or if stomatitis or oral ulceration develops. Severe diarrhoea and gastrointestinal bleeding may also limit its use.
5. Fluorouracil for intravenous infusion is prepared by dilution in glucose or sodium chloride solutions or mixtures thereof up to a final concentration not exceeding 1 g in 500 ml.

General notes
1. Fluorouracil preparations may be stored at room temperature but must be protected from light.
2. Solutions for infusion should be freshly prepared. Topical cream must not be diluted.

FLUPENTHIXOL (Depixol, Fluanxol)

Presentation
Tablets—0.5 mg and 1 mg (as dihydrochloride)
Injection—20 mg in 1 ml, 40 mg in 2 ml, 200 mg in 10 ml (all as decanoate)

Actions and uses
Flupenthixol is a neuroleptic and antidepressant drug used for its tranquillizing or calming effect in the management of patients with severe behavioural disorders including depression. It shares many of the actions and uses described for phenothiazine major tranquillizers in the section on phenothiazines.

Dosage
Adults:
1. 1–2 mg by the oral route once daily or up to 6 mg daily in two divided doses.
2. As a long-acting intramuscular depot injection it is administered every 2-4 weeks in doses of 20–40 mg or more.

Nurse monitoring
See the section on phenothiazines

General note
Flupenthixol tablets and injection should be stored at room temperature.

FLUPHENAZINE (Modecate, Moditen)

Presentation
Tablets—1 mg, 2.5 mg, 5 mg (as hydrochloride)
Elixir—0.5 mg in 1 ml (hydrochloride)
Injection—25 mg in 1 ml: 0.5 ml, 1 ml, 2 ml and 10 ml oil injection as the decanoate or enanthate

Actions and uses
Fluphenazine is a member of the phenothiazine group of drugs and its actions and uses are described in the section on these drugs. It may be taken orally or more frequently it is administered by deep intramuscular injection. The latter method of administration ensures a prolonged effect lasting several days to some weeks. The use of long-acting intramuscular preparations of fluphenazine allows many schizophrenic patients to be treated at home with their drug being administered at regular clinic visits.

Dosage
1. Adults:
   a. Orally: 1–4 mg daily as a single daily dose.
   b. By deep intramuscular injection: 25 mg is administered in a single dose at intervals varying between 10 days and 4 weeks according to clinical effect.
2. Children:
   a. Orally for behavioural disorders: 0.25–1 mg per day is given.

Nurse monitoring
1. The nurse monitoring points on fluphenazine are identical to those described for phenothiazines (q.v.).
2. The muscle twitching and tremors described in the section on phenothiazines which occur

as side-effects of phenothiazines are particularly likely to occur with this drug and usually require treatment with anti-Parkinsonian preparations.

General notes

1. Preparations containing fluphenazine may be stored at room temperature.
2. Oral liquid and solution for injection must be protected from direct sunlight.

FLURANDRENOLONE (Haelan)

Presentation
Cream and ointment—0.0125%

Actions and uses
A moderately potent corticosteroid (q.v.) which is applied topically for the treatment of inflammatory skin conditions, e.g. psoriasis, eczema, dermatitis etc.

Dosage
Apply sparingly two or three times daily to the affected area.

Nurse monitoring
Although applied topically, significant amounts of this drug may be absorbed to produce some or all of the side-effects described in the section on corticosteroids.

General notes

1. Flurandrenolone cream and ointment should be stored at room temperature.
2. If necessary these preparations may be diluted with aqueous cream B.P. (in the case of cream) or for ointment, white soft paraffin B.P.

FLURAZEPAM (Dalmane)

Presentation
Capsules—15 mg, 30 mg

Actions and uses
Flurazepam is a benzodiazepine drug (q.v.). Its marked sedative action makes it useful for use at night as an hypnotic.

Dosage
15–30 mg taken on retiring.

Nurse monitoring
See the section on benzodiazepines

General note
Preparations containing flurazepam may be stored at room temperature.

FLURBIPROFEN (Froben, Ocufen)

Presentation
Tablets—50 mg, 100 mg
Eye drops—0.03% in Polyvinyl alcohol film

Actions and uses

1. See the section on non-steroidal anti-inflammatory analgesic drugs.
2. Eye drops are administered to inhibit intraoperative miosis as a result of the anti-inflammatory action: the drug itself does not possess mydriatic properties.

Dosage
The usual adult oral dose is 150–200 mg daily in three or four divided doses.

Nurse monitoring
See the section on non-steroidal anti-inflammatory analgesic drugs.

General note
Flurbiprofen tablets may be stored at room temperature.

FLUTICASONE (Flixotide)

Presentation
Pressurized inhaler—25, 50, 125 and 250 microgram/metered dose
Dry powder for inhalation—50, 100, 250 and 500 microgram for use in a Diskhaler

Actions and uses
This drug is a new and potent corticosteroid for use by inhalation in the prophylaxis of asthma. Since chronic inflammation with hyperresponsiveness of the airways underlies asthma it follows that any

drug having potent anti-inflammatory activity can modify disease progression. Fluticasone is claimed to be more effective than beclomethasone dipropionate and may prove successful in patients who fail to respond adequately to that drug.

Dosage

1. Adults: Dosage varies between 100 and 1000 microgram twice daily depending upon that required to achieve control in the individual.
2. Children: Doses of between 50 and 100 microgram twice daily are generally required.

Nurse monitoring

1. Corticosteroids are important disease modifying drugs in asthma. They are intended to be used *regularly* as *preventatives* rather than on an as required basis to relieve bronchospasm. It is important that this is impressed upon patients who often fail to use steroids appropriately.
2. Patients should be instructed to keep their inhalers by their bedside and use them on awakening each morning and retiring at night.
3. High doses especially are preferably given via a large spacer device (Volumatic). This improves airways penetration and reduces local side-effects in the mouth and larynx (i.e. oral candidiasis and dysphonia).
4. Patients always require careful instruction in the use of their inhaler device in order to optimize therapy. Seek advice from the pharmacy, if necessary.
5. Patients should be advised to double their usual dose or use their inhaler four times daily in the event of worsening symptoms or development of a chest cold. Medical advice must be sought coincidentally.
6. Note that penetration of the airways by dry powder forms is generally poorer than with pressurized spray inhalers. Consequently, the dose using dry powder drug is generally double that of conventional inhalers.

General notes

1. Fluticasone preparations are stored at room temperature.
2. The powder form must be stored in a dry place.
3. Pressurized inhaler devices must not be incinerated after use.

FLUVOXAMINE (Faverin)

Presentation

Tablets—50 mg, 100 mg (both enteric-coated)

Actions and uses

Fluvoxamine is an antidepressant having some similarities to the tricyclic antidepressants. It appears to have a specific action on 5-hydroxytryptamine (serotonin) uptake by nerve fibres in the CNS and thus potentiates the action of this neurotransmitter at nerve endings. Such an effect is thought to be associated with mood elevation and increased activity and fluvoxamine is used in the treatment of depression characterized by persistent lowering of mood.

Dosage

Adults: 100 mg to 300 mg daily in a single or two divided doses.

Nurse monitoring

1. As a relatively new product there is a strong requirement to monitor response carefully and in particular to evaluate the safety of this drug.
2. Patients with disease of the liver and/or kidney should receive appropriately lower doses.
3. An elevation in plasma levels of propranolol and warfarin has been noted and caution is required when these drugs are co-prescribed.
4. Nausea is a common occurrence during the early treatment period and anorexia, constipation, agitation, and tremors have also been noted.
5. A decrease in heart rate may occur.

General note

Fluvoxamine tablets may be stored at room temperature.

FOLIC ACID

Presentation
Folic acid is available in a number of preparations either alone or in combination with iron and other vitamins.

Actions and uses
Folic acid is indicated for the treatment of megaloblastic anaemia (anaemia associated with large immature red cells in the blood). This type of anaemia may be produced by:
1. Nutritional deficiency
2. Pregnancy
3. Malabsorption.

Dosage
1. In the treatment of megaloblastic anaemia: Initially 10–20 mg a day for 14 days. Subsequently 5–10 mg per day.
2. For the prophylaxis of megalo-blastic anaemia in pregnancy: 200–500 microgram daily.

Nurse monitoring
1. No problems are encountered with the administration of this drug.
2. An important point to note which primarily concerns medical staff is that when a megaloblastic anaemia is identified, folic acid should never be instituted prior to the elucidation of its cause as administration of folic acid to patients with megaloblastic anaemia due to vitamin B_{12} deficiency (q.v.) may be highly dangerous and cause severe and irreversible neurological symptoms.

FORMESTANE (Lentaron)

Presentation
Injection—250 mg vial plus 2 ml diluent depot injection.

Actions and uses
Peripheral tissues are capable of metabolizing natural androgenic sex hormones to oestrogen by the action of an enzyme, *aromatase*. This provides a stimulus for continued growth of oestrogen-dependent tumours in advanced breast cancer in women after the menopause or in whom an early menopause has been induced. Formestane is a selective inhibitor of *aromatase* in peripheral tissues and so is effective in the treatment of post-menopausal women with advanced breast cancer.

Dosage
Adults: A single dose of 250 mg by deep intramuscular injection provides a depot effect for up to 2 weeks.

Nurse monitoring
1. Deep intramuscular injection into the gluteal region is advised using alternate buttocks for successive dosages. Avoid injecting close to the sciatic nerve which may otherwise be permanently damaged.
2. Local injection site reactions are common and include itching, pain and irritation, burning sensation, and appearance of lumps or granulomas. Haematomas are also reported and caution is advised if this drug is administered to an anticoagulated patient.
3. Skin rashes, pruritis and increased facial hair growth as well as alopecia may occur.
4. Other side-effects include lethargy, drowsiness, emotional upsets, headaches, dizziness, oedema of the lower leg, and thrombophlebitis.
5. Some patients complain of nausea, vomiting, constipation, hot flushes, vaginal bleeding, pelvic cramps, muscle cramps and arthralgia.
6. Note that this drug is intended for use in post-menopausal women only.

General notes
1. The unprepared injection is stored in a refrigerator.
2. Reconstitution with sodium chloride diluent provides a fine suspension from which the drug is gradually released into the

circulation. Gentle shaking facilitates dispersal of the drug. Prepare immediately before use or if necessary, store in a refrigerator for up to 24 hours.

FOSINOPRIL (Staril)

Presentation
Tablets—10 mg, 20 mg
Actions and uses
See section on ACE inhibitors.
Dosage
Range: 10–40 mg as a single daily dose.

Nurse monitoring
See section on ACE inhibitors

General note
Fosinopril tablets may be stored at room temperature.

FRUSEMIDE (Lasix)

Presentation
Tablets—20 mg, 40 mg, 500 mg
Injections——20 mg in 2 ml, 50 mg in 5 ml, 250 mg in 25 ml Paediatric liquid—1 mg in 1 ml
Actions and uses
All diuretics act on the kidney to increase excretion of water and electrolytes from the body. The functional unit of the kidney is called a nephron and is composed of a glomerulus and a tubule. The tubule has four sections, each of which has different functions. They are known as the proximal tubule, the loop of Henle, the distal tubule and the collecting tubule. Frusemide is the best known and most commonly used of the diuretics known as 'loop' diuretics. This particular group acts on the loop of Henle and inhibits electrolyte and therefore water reabsorption. Diuretics which act on the loop of Henle tend to have a rapid onset of action and a much more marked diuresis than diuretics acting at other parts of the tubule. The indications for use of frusemide therefore are in situations where a

rapid loss of body salt and water is necessary such as acute left heart failure with pulmonary oedema, or where milder diuretics have proved ineffective. It is worth noting that frusemide is not as effective in the management of hypertension as other thiazide-type diuretics (q.v.).
Dosage
1. Adults.
   a. Intravenous injection in emergency situations: The usual initial dose is between 40 and 250 mg depending on the severity of the problem and response to previous doses.
   b. Intramuscular: Frusemide may be given in emergency situations or where oral treatment is contraindicated, in equivalent doses to the intravenous dose.
   c. Oral dosage: Daily dosage is usually given once per day in the morning. Initial dosage is usually 40 mg, the dose being increased until an appropriate clinical response has been achieved. It is worth noting that doses of up to 2 g orally or 1 g intravenously may be given in patients with chronic renal failure.
2. Children's doses are as follows: 1 year or less—1–2 mg/kg; 1-5 years—10–20 mg; 6-12 years—20–40 mg. Intramuscular or intravenous doses should be half of the recommended oral dose.

Nurse monitoring
1. The nurse monitoring notes for thiazide diuretics (q.v.) are applicable to frusemide.
2. When high doses of frusemide are given transient deafness may occur.
3. Acute renal failure may be precipitated if frusemide and other 'loop' diuretics are used in combination with cephalosporin antibiotics.

General notes
1. Frusemide tablets, liquid and injection may be stored at room

temperature. The injection solution is sensitive to light and is therefore packed in amber coloured ampoules.
2. Other drugs must never be mixed with frusemide injection in the same syringe and the drug should not be added to dextrose solutions before infusion.
3. The recommended solutions for infusion are sodium chloride 0.9% injection or compound sodium lactate (Ringer's) injection: the rate of infusion must not exceed 4 mg/minute.

FUSIDIC ACID/SODIUM FUSIDATE (Fucidin)

(See Note 3, p. 362)
Presentation
Capsules—250 mg
Tablets—250 mg (enteric coated)
Suspension—250 mg in 5 ml
Injection—500 mg vials with 50 ml diluent
Ointment—2%
Gel—2%
Medicated gauze dressing—2%
Actions and uses
Fucidin is an antibiotic which has been found to be particularly effective against staphylococcal infections. It has the advantage that it may be given to patients who are sensitive to penicillin and in addition it is particularly good at penetrating most tissues including, importantly, bone. It has the disadvantage that when used alone bacteria rapidly become resistant to it and it is therefore often used in combination with other antibiotics such as erythromycin (q.v,) or novobiocin (q.v.). It is used in all types of staphylococcal infection including skin infection, wound infection, pneumonia, septicaemia, osteomyelitis and endocarditis.
Dosage
1. Oral:
   a. Adults: 500 mg–1 g three times a day.
   b. Children: Less than 1 year—50 mg/kg body weight in total daily in three divided doses; 1-5

years—250 mg three times per day; 5-12 years—500 mg three times per day.
2. Intravenous injection:
   a. Adults: 2 g in total per day in three or four divided doses.
   b. Children: 20 mg/kg per day in total usually given in three divided doses.
3. The ointment, gel or medicated gauze dressing should be applied to topical infections three or four times daily if uncovered and less frequently if covered.

Nurse monitoring
1. The drug itself is associated with very few side-effects other than some reports of jaundice. It is usually recommended that patients with liver dysfunction or those receiving high doses of the drug should have periodic liver function tests performed.
2. The major nurse monitoring aspects of this drug lie in the problems that may arise with the administration of fucidin in its various forms:
   a. Fucidin for injection should never be given intramuscularly or subcutaneously as severe local tissue reaction and injury may occur.
   b. Fucidin may be infused in sodium chloride and it has also been given safely in plasma and 5% dextrose. Higher concentrations of dextrose lead to an opalescence being formed by the infusion of the drug and it is recommended that such infusions be discontinued.
   c. Fucidin should not be infused with amino acid infusions or in whole blood.

General notes
1. The drug may be stored at room temperature.
2. Suspension should be protected from direct light.
3. After reconstitution the injection should be discarded if unused after 24 hours.

4. Powder for injections should be reconstituted with the diluent provided and it is customary to then dilute it in 500 ml of either normal saline or 5% dextrose and infuse over 2-4 hours or longer. Other problems with fucidin for infusion are discussed above.

F

G

GABAPENTIN (Neurontin)

Presentation
Capsules—100 mg, 300 mg, 400 mg

Actions and uses
Gabapentin is an anticonvulsant which chemicaly resembles the neurotransmitter, gamma-amino butyric acid (GABA) in the brain. As the importance of GABA as an inhibitory transmitter has become apparent, several newer anticonvulsants have been introduced which mimic or potentiate its action. The result is a 'dampening' of electrical discharge in the brain of which epilepsy is an extreme manifestation. Gabapentin is intended for add-on therapy (i.e. used with established anticonvulsants) and not as the sole agent.

Dosage
Adults: Titrate dosage to individual need using 300 mg daily increments to the usual range of 900–1200 mg. Up to a maximum 2400 mg daily may be given.

Nurse monitoring
1. The dose of gabapentin must be adjusted in patients with renal impairment. Guidelines should be available from the Pharmacy Department. Note also that the elderly often have reduced kidney function and may therefore require correspondingly lower doses.
2. This drug is not generally effective in absence seizures and indeed may activate absence seizures in some patients.
3. Likely side-effects of this drug include drowsiness, dizziness, ataxia, fatigue, nystagmus, headache, tremor, diplopia, rhinitis, nausea and vomiting.
4. The administration of antacids with gabapentin may reduce the amount absorbed by up to 25% and co-administration should be avoided.
5. Gabapentin is a member of a new range of anticonvulsants and it is unlikely that its true toxicity will emerge for some time. As with all new drugs therefore, extra vigilance is required and all suspected adverse events should be reported to the prescriber.

General note
Gabapentin capsules may be stored at room temperature.

GEMFIBROZIL (Lopid)

Presentation
Capsules—300 mg
Tablets—600 mg

Actions and uses
Gemfibrozil is a derivative of isobutyric acid: it is a lipid lowering substance which has actions and uses similar to those described for clofibrate. It is used in the management of familial hyperlipidaemias of types IIa, IIb, III, IV and V in cases where dietary measures alone are inadequate.

Dosage
Adults: 1200–1500 mg daily in three divided doses.

Nurse monitoring
1. Gastrointestinal upsets, skin rashes, dizziness, headaches and pain in fingers and toes and muscles are common side-effects.
2. It may produce sexual impotence in males.
3. Caution is required when prescribed for patients also receiving warfarin since anticoagulant control might be altered.
4. It should be avoided in patients with liver disease or gallstones.

General note
Gemfibrozil capsules may be stored at room temperature.

GENTAMICIN (Genticin, Cidomycin)
(See Note 3, p. 362)
Presentation
Injection—20 mg in 2 ml, 80 mg in 2 ml, 120 mg in 1.5 ml, 1 mg and 5 mg in 1 ml (intrathecal)
Powder—1 mg (sterile) for preparation of intrathecal injections
Ointment—3 mg in 1 g (0.3%)
Cream—3 mg in 1 g (0.3%)
Eye/ear drops—0.3% in 10 ml dropper
Actions and uses
1. The actions and uses of aminoglycoside antibiotics in general are discussed in the section on these drugs.
2. Superficial infections of the eye, ear and skin may be effectively treated by topical applications.
Dosage
1. For systemic infection:
   a. Adults. Usually 2-5 mg/kg/day divided into 8-hourly or 12-hourly doses. More recently high dose (e.g. 7 mg/kg) administered once daily has been used. The usual route of administration is intravenous bolus injection or rapid intravenous infusion.
   b. Children receive doses as above. Once daily dosing (3-4 mg/kg) is especially suitable for neonates who excrete the drug very slowly.

Blood levels of gentamicin are now measured in most centres and it is customary to adjust the dose according to the results of these investigations. By doing this the incidence of serious side-effects has been reduced.
2. Dosage of topical applications are as follows:
   a. Gentamicin cream and gentamicin ointment should be applied to the skin three to four times daily.
   b. Gentamicin eye and ear drops:
      i. 1–3 drops should be instilled into the affected eye 3-4 times daily or more frequently if required
      ii. 2–4 ear drops should be instilled 3-4 times per day and at night.

Nurse monitoring
1. See the section on aminoglycoside antibiotics.
2. The dosage should be adjusted so that the trough (immediate pre-dose) blood is less than 2 mg/litre. This is necessary in order to limit nephrotoxicity and ototoxicity. The pharmacist can advise on dosage adjustment in the individual patient when warranted.

General notes
1. Preparations containing gentamicin may be stored at room temperature.
2. The drug should never be mixed with other antibiotics prior to administration.

GLIBENCLAMIDE (Euglucon, Daonil)

Presentation
Tablets—5 mg, 2.5 mg
Actions and uses
See the section on hypoglycaemic drugs, oral (1)
Dosage
For adults: An initial dose of 2.5–5 mg is advised with gradual increments to a total of 20 mg as a single morning dose.

General note
Tablets may be stored at room temperature.

GLICLAZIDE (Diamicron)

Presentation
Tablets—80 mg
Actions and uses
See the section on hypoglycaemic drugs, oral (1).
Dosage
40–80 mg initially, increasing up to 320 mg daily.

Nurse monitoring
See the section on hypoglycaemic drugs, oral (1).

General note
Tablets may be stored at room temperature.

GLIPIZIDE (Glibenese, Minodiab)

Presentation
Tablets—2.5 mg, 5 mg
Actions and uses
See the section on hypoglycaemic drugs, oral (1).
Dosage
An initial dose of 2.5–5 mg is advised with gradual increments to a total of 30 mg daily. Daily doses above 10 mg are given in 2-3 divided doses.

Nurse monitoring
See the section on hypoglycaemic drugs, oral (1).

General note
Tablets may be stored at room temperature.

GLIQUIDONE (Glurenorm)

Presentation
Tablets—30 mg

Actions and uses
See the section on hypoglycaemic drugs, oral (1).
Dosage
45–60 mg daily (maximum 180 mg) taken before meals.

Nurse monitoring
See the section on hypoglycaemic drugs oral (1).

General note
Tablets may be stored at room temperature.

GLYCERYL TRINITRATE (Coro-Nitro, Nitrocine, Nitrocontin, Nitrolingual, Percutol, Suscard, Sustac, Transiderm-Nitro, Tridil)

Presentation
Sublingual tablets—500 microgram and 600 microgram
Slow release tablets—2.6 mg and 6.4 mg
Sublingual aerosol spray—400 microgram per metered dose
Buccal tablets—1 mg, 2 mg, 3 mg and 5 mg
Ointment—2%
Skin patches—5 mg and 10 mg
Injection—5 mg in 10 ml, 10 mg in 10 ml, 50 mg in 10 ml, 50 mg in 50 ml

Actions and uses
Glyceryl trinitrate reduces the work of the heart by a complex process. It would appear that its major action is the result of venous dilatation and reduction in the return of blood to the right side of the heart. This leads to a subsequent reduction in the amount of blood the heart pumps and therefore a reduction in the work that it performs. It is used to treat acute attacks of angina pectoris and also prophylactically particularly before exercise which would normally produce angina. The reduction in the venous return to the heart which glyceryl trinitrate produces gives the drug a further use in treatment of severe congestive cardiac failure

(often secondary to acute myocardial infarction) and for this purpose intravenous infusions are administered.

A bewildering range of different preparations are available, For acute attacks of angina a sublingual tablet is placed under the tongue and sucked vigorously in this position. Alternatively a metered dose is sprayed into the mouth.

For prophylaxis, the drug may be sucked or chewed, stuck to the gum, swallowed whole, sprayed into the mouth, smeared on the skin or stuck to the skin.

Dosage

1. Acute attacks of angina: One sublingual tablet (500 microgram or 600 microgram) administered as described above, or one metered dose (400 microgram) sprayed into the mouth.
2. Prophylaxis of angina:
   a. Sublingual route: One tablet held under the tongue immediately before exercise.
   b. Buccal route: One tablet (1, 2, 3 or 5 mg) stuck to the gum.
   c. Topical route: One dose of ointment (measured on a special ruler) smeared onto the skin or one skin patch applied to skin.
3. Intravenous route (for the treatment of heart failure): The dose range varies according to the individual response and is in the range 10–200 microgram/ minute infused in 5% dextrose or 0.9% sodium chloride.

Nurse monitoring

The nurse may contribute greatly towards the management of patients on this drug as follows:

1. Ensuring that the patient knows exactly how a particular form of the drug is administered, particularly when confusion exists due to the variety of alternatives available.
2. Patients may dislike using preparations containing glyceryl

trinitrate because of the side-effects of flushing, headaches, syncope and hypotension which are all due to an extension of the pharmacological activity of the drug. Often, however, these effects diminish with continued use of the drug. If they occur after sublingual tablets are sucked during an acute attack of angina, patients should be instructed to terminate the action of the drug by spitting out or swallowing the tablet once the angina is relieved.

3. Should an attack of angina be unresponsive to one or two doses of glyceryl trinitrate and should its duration exceed 15 minutes, a myocardial infarction should be suspected and medical assessment and appropriate treatment must be organized.
4. Tablets deteriorate with age, and may become ineffective. Loss of a bitter taste in the mouth may give an indication that this has occurred. This is especially important to note in patients who only rarely require to use the drug.

GLYCOPYRROLATE (Robinul)

Presentation

Tablets—2 mg
Powder—for reconstitution with saline solution

Actions and uses

1. It has an anticholinergic effect identical to that described for poldine sulphate (q.v.) and is used in the treatment of peptic ulceration.
2. This drug may be given as an application to the skin to reduce excess sweating.

Dosage

1. Peptic ulceration: The adult dose is 1–4 mg two to three times per day.
2. For hyperhydrosis a 0.05% solution in distilled water is used.

Nurse monitoring
> The nurse monitoring notes on this anticholinergic drug are identical to those for hyoscine-N-butylbromine (Buscopan) (q.v.).

General note
> Preparations containing glycopyrrolate may be stored at room temperature.

GOSERELIN (Zoladex)

Presentation
> Depot injection—3.6 mg in a solid, biodegradable base

Actions and uses
> Goserelin is a chemical analogue of the hypothalamic hormone LHRH (GnRH) with actions and uses as described for the related agent buserelin (see p. 56). Goserelin has a major advantage in that it is easily administered as a single dose at intervals of 28 days.

Dosage
> The 3.6 mg implant is injected subcutaneously into the anterior abdominal wall every 4 weeks. The base or matrix is biodegradable and designed to release the drug in a gradual, controlled manner.

Nurse monitoring
> The nurse monitoring aspects described for buserelin also apply to this agent.

General note
> The goserelin implant is supplied in a single unit sealed package which should be stored in a refrigerator.

GRANISETRON (Kytril)

Presentation
> Tablets—1 mg
> Injection—3 mg in 3 ml

Actions and uses
> Granisetron is a member of the group of drugs including ondansetron and tropisetron which selectively inhibit the effects of 5-hydroxytryptamine (5-HT, serotonin) at specific binding sites called 5-HT$_1$ receptors. Stimulation of these receptors in the gastrointestinal tract and chemoreceptor trigger zone induces nausea and triggers the vomiting reflex. Drugs of this type are therefore used to prevent and treat nausea and vomiting in patients who are exposed to various emetogenic stimuli including anticancer drugs and radiotherapy. More recently they have been shown to be similarly effective in the control of post-operative nausea and vomiting.

Dosage
> 1. Adults:
>   a. Oral: 1 mg twice daily for the duration of cytotoxic chemotherapy with the first dose administered 1 hour before the start of the chemotherapy course.
>   b. Intravenous: 3 mg administered in 20–50 ml sodium chloride or glucose injection over 5 minutes prevents nausea and vomiting for 24 hours in the majority of cases. Up to two further doses can however be given if necessary but administered at least 10 minutes apart.

Nurse monitoring
> The nurse monitoring aspects for ondansetron also apply to this drug.

General notes
> 1. Granisetron tablets and injection are stored at room temperature but must be protected from light during storage.
> 2. The drug may be injected slowly via the drip tubing of a running infusion fluid or added to 100 ml sodium chloride 0.9% or glucose 5% injection and administered over 30 minutes.
> 3. Once reconstituted, solutions for injection should be used immediately and any remaining discarded after 24 hours.

GRISEOFULVIN (Fulcin, Grisovin)

Presentation
Tablets—125 and 500 mg
Suspension—125 mg in 5 ml

Actions and uses
Griseofulvin is an effective anti-fungal agent which in clinical practice is used most commonly for the treatment of fungal infections of skin, scalp and nails.

Dosage
1. Adults: 500 mg per day which may be given once daily or divided into four doses. Severe infections may be treated by doubling the dose.
2. Children: A total daily dose of 10 mg/kg may be administered as a single dose or in four divided doses.

Nurse monitoring
1. Headache and gastrointestinal upset may occur especially during the early stages of treatment. The nurse may make a positive contribution by encouraging the patient to persist with treatment despite these effects.
2. Urticaria, erythematous rashes and photosensitivity reactions may occur.
3. Patients suffering from severe liver disease should not receive this drug.
4. Patients suffering from the rare condition of porphyria should not receive this drug.
5. The dosage of warfarin required for anticoagulation may have to be altered if griseofulvin is given.

General note
The drug may be stored at room temperature.

GUANETHIDINE (Ismelin)

Presentation
Tablets—10 mg, 25 mg
Injection—10 mg in 1 ml
Eye drops—5%

Actions and uses
A simplified description of the action of guanethidine is as follows: Arterioles are small arteries present throughout the body. The degree to which these arterioles are constricted is one of the major determinants of blood pressure and depends on stimuli which pass to the arterioles from the brain via the sympathetic nervous system. Stimuli are transmitted between nerves in this system by the release of noradrenaline. Any drug which reduces the activity along the adrenergic neurone will reduce the amount of noradrenaline present, or block its release, leading to vasodilation and the lowering of blood pressure. Guanethidine is one such drug: it is known as an 'adrenergic neurone blocker.' The drug is usually given orally but may be given intramuscularly if required in an emergency situation.

The adrenergic neurone blocking action of guanethidine in the eye enhances and prolongs the effect of adrenaline. Used alone this drug initially causes mydriasis so increasing aqueous humour outflow and subsequently it reduces aqueous production. This results in a fall of intraocular pressure in patients with open-angle (simple) glaucoma.

Dosage
1. Hypertensive emergency: The intramuscular dosage for emergency use is 10–20 mg repeated every 3-4 hours if necessary. Intramuscular doses for children are the same as oral doses outlined below.
2. Hypertensive oral maintenance:
   a. Adults: Doses vary widely. Normally 20–40 mg per day is sufficient, but up to 100 mg may be given for severe degrees of hypertension. Initial dosages do not usually exceed 10 mg. As guanethidine has a long duration of action it may be given as a single daily dose.
   b. Children: Up to 1 year old—0.2 mg/kg orally; Between 1-6 years—2.5 mg orally; Above 7 years—5 mg or as a single daily dose.

These are initial children's doses and, as in the case of adults, they may be increased gradually up to 20 times the dose stated.
3. Open-angle glaucoma: 1 drop once or twice daily.

Nurse monitoring
Guanethidine and the other adrenergic neurone blockers have a number of serious side-effects:
1. Bradycardia may commonly be produced.
2. Postural hypotension occurs frequently. The nurse may be the first to notice this, when patients may complain of dizziness or fainting when rising from a chair, or more commonly getting out of bed.
3. Diarrhoea, nasal congestion, weakness, paraesthesia, myalgia and impotence may all occur.

4. Adrenergic neurone blocking drugs interact with tricyclic antidepressants such as imipramine or amitryptyline and control of blood pressure may be lost.
5. The antihypertensive action of guanethidine is increased by alcohol and patients should be advised to restrict their alcohol intake when on these drugs.
6. Guanethidine is contraindicated in closed-angle glaucoma.

General notes
1. Guanethidine tablets, eye drops and solution for injection may be stored at room temperature.
2. In hospital wards, eye drops should be discarded one week after opening or after 4 weeks in the community.

H

HALCINONIDE (Halciderm)

Presentation
Cream—0.1 %
Actions and uses
This is a very potent corticosteroid
(q.v.) which is used most frequently
as a topical preparation for the
treatment of inflammatory skin
conditions such as eczema,
dermatitis and psoriasis.
Dosage
The cream is applied sparingly to the
affected area two or occasionally
three times per day.

Nurse monitoring
1. Although halcinonide is applied
to the skin only, it is important to
remember that prolonged
excessive use can result in
significant absorption and all the
effects described under the nurse
monitoring section of
corticosteroids (q.v.) can occur.

General notes
1. Halcinonide creams may be
stored at room temperature.
2. The creams should not normally
be diluted as chemical stability
may be affected.

HALOPERIDOL (Haldol, Serenace)

Presentation
Tablets—0.5 mg, 1.5 mg, 5 mg, 10
mg, 20 mg
Oral liquid—10 mg and 50 mg in 5ml
Injection—5 mg/ml, 1 and 2 ml
ampoules, 100 mg in 1 ml (as
decanoate) depot injection.

Actions and uses
Haloperidol is a neuroleptic drug
which is used for its tranquillizing or
calming effect in severely agitated
patients with a range of behavioural
disorders including schizophrenia,
mania and other psychoses. In this
respect haloperidol possesses
many of the properties of the
phenothiazine tranquillizers which
are discussed in the section on
phenothiazines. For example, it has
pronounced anti-emetic effects which
are usefully employed in the control
of nausea and vomiting in cancer
patients receiving morphine or
diamorphine analgesia.
Dosage
1. Adults: The dosage varies widely
according to the nature and
severity of the disorder under
treatment. Initially 1–15 mg daily
in single or divided doses with
gradual increments up to 200 mg
until control is achieved.
Thereafter maintenance doses are
tailored to individual patients.
2. Emergency control of severely
disturbed patients may be
treated by an intramuscular or
intravenous injection 5–30 mg
repeated at 6-hourly intervals.
3. Haloperidol decanoate is a depot
injection for long-term control
administered as 100–300 mg by
deep intramuscular injection each
month.

Nurse monitoring
1. Adverse effects which are
associated with the phenothiazine tranquillizers are also
commonly encountered with
haloperidol. In particular a

degree of unwanted sedation, extrapyramidal (Parkinsonian) symptoms and tardive dyskinesia occur. See the section on phenothiazines.
2. Photosensitivity reactions occasionally occur and patients should be warned to avoid excessive exposure to strong sunlight.
3. The endocrine side-effects of the phenothiazines are also associated with haloperidol as is the depressant action on the bone marrow affecting the production of white blood cells. Since this latter effect makes the patients more susceptible to infection, patients developing even simple symptoms such as sore throat should have their white blood cell count checked.

General notes
1. All preparations containing haloperidol should be stored at room temperature.
2. The drug is very sensitive to light and accordingly oral solution or solutions for injections should be suitably protected during storage.
3. Note that haloperidol decanoate injection, if stored for long periods in the cold, may precipitate (turn cloudy), though the injection should clear on re-storage at room temperature.

HEPARIN (Calciparine, Hep-Flush, Heplok, Hepsal, Minihep, Monoparin, Multiparin, Uniparin, Unihep)

Note 1. See section on Low Molecular Weight Heparin/ Heparinoid for a separate account of this new group which are also under their individual approved names.
Note 2. Heparin is available as both the sodium and calcium salt.

Presentation
Injection (intravenous)—5 ml vials contain 1000, 5000 and 25 000 units in 1 ml
Injection (subcutaneous)—5000

units in 0.2 ml, 12,500 units in 0.5 ml, 20,000 units in 0.8 ml
Solution (for addition to intravenous catheters)—50 units in 5 ml, 200 units in 2 ml

Actions and uses
Heparin is a naturally occurring antithrombin—a specialized protein which prolongs the bleeding time in the presence of a plasma co-factor (antithrombin III). Various clotting factors and hence blood clot formation are inhibited, as follows:
1. Thrombin (Factor IIa) is bound in an inactive complex so preventing the conversion of fibrinogen to fibrin.
2. Activated Factor X (or Xa) is similarly neutralized with the result that the conversion of prothrombin to thrombin is prevented.
3. Other effects of heparin include inhibition of platelet aggregation and the binding of fibrinogen to platelet aggregates.
Heparin is given by intravenous injection in the treatment of arterial and venous thrombosis and by subcutaneous injection for the prophylaxis of thromboembolic complications following surgery and myocardial infarction.

Dosage
1. For the treatment of arterial and venous thrombosis: Heparin may be administered by continuous or intermittent intravenous infusion:
   a. Continuous intravenous infusion: It is normal to administer 1000 units/hour and regularly check the thrombin time which is the test of choice for anticoagulant effect in patients on heparin.
   Depending on the results of this test the dose may be adjusted up or down until appropriate anticoagulation is obtained.
   b. Intermittent intravenous infusion: 5000–10 000 units is administered intravenously by bolus injection 4 to 6-hourly and individual requirements are then adjusted according to the results of the thrombin time.
2. For the prevention of thrombo-embolic complications following

surgery or myocardial infarction: The drug is administered subcutaneously in a dose of 5000 units 8-12 hourly. Clotting studies are not usually estimated when heparin is given by this route as it does not achieve a full anticoagulant effect but still proves useful in the prevention of thromboembolism.
3. For prevention of clotting in intravenous catheters and cannulae: Flush through with low strength (10–100 units/ml) solution regularly, e.g. 2-4 times daily and after use of the line.

Nurse monitoring
1. As with all anticoagulant therapy the two major risks to the patients are:
   a. Overcoagulation with resultant bleeding.
   b. Undercoagulation with failure to treat or prevent problems of thrombosis or embolism. The nurse may play a very important role in the successful administration of heparin by ensuring that intravenous infusions proceed at the appropriate rate and intermittent intravenous treatment or subcutaneous treatment is administered at appropriate times and in the appropriate dosage.
2. It is important to note that subcutaneous injections may be very painful.
3. Occasional urticaria, fever and thrombocytopenia may be produced by heparin.
4. The drug should never be administered by bolus injection by the intramuscular route.
5. Heparin is contraindicated for administration to patients with blood clotting disorders such as haemophilia and patients who have a history of active peptic ulceration or severe, uncontrolled hypertension.
6. When symptoms of overcoagulation occur the effect of heparin may be rapidly reversed by the administration of protamine sulphate.

General notes
1. Heparin preparations are stored at room temperature.
2. Intravenous infusions, which are delivered continuously via a volumetric pump or other infusion device, are prepared in sodium chloride or glucose injections.

HISTAMINE H$_2$-RECEPTOR ANTAGONISTS

Actions and uses
Drugs of this class are so-called because they competitively inhibit (block) the action of histamine, a naturally occurring substance, on the acid producing cells of the stomach resulting in reduced acid output and a corresponding rise in intragastric pH. This is associated with (i) increased healing rates for gastric and duodenal ulcers, (ii) mainten- ance of remission (or non- recurrence) in peptic ulcer disease, (iii) symptomatic improvement in reflux oesophagitis, (iv) enhanced activity of pancreatin preparations and (v) prevention of gastric aspiration during anaesthesia (Mendelson's syndrome).
The success of the H$_2$-blockers is such that a proliferation of agents has followed the introduction of the first, cimetidine, over 15 years ago. Presently the following are available:
1. Cimetidine
2. Ranitidine
3. Nizatidine
4. Famotidine.
Dosage
See individual drugs.

Nurse monitoring
1. The dosage regime for individual drugs may vary and patients require careful instruction in order to derive maximum benefit from therapy. Many patients, for example, are required to take H$_2$-blockers continuously to prevent ulcer relapse but, in the absence of symptoms, they may discontinue treatment without medical consultation. Also these

drugs are so effective that they are liable to misuse and there are many instances where patients have decided, without medical advice, to start treatment for vague symptoms of indigestion.

2. Cimetidine, but probably not other drugs, may interfere with anticoagulant control, and bleeding episodes have followed the administration of cimetidine to patients treated with warfarin. Close monitoring of blood clotting, with possibly an adjustment in warfarin dosage, is therefore essential.

3. All drugs are primarily excreted by the kidney and will accumulate in patients with renal impairment in whom reduced dosages are therefore necessary.

4. Common side-effects of the H_2-blockers include gastrointestinal upsets (nausea, constipation, diarrhoea), headaches, dizziness, mental confusion, and skin rashes. Cimetidine is widely reported to produce breast enlargement and tenderness (gynecomastia) in males and also male impotence, as a result of its anti-androgenic action.

General note
See specific drugs.

HORMONES (1) OESTROGENS AND DRUGS WITH MAINLY OESTROGENIC ACTIONS

Introduction
This group of drugs includes: Stilboestrol, Dinoestrol, Ethinyloestradiol, Mestranol, Oestradiol/Oestradiol valereate; Oestrogens conjugated (equine), Oestriol, Quinestrol, Piperazine oestrone sulphate, Quinestradiol.

Presentation
See individual drugs.

Actions and uses
1. The contribution of oestrogens to oral contraceptive therapy is discussed in the section on contraceptives—oral.

2. Oestrogens are used widely for a number of disorders including:
   a. Obstetric problems:
      i. Habitual and threatened abortion
      ii. Suppression of lactation
      iii. Puerperal depression
   b. Gynaecological problems:
      i. Menstrual irregularities
      ii. Functional uterine bleeding
      iii. Endometriosis
      iv. Menopausal symptoms
      v. Premenstrual tension
      vi. Endometrial carcinoma
      vii. Atrophic or senile vaginitis
   c. Treatment of cancer:
      i. Mammary carcinoma
      ii. Endometrial carcinoma
      iii. Prostatic carcinoma
   d. Prevention of bone resorption: Oestrogens are used for the prevention and treatment of osteoporosis in post-menopausal women.

Dosage
See specific drugs.

Nurse monitoring
1. The nurse monitoring aspects of the oestrogen component of contraceptive therapy are discussed in the section on contraceptives.

2. The use of oestrogens in other clinical situations is associated with the following problems:
   a. In females, increased uterine growth, withdrawal bleeding and amenorrhoea may occur.
   b. Breast tenderness, gynaecomastia and loss of sexual characteristics in males.
   c. Nausea, vomiting, depression, headache and dizziness may commonly occur.
   d. Salt and water retention leading to hypertension and weight gain may occur.
   e. Treatment with oestrogens occasionally produces jaundice due to liver damage.
   f. Rare side-effects include hypercalcaemia, skin rashes, e.g. urticaria and erythema multiforme.

H

3. Oestrogens may stimulate the growth of malignant tumours and are contraindicated in patients with a history of neoplastic disease of the breast or genital tract.
4. Oestrogens should not be administered to patients with a history of liver disease or previous thromboembolic disorders.
5. The administration of oestrogens to diabetic patients may alter insulin or oral hypoglycaemic requirements.
6. The administration of oestrogens to epileptics may lead to an increase in fit frequency and the need to alter their anticonvulsant regime.

General note
See specific drugs.

HORMONES (2) PROGESTOGENS AND DRUGS WITH PROGESTATIONAL ACTION

Introduction
This group of drugs includes: Allgloestrenol, Medroxyprogesterone, Hydroxyprogesterone, Progesterone, Dydrogesterone.
Presentation
See individual drugs.
Actions and uses
1. The contribution of progesterone to oral contraceptive therapy is discussed in the section on contraceptives.
2. Progesterones are used widely for a number of disorders including:
a. Obstetric problems:
i. Habitual and threatened abortion
ii. Suppression of lactation
iii. Puerperal depression
b. Gynaecological problems:
i. Menstrual irregularities
ii. Functional uterine bleeding
iii. Endometriosis
iv. Menopausal symptoms
v. Premenstrual tension
vi. Endometrial carcinoma
vii. Atrophic or senile vaginitis

c. Treatment of cancer:
i. Mammary carcinoma
ii. Endometrial carcinoma
iii. Prostatic carcinoma.

Nurse monitoring
1. The administration of progestogens can lead commonly to symptoms of gastrointestinal upset, headache, depression, urticaria, pruritus vulvae and change in menstrual function.
2. Acne, weight gain and hypertension due to salt and water retention, gynaecomastia, vaginal candidiasis and vaginal discharge may occur when patients receive this drug.
3. Less frequently jaundice and liver damage have been produced.
4. Progestogen drugs should be used with caution in patients with heart and kidney disease due to their salt and water retaining effects.
5. Progestogens should not be given to pregnant women as they cause masculinization of the female fetus.
6. The administration of progestogens to asthmatics and epileptics may lead to an exacerbation of their symptoms.

HORMONES (3) DRUGS WITH MIXED OESTRO-GENIC AND PROGESTOGENIC ACTIONS

Introduction
Norethisterone is the commonest drug in use with mixed oestrogenic and progestogenic actions.
Presentation
See individual drugs.
Actions and uses
The actions and uses of this group of drugs are identical to those described for oestrogens (q.v.).

Nurse monitoring
The nurse monitoring aspects of this drug are identical to those described for oestrogens (q.v.) and progestogens (q.v.)

HORMONES (4)
DRUGS WITH ANDROGENIC AND ANABOLIC ACTIONS

Introduction

This group of drugs includes: Fluoxymesterone, Testosterone preparations, Mesterolone. Methyltestosterone.

Presentation

See individual drugs.

Actions and uses

Drugs with androgenic and anabolic actions have a limited number of uses. They include:

1. The treatment of male patients with deficiency states involving these hormones.
2. The treatment of mammary carcinoma in females.
3. These drugs are occasionally used to treat rare haematological disorders including aplastic anaemia and haemolytic anaemia.

Dosage

See individual drugs.

Nurse monitoring

1. All patients receiving these drugs may experience an increase in weight, an increase in muscle bulk and salt and water retention with resultant hypertension and oedema.
2. When these drugs are given to female patients menstrual function is suppressed and virilization may occur character-ized by deepening of the voice, hirsutism (excess body hair) and atrophy of the breasts. Increased libido is a further feature.
3. Prolonged treatment with these drugs has been noted to cause an increased incidence of tumours of the liver.
4. These drugs should never be given to patients with carcinoma of the prostrate as they appear to stimulate the tumour growth.
5. These drugs should be used with great caution in patients with cardiac failure, renal failure or liver impairment as they may lead to a worsening of the patient's condition.

---

6. They should be used with great caution in patients suffering from epilepsy as an increased frequency of seizures may be precipitated.
7. They should be used with caution in patients with migraine as symptoms may be aggravated.

HORMONES (5)
DRUGS OF THE ANDROGEN GROUP WHICH HAVE MAINLY ANABOLIC ACTIVITY

Introduction

This group of drugs includes: Drostanolone, Nandrolone, Oxymethalone, Stanazolol, Norethandrolone.

Presentation

See individual drugs.

Actions and uses

1. These drugs stimulate skeletal growth by affecting protein metabolism. They may rarely be used in clinical situations for this effect.
2. This group of drugs is also occasionally used for the treatment of rare disorders involving bone marrow function including aplastic anaemia and haemolytic anaemia.
3. These drugs inhibit bone resorp-tion in the elderly male and are used therefore in the treatment of senile osteoporosis in males.

Dosage

See individual drugs.

Nurse monitoring

The nurse monitoring notes for these drugs are identical to those described for androgen and anabolic steroids (q.v.).

General note

See individual drugs.

HYALURONIDASE (Hyalase)

Presentation

Ampoules containing 1500 international units of hyaluronidase.

Actions and uses

This substance breaks down hyaluronic acid which is a substance concerned with maintaining structure in cells. It is used in clinical practice as an aid to the dispersal of infusions administered subcutaneously or intramuscularly. It may also be used to reduce local inflammation and oedema.

Dosage

Adults: In general 1500 international units are sufficient for the administration of 500–1000 ml of most fluids.

Nurse monitoring

1. This drug should never be administered to the site of bites or stings or at sites where infection or malignancy are present.
2. The drug should never be given intravenously.
3. Side-effects are due to sensitization and may be severe enough to produce anaphylactic shock.

General note

The drug should be stored in a cool, dry place.

HYDRALAZINE (Apresoline)

Presentation

Tablets—25 mg, 50 mg
Injection—20 mg powder in
2 ml ampoule

Actions and uses

Hydralazine has a direct action on the small arteries (arterioles) causing them to dilate. The effect of this is to reduce the blood pressure in hypertension and heart work in cardiac failure. Administration of the drug often leads to a degree of fluid retention and tachycardia and is often therefore given along with thiazide diuretics and/or beta-blocking drugs.

Dosage

1. It may be given by slow intra-venous injection or intravenous infusion for hypertensive emergencies and acute heart failure. The usual dose is 20–40 mg.

2. The adult oral maintenance dose is 25–50 mg two to three times daily. The maximum dose advisable is 200 mg per day in hypertension and 300 mg daily in heart failure.

Nurse monitoring

1. The nurse should be aware that the presence of tachycardia in a patient on hydralazine may be due to the drug therapy.
2. Fluid retention and heart failure may develop if patients who are on hydralazine are not on a diuretic.
3. Headache and flushing may be caused by the vasodilator action of the drug. As these side-effects are often poorly tolerated there may be a reduction in compliance with treatment and patients should always be asked therefore whether they are suffering from these effects.
4. A serious side-effect usually seen only with high dosage, is a development of a syndrome similar to systemic lupus erythematosus which is associated with widespread damage to the arterial system reflected in skin rashes, renal and hepatic dysfunction etc. The development of the features of this syndrome are an indication for immediate withdrawal of drug therapy.

General notes

1. Hydralazine tablets and powder for injection may be stored at room temperature.
2. Solutions for injection are prepared by adding 1 ml of water for injection to each ampoule which is then further diluted with sodium chloride 0.9% (normal saline) injection.
3. It is given by slow intravenous injection or added to an infusion of sodium chloride 0.9% or compound sodium lactate (Ringer's) injection.
4. Any unused solution must be immediately discarded.

HYDROCHLOROTHIAZIDE (Hydrosaluric)

Presentation
Tablets–25 mg, 50 mg
Actions and uses
See the section on thiazide and related diuretics.
Dosage
The daily adult dose range is 25–50 mg twice daily. Hydrochlorothiazide is effective for 6-12 hours after an oral dose.

Nurse monitoring
See the section on thiazide and related diuretics.

General note
Hydrochlorothiazide tablets may be stored at room temperature.

HYDROCORTISONE (Hydrocortone, Efcortesol, Efcortelan, Solu-cortef)

Numerous other preparations containing hydrocortisone (often combined with other substances) are available.
Presentation
Tablets—10 mg, 20 mg
Injection—intravenous or intramuscular—100 mg in 1 ml and 2 ml; —500 mg in 5 ml
Injection—intra-articular—25 mg in 1 ml
Ointment and cream—0.5%, 1% and 2.5%
Eye drops—1%
Eye ointment—2.5%
Actions and uses
See the section on corticosteroids.
Dosage
Dosages vary considerably with the nature and severity of the illness being treated and it is not therefore appropriate to quote specific instances.

Nurse monitoring
See the section on corticosteroids.

General notes
1. Preparations containing hydrocortisone may be stored at room temperature.

2. Intravenous use: Sodium succinate or sodium phosphate salts only should be used. Hydrocortisone acetate is for intra-articular injection only.
3. Intravenous injections are given slowly over a period of one minute to several minutes.
4. Intravenous infusions are prepared by adding the required dose to a volume of 5% dextrose or 0.9% sodium chloride injection. The volume of diluent varies from 100 ml to 1 litre.

HYDROFLUMETHIAZIDE (Hydrenox)

Presentation
Tablets—50 mg
Actions and uses
See the section on thiazide and related diuretics.
Dosage
The adult dose range is 25–100 mg daily in divided doses. The duration of action of hydroflumethiazide is about 4-6 hours.

Nurse monitoring
See the section on thiazide and related diuretics.

General note
Hydroflumethiazide tablets may be stored at room temperature.

HYDROXOCOBALAMIN—VITAMIN B_{12} (Neo-Cytamen)

Presentation
Injection—250 microgram in 1 ml, 1000 microgram in 1 ml
Actions and uses
Hydroxocobalamin (vitamin B_{12}) is indicated for the treatment of megaloblastic anaemia where this has been shown to be due to a deficiency of vitamin B_{12} by the appropriate laboratory test. Deficiency of vitamin B_{12} occurs either where there is a deficiency in the gut of a substance (intrinsic factor) normally produced by the stomach which is essential for the

absorption of Vitamin B$_{12}$, this condition being known as pernicious anaemia, or it may be due to other forms of malabsorption. More rarely vitamin B$_{12}$ deficiency may be seen in people who have a strict vegan diet.

Dosage

1. For pernicious anaemia: Initially 250–1000 microgram intramuscularly on alternative days for 1-2 weeks, and then 1000 microgram every 2-3 months.
2. For the prophylaxis of megalo-blastic anaemia due to gastrectomy or malabsorption syndromes or strict veganism: 250–1000 microgram monthly.

Nurse monitoring

1. Sensitization to vitamin B$_{12}$, is extremely rare, It may present as an itching skin rash and very exceptionally as anaphylactic shock.
2. Hydroxocobalamin is preferable as the form of vitamin B$_{12}$ for replacement therapy as it has the advantage over cyanocobalamin in that it does not contain cyanide. This is especially important when vitamin B$_{12}$ is being given to patients with either tobacco amblyopia or optic atrophy and optic neuritis due to Leber's optic atrophy when cyanide containing compounds are specifically contraindicated.
3. Hydroxocobalamin has an additional advantage over cyanocobalamin in that it is longer acting and therefore the interval between injections can be at least monthly.

General note

Ampoules should be protected from light.

HYDROXYCHLOROQUINE (Plaquenil)

Presentation

Tablets—200 mg

Actions and uses

This anti-malarial drug has been found to be useful in the treatment of the following conditions:
1. Malaria
2. Giardiasis
3. Rheumatoid disease
4. Lupus erythematosus.

The mechanism of action in 3 and 4 above is not clearly understood but hydroxychloroquine belongs to the group of drugs which have autoimmune disease modifying activity. It is not an anti-inflammatory analgesic drug.

Dosage

1. Malaria:
   a. Prophylactically 400 mg once per week during the period of exposure and for 4-8 weeks afterwards.
   b. Treatment of an acute attack of malaria: Initial dose of 800 mg followed by 400 mg after 6-8 hours and then 400 mg on two successive days.
2. Giardiasis: 200 mg three times daily for 5 days.
3. Rheumatoid disease and lupus erythematosus: 400–500 mg per day are given initially usually at mealtimes and if a response is obtained the dose is reduced after several weeks to a maintenance dosage of 200–400 mg per day.

Note: All the above doses are for adults only.

Nurse monitoring

The nurse monitoring notes on chloroquine (q.v.) are entirely similar to those for hydroxychloroquine.

General note

Hydroxychloroquine tablets may be stored at room temperature.

HYDROXYPROGESTERONE HEXANOATE (Proluton Depot)

Presentation

Injection—250 mg/ml

Actions and uses

1. See the section describing the actions and uses of progestational

hormones in general in hormones (2).

2. Proluton Depot in clinical practice is used for the treatment of threatened abortion and habitual abortion.

Dosage
1. For the treatment of habitual abortion: 250–500 mg at weekly intervals during the first half of pregnancy.
2. For the treatment of threatened abortion: 500 mg of Proluton Depot intramuscularly daily until bleeding has stopped. Subsequently 250–500 mg intramuscularly every three days for three doses and then weekly throughout the first half of pregnancy.

Nurse monitoring
1. See the section describing the nurse monitoring aspects of progestational hormones in general in hormones (2).
2. Rarely local reactions may occur at the site of injection.

General note
The drug may be stored at room temperature.

HYDROXYZINE (Atarax)

Presentation
Tablets—10 mg and 25 mg
Syrup—10 mg in 5 ml

Actions and uses
Hydroxyzine is a depressant affecting the CNS. It has a calming effect in anxious patients, an anti-emetic activity and via its antihistamine action, an antipruritic action. In clinical practice the drug is used mainly for its ability to suppress itch in various dermatological conditions, particularly in patients who have an associated anxiety.

Dosages
1. Adults: 25–100 mg taken three or four times daily.
2. Children:
   a. Under 6 years: 30–50 mg daily in divided doses
   b. Over 6 years: 50–100 mg daily in divided doses

Nurse monitoring
1. Hydroxyzine is a CNS depressant drug and marked sedation may follow its use, particularly if other sedative drugs are taken.
2. In the above context patients should be warned of the dangers of taking alcohol, even in moderate amounts, concurrently with hydroxyzine.
3. Some patients may complain of dryness of the mouth with this drug.
4. Rarely tremor or abnormal muscle activity is produced. This symptom is indicative of excessive dosage and if it occurs, should be brought to the attention of the doctor.

General note
Tablets and syrup containing hydroxyzine should be stored at room temperature.

HYOSCINE-N-BUTYLBROMIDE (Buscopan)

Presentation
Tablets—10 mg
Injection—20 mg in 1 ml

Actions and uses
Hyoscine-N-butylbromide is an anticholinergic drug. It has a specific antispasmodic action on the smooth muscle of the gut, renal and biliary tracts and female genital tract. It is therefore used to relieve pain associated with acute spasm, i.e. renal colic, biliary colic, dysmenorrhoea and spasm produced by diagnostic procedures such as gastric or duodenal endoscopy.

Dosage
1. Adults:
   a. Oral: 20 mg four times a day. Courses lasting 5 days and commencing 2 days before the onset of menstruation are used in the treatment of dysmenorrhoea.
   b. By injection: 20 mg intramuscularly or intravenously

H

repeated at half-hourly intervals as required.

2. Children:
   a. Oral: 10 mg three times daily is the ideal dose range for the 6-12 year age group.

Nurse monitoring

1. Patients may frequently suffer the common anticholinergic side-effects of dryness of the mouth, visual disturbance and tachycardia.
2. More serious side-effects which may be encountered are:
   a. Intra-ocular pressure may be raised, thus the drug is contraindicated in patients with glaucoma and may on occasions precipitate glaucoma in patients who had not previously had this problem recognized.
   b. Patients may have difficulty in initiating micturition and occasionally urinary retention may result.
   c. The drug should not be used in patients with heart disease or intestinal obstruction.

General notes

1. Hyoscine-N-butylbromide tablets and injection may be stored at room temperature. The injection solution however should be protected from light.
2. Should it be necessary to dilute the injection solution, dextrose 5% injection may also be mixed with commonly used radiological contrast media, e.g. diodone, sodium diatrizoate, before intravenous pyelography when spasm and pain in the urinary tract may be produced.

HYPOGLYCAEMIC DRUGS, ORAL (1) SULPHONYLUREAS

Presentation
See individual drugs.
Actions and uses
Sulphonylurea drugs stimulate the islet cells of the pancreas to produce more insulin. They are, therefore,

useful in the management of patients who have been found to have diabetes mellitus which is not adequately controlled by diet only but which is not sufficiently severe to require insulin. It should be pointed out that as they stimulate production of insulin by the pancreas, at least some degree of insulin production by the pancreas must already be present.

Dosage
The dosage required for each of the drugs in this group should be tailored to individual patient requirements and should be monitored by regular estimation of plasma glucose and urine glucose. For specific doses see individual drugs.

Nurse monitoring

1. Sulphonylurea drugs should be avoided if possible in patients who are overweight as their stimulation of insulin production may lead to further gain in weight.
2. With the longer acting members of this group of drugs such as chlorpropamide, hypoglycaemia may be produced especially in the early hours of the morning and in elderly patients. The nurse should be alerted to the possibility of this by noting the occurrence of any faintness, dizziness or confusion in elderly patients at the appropriate time.
3. Common side-effects include gastrointestinal upset manifest by nausea, vomiting and epigastric pain, neurological side-effects including dizziness, weakness, paraesthesia and headache.
4. Less common side-effects include hypersensitivity reaction such as fever, skin rash and jaundice and blood dyscrasias such as leucopenia, thrombocytopenia, aplastic anaemia and agranulocytosis.
5. A proportion of patients receiving sulphonylureas will experience facial flushing, tachycardia, sweating, breathlessness, headache, vomiting and

dizziness if they take alcohol. Patients should be warned of the potential development of these effects and if they occur the only alternatives are to change to another drug or to avoid alcohol.

6. A number of important problems may arise when diabetic patients on sulphonylurea drugs receive other drugs. These are as follows:

a. Beta blockers: These may be dangerous because patients on beta-blocking drugs may not experience the early symptoms which normally warn them that they are about to become hypoglycaemic, and they might then proceed to sudden hypoglycaemic coma.

b. Corticosteroids: These may affect glucose metabolism in the body in such a way that increased requirements for insulin or oral hypoglycaemics are necessary.

c. Diuretics: These have two effects:
   i. They may raise blood glucose levels and result in the need for change in dosage.
   ii. They may potentiate hyperosmolar diabetic states.

d. Alcohol: Alcohol has two actions:
   i. It may produce symptoms with sulphonylurea drugs described in the section above.
   ii. Alcohol itself may produce hypoglycaemia of a transient nature.

e. Monoamine oxidase inhibitors: These drugs enhance and/or prolong the hypoglycaemic response to oral hypoglycaemic drugs and a reduction in dosage may be necessary.

f. Phenylbutazone: This drug interferes with the liver meta-bolism of oral hypoglycaemic drugs and a change in dosage may be necessary.

g. Salicylates: These may displace oral hypoglycaemic drugs from the proteins to which they bind in blood and a change in dosage may be necessary.

h. Sulphonamides: These may affect both the metabolism and protein binding of the sulphonylureas, making a change in dosage necessary.

7. When dealing with diabetic patients, the nurse may be faced with the problem of a patient presenting with coma or altered level of consciousness. This is further discussed in the nurse monitoring section (7) on insulins (q.v.)

General note
Sulphonylurea drugs may be stored at room temperature.

HYPOGLYCAEMIC DRUGS, ORAL (2) BIGUANIDES

Note: Since the withdrawal of phenformin due to its potential to produce serious and life-threatening side-effects, metformin is currently the only drug of this type available.

Presentation
See individual drugs.

Actions and uses
Biguanide drugs do not stimulate insulin secretion. Their precise mechanism of action is not clearly understood but they appear to increase the utilization of glucose in the tissues.

Dosage
See individual drugs.

Nurse monitoring
1. Biguanide drugs would appear to be the treatment of choice in obese diabetics who do not require insulin.
2. Metformin (though to a lesser extent than phenformin) may cause a serious alteration in the blood biochemistry known as lactic acidosis. For this reason

phenformin has now been withdrawn from clinical use. It remains, however, that there is still a risk of this effect occurring with metformin. The clinical features of lactic acidosis are of general malaise, impaired consciousness and other symptoms suggestive of diabetic ketoacidosis, but ketones are not detectable on the breath or in the urine, and this gives the clue to the diagnosis.

3. Gastrointestinal upsets are relatively common and symptoms include nausea, vomiting and diarrhoea.

4. A metallic taste may be produced by these drugs.

5. Less common side-effects include muscle weakness, lassitude and skin rash.

6. The coincident administration of other drugs may affect patients on biguanide therapy in varying ways:

   a. Beta-blockers: These may be dangerous because patients on beta-blocking drugs may not experience the early symptoms which normally warn them that they are about to become hypoglycaemic and they might then proceed to sudden hypoglycaemic coma.

   b. Corticosteroids: These may affect glucose metabolism in the body in such a way that increased requirements for insulin or oral hypoglycaemics are necessary.

   c. Diuretics: These have two effects:
      i. They may raise blood glucose levels and result in a need for change in dosage
      ii. They may potentiate hyperosmolar diabetic states.

d. Alcohol: Alcohol has three effects:
   i. It may produce symptoms with biguanide drugs as described under section (5) of the nurse monitoring notes on sulphonylurea drugs (q.v.).
   ii. Alcohol itself may produce hypoglycaemia of a transient nature.
   iii. Patients who take alcohol are at an increased risk of developing the metabolic complication of lactic acidosis (see above).

e. Monoamine oxidase inhibitors: These drugs enhance and/or prolong the hypoglycaemic response to oral hypoglycaemic drugs and a reduction in dosage may be necessary.

f. Phenylbutazone: This drug interferes with the liver metabolism of oral hypoglycaemic drugs and a change in dosage may be necessary.

g. Salicylates: These may displace oral hypoglycaemic drugs from the proteins to which they bind in blood and a change in dosage may be necessary.

h. Sulphonamides: These may affect both metabolism and protein binding of the biguanides, making a change in dosage necessary.

7. When dealing with diabetic patients, the nurse may be faced with the problems of a patient presenting with coma or altered level of consciousness. This is further discussed in the nurse monitoring section (7) on insulins (q.v.).

General note

Biguanide hypoglycaemic drugs may be stored at room temperature.

I

IBUPROFEN (Brufen)

Presentation
Tablets—200 mg, 400 mg, 600 mg
and 800 mg (sustained-release)
Suspension—100 mg in 5 ml

Actions and uses
See the section on non-steroidal
anti-inflammatory analgesic drugs.

Dosage
1. Adults.
   a. Initial dosage is 1200 mg per
      day in three or four divided
      doses.
   b. Maintenance dosage is 600–
      1200 mg per day in divided
      doses.
   c. Alternatively 1600 mg may be
      taken at night in sustained-
      release form, or up to 2400 mg
      daily in two divided doses.
2. Children: A dosage of 20 mg/kg
   has been used but the total daily
   dose should not exceed 500 mg in
   those weighing less than 30 kg.

Nurse monitoring
See the section on non-steroidal
anti-inflammatory analgesic drugs.

General note
Ibuprofen tablets and suspension
may be stored at room temperature.

IDOXURIDINE (Herpid, Dendrid)

Presentation
Paint—5% in dimethylsulphoxide
(DMSO)
Eye drops—0.1%
Eye ointment—0.5%

Actions and uses
This compound is effective against
viral infections. Unfortunately, it is
only available for topical use and in
clinical practice it may be used to
treat the following diseases:
1. Cutaneous herpes zoster
   (shingles)
2. Ocular herpes zoster
3. Skin infections due to herpes
   simplex
4. Acute dendritic ulcer.

Dosage
1. If the paint is used it should be
   applied carefully and sparingly to
   the skin lesion and the immediate
   surrounding erythematous area
   four times per day for 4-5 days.
2. Eye drops should be administered
   at the rate of one drop each hour
   during the day and one drop 2-
   hourly throughout the night.
3. Eye ointment should be applied
   sparingly 4-hourly.
4. Idoxuridine 0.1% (using eye drop
   solution) is applied to oral or
   perioral lesions (the 5% paint is
   not suitable in this case). Adults
   and children should hold
   approximately 2 ml in the mouth in
   contact with the lesion for 2-3
   minutes at least three times a day.
   Alternatively the solution may be
   applied 4-5 times daily.

Nurse monitoring
1. The dimethylsulphoxide component of the paint preparation will
   damage normal skin and care
   should be taken to apply the
   paint only to the infected area.
2. The paint may produce stinging
   and an unpleasant taste if
   applied to the mouth.

3. Irritation, pain, itching and inflammation may follow the use of ophthalmic preparations.
4. It is worth noting that topical corticosteroid preparations should never be used where viral infection is suspected.

General notes
1. The paint preparation may be stored at room temperature.
2. Ophthalmic preparations should be refrigerated.

IMIPENEM (Primaxin)

(See Note 3, p 362)

Presentation
Injection (intramuscular)—500 mg + Cilastatin 500 mg
Injection (intravenous)—250 mg + Cilastatin 250 mg
Injection (intravenous)—500 mg + Cilastatin 500 mg

Actions and uses
Imipenem is a new chemical derivative of the beta-lactam series of antibiotics which includes the penicillins and cephalosporins. It is described as a thienamycin beta-lactam antibiotic.

This drug is administered in combination with cilastatin, a substance which inhibits its enzymic destruction by the kidney. This has two important consequences. Firstly, it enhances the antibacterial effect of imipenem and provides a notably broad spectrum of activity and, secondly, it prevents the formation of a degradation product which is itself toxic to the renal tissues.

Imipenem is active against a wide range of aerobic and anaerobic Gram-positive and Gram-negative bacteria which is reflected in its many indications. These include septicaemia, pneumonia, intra-abdominal and pelvic sepsis and infections of bone, skin and soft tissue and the genito-urinary tract. Because of its broad spectrum imipenem may be used on an empirical basis when the infecting organism cannot be readily predicted and the results of bacteriological screening are awaited.

Dosage
1. Adults: Doses range from 250 mg to 1 g 6-8 hourly by i.v. infusion depending upon the severity of infection and sensitivity of the specific pathogen. Alternatively 500–750 mg 12-hourly may be given by deep intramuscular injection for less serious infections and as a single dose in the treatment of gonococcal urethritis.
2. Children (over 3 months): 15 mg/kg body weight 6-hourly up to a maximum daily dose of 2 g.

Nurse monitoring
1. Although some chemical differences exist between imipenem and the penicillins and cephalosporins, cross-reactivity in patients with hypersensitivity to these agents may exist.
2. Gastrointestinal upsets (nausea, vomiting, diarrhoea), blood dyscrasia and altered liver and kidney function are relatively common side-effects. Excessive dosage may produce CNS disturbances: convulsions have been reported.
3. Patients with inflammatory bowel disease may develop acute flares during treatment with this and other broad spectrum antibiotics.
4. Blood levels of imipenem are increased in patients treated concurrently with probenecid. This is in fact useful in prolonging its action when single doses are used in the treatment of gonococcal urethritis.

General notes
1. Imipenem injection vials are stored at room temperature.
2. Solutions for i.v. infusion are prepared in sodium chloride 0.9% or glucose 5% injection: 500 mg in 100 ml and administered over 30 minutes (up to 1 hour for 1 g dose).

IMIPRAMINE (Tofranil)

Presentation
Tablets—10 mg, 25 mg
Syrup—25 mg in 5 ml
Injection—25 mg in 2 ml

Actions and uses
Imipramine is a tricyclic antidepressant drug. Its actions and uses are described in the section dealing with these drugs.

Dosage
1. For the treatment of depression:
   a. Oral doses range from 75–200 mg daily in total usually given in three or four divided doses. Lower doses, i.e. up to 30 mg daily may be sufficient in older patients who often have difficulty in tolerating the standard doses described.
   b. In patients who require injection, i.e. those who are uncooperative or have severe depression which requires rapid control, intramuscular injections of 25 mg up to six times daily may be administered.
2. For the treatment of enuresis in children dose ranges are as follows: 5-12 years—25 mg taken as a single dose at bed time; Over 12 years—50 mg taken as a single dose at bed time.

Nurse monitoring
See the section on tricyclic antidepressant drugs.

General notes
1. Preparations containing imipramine should be stored at room temperature.
2. Solution for injection and syrup should be protected from light.

INDAPAMIDE (Natrilix)

Presentation
Tablets—2.5 mg

Actions and uses
1. When given in a dosage of 2.5 mg per day, the drug has a weak diuretic but much more pronounced hypotensive action. It is therefore useful in the treatment of hypertension.
2. Higher doses have a more pronounced diuretic action and therefore it may be used as such.

Dosage
For adults the usual dose is 2.5 mg taken once daily in the morning.

Nurse monitoring
1. When given in the above dosage for hypertension side-effects may be seen in the form of nausea, vomiting and headache. Hypotension and its clinical features may also be produced.
2. If higher doses are used the diuretic effect becomes more pronounced and all the adverse effects associated with thiazide diuretics (q.v.) may occur.

General note
Indapamide tablets may be stored at room temperature.

INDOMETHACIN (Indocid)

Presentation
Capsules—25 mg, 50 mg, 75 mg (sustained release)
Suspension—25 mg in 5 ml
Suppositories—100 mg

Actions and uses
See the section on non-steroidal anti-inflammatory analgesic drugs.

Dosage
1. Adults:
   a. The usual adult dose range is 25 mg twice or three times daily up to 200 mg per day in divided doses.
   b. A sustained release capsule on a once or occasionally twice daily dosage regime can be used.
   c. One suppository (100 mg) inserted at night is often useful in relieving the troublesome morning stiffness in joints affected by rheumatoid arthritis.

General note
Indomethacin capsules, suspension and suppositories may be stored at room temperature.

INOSITOL NICOTINATE (Hexopal)

Presentation
Tablets—500 mg, 750 mg
Suspension—1 g in 5 ml

Actions and uses
The actions and uses of this drug are identical to those described for nicofuranose (q.v.).

Dosage
Adults: 500 mg–1 g two or three times per day.

General note
The drug should be stored at room temperature.

INSULIN

Changes in the availability of commercial insulins continue to take place. Information provided in the accompanying Table will therefore require frequent revision.

1. **Source of insulin:** Insulins available in the United Kingdom will, in time, be based only on the 'human' variety, i.e. they will contain the precise amino acid sequences on both the A and B chains of the human peptide. Thus beef insulins are expected to disappear completely during the 1990s and similarly pork insulins will probably be phased out before the end of the century. Human insulin is derived from two sources in the laboratory; it is obtained by chemical manipulation of pork insulin after extraction from pig pancreas (enzymatically modified pork or 'emp' insulin) or it can be manufactured biosynthetically using a DNA-modified bacterium (recombinant DNA or 'crb' insulin). See special considerations for transfer of patients to human insulin in the nurse monitoring section.

2. **Concentration:** Since 1983 all manufacturers of insulins have produced only a single strength containing 100 units in 1 ml or U100.

3. **Insulin syringes:** At the time of introduction of insulin U100 two new standard syringes of 0.5 ml and 1 ml were also introduced. These were graduated in insulin 'units' and the earlier practice of using a 'marks' system which required prior conversion to units was discontinued, thus eliminating a common source of dosage error. A further important development followed in 1986 when the authorities permitted the supply, free of charge, on NHS prescription of disposable insulin syringes. Thus patients are likely to have reverted completely to these syringes and glass, non-disposable syringes will be encountered only rarely, if ever. The practice of re-using disposable insulin syringes in the short-term, as a means of saving money for those who previously had to buy them, should cease. They are intended for single dose use and re-use carries a risk, albeit slight, of contamination and subsequent infection.

4. **Insulin pens:** Pen injection devices facilitate the setting of variable doses and insulin injection from an insulin cartridge and are especially useful for active diabetics who use frequent daily doses adjusted to lifestyle.

The device is not however available on NHS prescription but can be readily purchased: insulin pen cartridges can however be prescribed.

5. **Soluble insulin:** The old fashioned acid soluble insulin which frequently caused local irritation at injection sites has now disappeared and the term 'Soluble Insulin' is now synonymous with neutral (neutral pH) soluble insulin which is better tolerated and less likely to cause local reactions.

6. **Preservatives:** Insulin, being available in multi-dose vials, requires the addition of a preservative (antiseptic) agent to prevent the growth of micro-organisms which may be accidentally introduced to the vial during repeated use. Modern

Available 'human' insulins (all 100 units/ml)

Insulin	Proprietary name	Action (hours)	
		Onset	Duration
Soluble (Neutral)	Human Actrapid	$1/_2$	6-8
	Human Velosulin		
	Humulin S		
	Pur-in Neutral		
Isophane	Human Insulatard	$1-1^1/_2$	20-24
	Human Protaphane		
	Humulin I		
	Pur-in Isophane		
Insulin Zinc Suspension (Crystalline)	Humulin Zn	3	24
	Human Ultratard	4	28
Insulin Zinc Suspension (Mixed)	Human Monotard	3	24
	Humulin Lente	$2^1/_2$	24
Biphasic Insulin* Human Initard + Isophane)	Human Actraphane	$1/_2$	15-24 (Neutral Soluble)
	Human Mixtard		
	Humulin M1	–	18
	Humulin M2	–	16
	Humulin M3	_	15
	Humulin M4	_	15
	Penmix 10/90	_	24
	Penmix 20/80	_	24
	Penmix 30/70	_	24
	Penmix 40/60	_	24
	Penmix 50/50	_	24
	Pur-in Mix 50/50	_	16
	Pur-in Mix 25/75	_	18
	Pur-in Mix 15/85	_	20

* Ready mixtures of neutral soluble insulin and isophane insulin (fixed proportions) are used for patients who experience difficulty in mixing insulins from separate containers. The proportions of soluble and isophane insulin in each make varies and therefore so too does the activity profile, albeit within a similar duration of action overall for certain mixtures. Thus a range of mixes allows optimum choice for precise control in the individual patient. Note that such mixtures (Penmix) are also available for use with the pen injector.

preservatives include cresols, phenols and hydroxybenzoates (parabens) and some patients may display allergy to one or other of these. Persistent allergic reactions (usually reddening or itchy rash) at injection sites might develop and necessitate a change of insulin, since the type of preservative varies between manufacturers. Note that the nature and concentration of preservative is always indicated on the insulin package.

Actions and uses

Insulin is the hormone produced by the islet cells of the pancreas which regulates blood glucose levels. Exogenous (injected) insulin is essential in the management of diabetes mellitus, in which exists a failure of these endocrine cells to produce natural (endogenous) hormone. Many patients with diabetes controlled by diet alone or a combination of diet and oral hypoglycaemic drug therapy (non-insulin dependent diabetes) may also require insulin injections during an acute illness or at the time of surgery or if they develop ketosis.

Dosage

The dose of insulin varies considerably from patient to patient but with the introduction of more highly purified insulins, particularly of the human type, it is likely that most patients will be controlled on a total daily dose of less than 50–100 units. The dosage may be administered by intramuscular or subcutaneous routes. Usually a twice daily regime is used but single daily doses of long-acting types, more frequent doses with meals and snacks, and even continuous infusions, have also been employed.

Nurse monitoring

1. The nurse plays an invaluable role in many aspects of patient education; good control of diabetes mellitus can only be achieved by highly motivated well-informed patients. It is therefore important that those nursing diabetic patients understand dosage calculations and injection techniques and also that they are well acquainted with modern methods of blood and urine glucose estimation and their relation to dosage.

2. a. When mixing soluble and longer-acting insulins it is important that the soluble (clear) insulin be drawn up into the syringe first. In this way the soluble insulin should never be contaminated by the longer-acting (cloudy) insulin, the consequences of which may adversely affect diabetic control.

   b. Soluble insulin can be mixed with other insulin types, with the exception of Protamine Zinc Insulin (though now rarely used), without affecting the duration of action of either preparation.

   c. Mixing of insulins from different sources, e.g. beef, pork and human, is irrational and should be avoided.

   d. When insulins containing different preservatives are mixed, the risk of local or general reactions is increased.

   e. Insulins mixed in a syringe should be injected immediately or if not used, promptly discarded.

3. Transferring patients from beef to human insulins is likely to result in a reduction in daily insulin requirement, since levels of insulin-binding (inactivating) antibodies will rapidly recede. In general a dose reduction of between 10–20% of the total daily dose is likely with the greatest reduction arising in those who were previously controlled on high doses of beef insulin, e.g. greater than 50 units daily.

Patients who transfer from pork to human insulin should be carefully monitored for a changing requirement but, in general, a major reduction in dosage of human insulin is less likely than it is when beef insulin was previously used.

4. In the early 1990s there was an increase in the numbers of diabetics developing serious and life threatening hypoglycaemia. Of particular concern was the fact that many such patients failed to detect early signs of their hypoglycaemia (i.e. they had hypoglycaemic unawareness) and it was initially thought that wholesale transfer to human-type insulin was the significant event. However, after further investigation, it is now generally accepted that hypoglycaemic unawareness is not related to human insulin per se but rather it is a problem which has arisen as more and more tighter control of diabetes has been attempted. Accordingly the target blood glucose levels and glycosylated haemoglobin levels (indicators of how tight control is) have been set at less demanding values.

5. Local reactions at injection sites due to the insulin itself and not the preservative, may occur during the early treatment period, but are now rare with modern high purity insulins.

6. High purity insulins are also much less likely than the older types to be associated with fat atrophy at injection site which may be of cosmetic importance, particularly among young female diabetics. If fat atrophy does occur, however, it is advisable to limit this by regularly varying injection sites.

7. When dealing with diabetic patients, the nurse may be faced with the problems of a patient presenting with coma or an altered level of consciousness, which may be due to either hyperglycaemia or hypoglycaemia, and differentiation may prove difficult. A recent history of weight loss, malaise, thirst and polyuria, a recent intercurrent infection, along with signs of dry, lax skin, a dry tongue and ketotic (deep and rapid) breathing would suggest hyperglycaemia. Hypoglycaemia would be suggested by recent good health, recent alcohol consumption, a missed meal, rapidity of onset of coma, and tachycardia, sweating and pallor. If still in doubt, and while awaiting emergency medical assessment, the administration of oral or intravenous glucose (dextrose) while correcting hypoglycaemia will not significantly worsen hyperglycaemia. On the other hand, if insulin were administered in such doubtful cases, death might result if hypoglycaemia existed and such a practice is contraindicated.

General notes

1. Insulins should be stored in a cool place. In hospital a refrigerator should be used since everyday ward temperatures tend to be too high for optimum stability.

2. It is also good practice in hospital wards to add the date of first use to the label of a multidose vial of insulin and to discard any drug remaining after three months.

INTERFERON (Intron A, Roferon-A, Wellferon)

Presentation

Injection-3, 5, 9, 10, 18 and 30 mega (million) international units.

Actions and uses

Interferon is the collective name given to a group of naturally occurring proteins produced by all cells which have both antiviral and tumour-inhibiting properties. The interferons do not act directly on viral or cancer cells but trigger normal functions which counter viral and tumour cell invasion and proliferation. Although human interferon was discovered about 30 years ago, it has only recently become possible to produce the substance in the laboratory.

Theoretically at least Interferon could be used to treat a host of viral infections or malignancies but its cost is prohibitive and it is used only when benefit can be clearly established. At present it is used in the treatment of hairy cell leukaemia, chronic myeloid leukaemia, venereal wart infection (condyloma acuminata), and Kaposi's sarcoma in patients with AIDS (see Note 7).

Dosage

1. Hairy cell and chronic myeloid leukaemia: A series of subcutaneous injections of 2 mega units/m^2 body surface area given alternate daily (three times per week). A course of injections lasts for 1-2 months and possibly as long as 6 months.
2. Condyloma acuminata: Single doses of 1 mega unit are injected directly into the lesion on alternate days or multiple injections up to 5 mega units for large lesions.
3. AIDS-related Kaposi's sarcoma: An induction dose of 36 mega units is given daily for up to 10 days with maintenance doses of 36 mega units on alternate days thereafter.

Nurse monitoring

1. It should be noted that injection of any foreign protein including interferon may be associated with flu-like symptoms, occasionally severe enough to warrant co-administration of an antipyretic such as aspirin or paracetamol.
2. Also, as a foreign protein, interferon might produce an acute allergic reaction in susceptible individuals. Hypotension and cardiac arrhythmias have been reported and patients with ischaemic heart disease or recent myocardial infarction must be carefully monitored during treatment.
3. Some patients may experience central side-effects, usually confusion, which can take several weeks to resolve on stopping treatment.
4. A modified dose is required for patients with kidney impairment.

General notes

1. Vials containing interferon must be stored in a refrigerator.
2. Injections are normally prepared by reconstitution with water for injection immediately before use but may also be stored in a refrigerator if used within 24 hours.

IPRATROPIUM BROMIDE (Atrovent, Rinatec)

Presentation

Metered aerosol—20 microgram and 40 microgram per dose
Nebulizer solution—250 microgram in 1 ml
Nasal spray—20 microgram per dose

Actions and uses

Ipratropium bromide is a drug with anticholinergic actions. When inhaled via an aerosol it exerts a direct effect on the airways causing bronchodilation and relief from the symptoms of wheeze and breathlessness due to airways obstruction in diseases such as asthma, emphysema and chronic bronchitis. The drug also has antisecretory activity and in particular reduces secretory excess in patients with rhinorrhoea associated with perennial rhinitis.

Dosage

1. Obstructive airways disease:
   a. Adults: One or two inhalations (20–40 micrograms) three or four times daily. If necessary up to four inhalations may be given four times daily to obtain maximum benefit.
   b. Children: Under 6 years: One inhalation three times daily. 6-12 years: One or two inhalations three times daily. There is limited evidence that this drug causes useful bronchodilatation in asthmatic babies and infants, who are otherwise generally unresponsive to salbutamol and related beta-agonists.
2. In severe breathlessness solution may be administered via a nebulizer in which case it

supplements the action of salbutamol or other beta-agonists when nebulized together: The usual dose is 0.4–2 ml administered up to three times a day in children or four times a day in adults.
3. Rhinorrhoea: Adults only: 1–2 sprays into the nostrils up to four times daily.

Nurse monitoring
1. This drug has minor anticholinergic side-effects and may produce a dry mouth.
2. Systemic toxic effects rarely occur.

General notes
1. Ipratropium bromide inhaler may be stored at room temperature.
2. As with all pressured aerosols the container should never be punctured or incinerated after use.

IPRINDOLE (Prondol)

Presentation
Tablets—15 mg
Actions and uses
Iprindole is a tricyclic antidepressant drug. Its actions and uses are described in the section dealing with these drugs.
Dosage
15–30 mg three times daily is the normal oral dosage for the treatment of depression in adults. If necessary a maximum daily dose of up to 180 mg may be used.

Nurse monitoring
See the section on tricyclic antidepressant drugs.

General note
Iprindole tablets may be stored at room temperature.

IRON (Parenteral)
Iron Sorbitol injection BP (Jectofer)

Presentation
Intramuscular injection—100 mg elemental iron in 2 ml

Actions and uses
The indications for parenteral iron are identical to those described for oral iron but it is a potentially toxic form of therapy and must only be given when the oral route has failed e.g. due to malabsorption, persistent non-compliance, disabling gastrointestinal upsets, or when there is continuing severe blood loss. Intravenous injection is notably hazardous and therefore no longer used.
Dosage
The total replacement dose required is determined by reference to tables produced by the manufacturer and related to body weight and observed haemoglobin. The total dose may then be administered as a series of daily or alternate day intramuscular injections of 1.5 mg/kg body weight (maximum 100 mg per dose) administered in alternate muscle sites.

Nurse monitoring
1. Parenteral iron is potentially toxic and should only be used when the oral route has been tried and found to be totally unsuccessful.
2. The administration of parenteral iron may lead to hypersensitivity reactions including fever, urticaria, skin rash, muscle pain, lymphadenopathy and occasionally anaphylactic shock which is potentially fatal.
3. Test doses should always be given and facilities for emergency resuscitation and the administration of intravenous adrenaline, antihistamines and corticosteroids should be available.

General note
Iron for injection may be stored at room temperature.

IRON (Oral)

Presentation
A wide range of preparations contain iron, either on its own or in combination with folic acid or in combination

with vitamins. Iron is available for administration either as the fumarate, succinate, gluconate or sulphate.

Actions and uses

Iron may be administered usefully in two situations:

1. Where patients, due to inadequate diet or disease of the gut, have been shown by laboratory testing to be deficient in iron.
2. Where patients are known to be at risk of developing iron deficiency anaemia such as in pregnancy.

Dosage

The dosage of any iron preparation may be expressed in terms of the elemental iron which it supplies, i.e.:

1. For the treatment of iron deficiency anaemias: 100–200 mg of elemental iron daily is required in adults for 3-6 months.
2. For the prevention of iron deficiency anaemias during pregnancy: 100 mg of elemental iron (Fe) per day is recommended.

The four major salts of iron available, i.e. ferrous sulphate, ferrous fumarate, ferrous gluconate and ferrous succinate are discussed individually in the text and the tablet dosage equivalent to the elemental iron requirements is given.

Nurse monitoring

1. Iron is irritant to the gastrointestinal tract. It may produce nausea, vomiting, constipation or diarrhoea. These symptoms may be so troublesome that patients may not take their treatment. The nurse may play an important role in identifying whether patients are complying with their therapy in emphasizing to them the importance of continuing with therapy. The nurse may advise them to seek alternative preparations of iron from their doctor should the particular preparation they are taking be causing severe side-effects. Patients may find their symptoms are reduced if they take iron with food.

2. The gastrointestinal side-effects described above vary and therefore where side-effects are troublesome different types of iron salts may be administered until one with lesser effects is obtained.
3. Iron always produces a black stool, This may alarm patients and the nurse may play an important role in patient management by warning them of the possible occurrence of black stools and reassuring them of its innocence.
4. In excessive dosage iron is an extremely dangerous compound, especially in children. The nurse may contribute to the management of this problem by emphasizing to patients the importance of keeping iron preparations out of the reach of children and also by warning patients to take their children immediately to hospital for treatment should they accidentally swallow any number of iron tablets.

General note

Most iron tablets may be stored safely at room temperature.

IRON SORBITOL INJECTION BP (Jectofer)

Presentation

100 mg of elemental iron (Fe) in 2 ml ampoules for intramuscular injection.

Actions and uses

See the section on iron (parenteral).

Dosage

See the section on iron (parenteral).

Nurse monitoring

See the section on iron (parenteral).

General note

Iron for injection may be stored at room temperature.

ISOCARBOXAZID (Marplan)

Presentation

Tablets—10 mg

Actions and uses

Isocarboxazid is a monoamine oxidase inhibiting drug. Its actions and uses are described in the section on these drugs.

Dosage

10—30 mg daily.

> **Nurse monitoring**
> See the section on monoamine oxidase inhibitors.

General note

Isocarboxazid tablets may be stored at room temperature.

ISONIAZID

Presentation

Tablets—50 mg, 100 mg
Injection—50 mg in 2 ml

N.B. Isoniazid is generally used in combinations containing other drugs. These are as follows:

1. Isoniazid and sodium aminosalicylate (Inapasade)
2. Isoniazid and ethambutol (Mynah)
3. Isoniazid and rifampicin (Rifinah, Rimactazid)

Actions and uses

Isoniazid is an antibacterial drug which is of use only for the treatment of tuberculosis caused by the organism *Mycobacterium tuberculosis*. Its action may be either bacteriostatic (inhibiting growth and replication of the organism) or bacteriocidal (killing the organism), depending on the concentration achieved in the tissues. If used on its own for the treatment of tuberculosis it will be, in a large number of cases, ineffective as the organism gradually develops resistance to it and therefore it is usually used in combination with other antituberculous drugs (q v.).

Dosage

For oral or intramuscular administration:

1. Adults: 300–600 mg daily in total given in three divided doses.
2. Children: 16 mg/kg body weight daily in two divided doses.

Nurse monitoring

1. Patients undergoing treatment for tuberculosis receive their drugs for considerable periods of time. The nurse may play an important role in reminding patients that their drug therapy must be taken regularly for as long as recommended by medical staff, whether or not they themselves feel that they have recovered.
2. Gastrointestinal upset including nausea and vomiting commonly occur in patients receiving this drug.
3. Isoniazid is associated with a high incidence of neurological side-effects, the most common of which is peripheral neuropathy (altered sensation and motor function of the limbs). Peripheral neuropathy may be treated by giving pyridoxine 50–100 mg orally per day in addition to the isoniazid. Other neurological side-effects include mental disturbance, convulsion, inco-ordination, encephalopathy and alcohol intolerance. If the patient is not receiving too high a dose of the drug then the occurrence of these side-effects is an indication for change of treatment to alternative drugs.
4. Isoniazid interferes with the metabolism of naturally occurring pyridoxine. This may cause peripheral neuropathy and more rarely anaemia or a deficiency syndrome known as pellagra which is characterized by diarrhoea, dementia and dermatitis of the light exposed areas of the skin.
5. Other side-effects include disorders of the blood such as haemolytic anaemia, aplastic anaemia or agranulocytosis, skin rashes and metabolic disturbances such as hyperglycaemia and acidosis.
6. The drug should be used with caution in patients with liver disease, epilepsy or those with reduced renal function.
7. The drug should be given with caution to patients receiving phenytoin as it increases the effects of phenytoin and may precipitate phenytoin toxicity (q.v.).

General note

The drug may be stored at room temperature.

ISOPRENALINE (Saventrine)

Presentation

Tablets—30 mg
Injection—2 mg in 2 ml
Isoprenaline is included in several proprietary aerosol preparations for inhalation therapy.

Actions and uses

Isoprenaline is a powerful stimulant of the beta-adrenergic receptors which form a part of the sympathetic branch of the autonomic nervous system. It is sufficient to note that the stimulation of these beta-receptors will result in dilation of the bronchioles (small airways) in the lungs, and increase in heart rate and cardiac output. Isoprenaline therefore has a number of possible actions.

1. If given by inhalation it may reverse the constriction of bronchioles in bronchial asthma. Because of its effects on heart rate and because there are other drugs now available which have the same effect on the lungs but do not have the effect on heart rhythm the drug is rarely used for this purpose nowadays.
2. It may be used orally or intravenously to stimulate the heart rate in patients with bradycardia due to disease of the tissues which conduct electrical impulses through the heart. It is however only a second choice after electrical pacing.
3. The effect of stimulation of both heart rate and cardiac output makes it a potentially useful drug when given intravenously for the state of cardiogenic shock.

Dosage

1. The dose administered via aerosol depends on the proprietary preparation used.
2. When used in the treatment of bradycardia the dose range is

90–270 mg in three divided doses orally. It may be given by intravenous infusion at a rate of 0.5–40 microgram/minute. The intravenous dosage is usually titrated by observing the effect on blood pressure and pulse.

Nurse monitoring

1. As mentioned above, isoprenaline has the potentially serious side-effect of tachycardia when given by aerosol. Other preparations such as salbutamol (ventolin) which do not have this effect are more suitable. However, should nurses encounter patients on this drug, they should be aware that it may cause tachycardia, and in extreme cases, cardiac arrest due to ventricular fibrillation may occur.
2. When given orally or intravenously for bradycardia there is still a risk of the production of a serious tachycardia or other cardiac dysrhythmia should an excessive dose be given. Patients on oral treatment should have their pulse checked regularly and intravenous treatment should never be given unless facilities are available for ECG monitoring or unless the drug is given as an emergency treatment to sustain the patient while transfer to hospital for further treatment is effected.
3. Side-effects other than tachycardia are palpitations, tremor, precordial pain, sweating, facial flushing and headache.

General notes

1. Isoprenaline tablets may be stored at room temperature. The solution for injection should be stored in a refrigerator and protected from light.
2. When given by intravenous infusion the injection solution should be added to 5% dextrose.

ISOSORBIDE DINITRATE
(Cedocard, Imtak, Isoket, Isordil, Soni-slo, Sorbichew, Sorbid SA, Sorbitrate)

Presentation
Tablets—10 mg, 20 mg, 30 mg, 40 mg
Tablets—5 mg (sublingual and chewable)
Tablets—20 mg, 40 mg (sustained release)
Capsules—20 mg, 40 mg, (sustained release)
Buccal spray—1.25 mg/metered dose
Injection—10 mg in 10 ml, 25 mg in 50 ml, 50 mg in 50ml.

Actions and uses
This drug reduces heart work in a similar manner to glyceryl trinitrate (q.v.). It is sprayed into the mouth, chewed or allowed to dissolve under the tongue in the treatment of angina pectoris or taken orally as prophylaxis. Its advantage over glyceryl trinitrate is that it has a longer duration of action (up to 12 hours with slow release preparations).
In acute unstable angina and myocardial infarction in which there is a risk of development of heart failure, isosorbide may be administered by continuous intravenous infusion.

Dosage
1. The usual oral adult dose for prevention of angina is 10 mg three or four times a day or 20 mg twice daily of the sustained release preparation. In an acute attack 1–3 doses may be sprayed into the mouth or 5 mg taken sublingually or chewed.
2. Continuous intravenous infusions are administrated in acute unstable angina and after myocardial infarction to reduce the possibility of cardiac failure (a frequent cause of late mortality).
The dose must be carefully titrated against the individual's cardiac output.

Nurse monitoring
See the section on glyceryl trinitrate.

General note
Isosorbide dinitrate tablets and injection may be stored at room temperature.

ISOSORBIDE MONONITRATE
(Elantan, Imdur, Isomo, Monit, Mono-Cedocard)

Presentation
Tablets—10 mg, 20 mg, 40 mg
Tablets—40 mg, 60 mg (sustained release)
Capsules—25 mg, 50 mg (sustained release)

Actions and uses
This drug is one of the active metabolites of isosorbide dinitrate, the difference being that it passes through the liver after absorption without being substantially metabolized. It is often preferred therefore to isosorbide dinitrate for oral use i.e. for the prophylaxis of angina pectoris, because its effects are more predictable.

Dosage
Usually 20–40 mg is taken three times a day.
Alternatively a single daily dose of from 25 mg up to 60 mg carefully titrated against individual need may be taken using sustained release preparations.

Nurse monitoring
See the section on glyceryl trinitrate.

General note
Isosorbide mononitrate tablets and capsules may be stored at room temperature.

ISOTRETINOIN (Roaccutane)

Presentation
Capsules—5 mg, 20 mg

Actions and uses
Isotretinoin is a chemical derivative of vitamin A and, like etretinate and acitretin, belongs to the family known as the retinoids. However its major use is in the treatment of severe acne which is unresponsive to antibiotic therapy.

Dosage

Adults only: An initial dose of 0.5 mg/kg/day is taken once or twice daily for a few weeks then adjusted according to the response. The maintenance dose is usually in the range 0.1–1.0 mg/kg/day. Single courses of up to four months are given.

Nurse monitoring

1. Vitamin A derivatives are strongly teratogenic and fetal malformations are highly likely in the event of pregnancy. Pregnancy must be excluded in women of childbearing age at the outset and patients actively counselled thereafter to ensure that adequate contraceptive measures are always taken. Therapeutic abortion is offered if pregnancy occurs.
Furthermore, pregnancy must be avoided for at least 4 weeks after treatment is discontinued since isotertinoin is stored for prolonged periods in the body tissues.

2. It is important to note that treatment with isotretinoin must be arranged through a specialist clinic and supplies of the drug are restricted to hospitals only.

3. Vitamin A compounds are poorly tolerated by some patients (hence the need for careful dosage adjustment). Dryness of the skin, erythema, pruritis and alopecia are common and erosion of mucous surfaces is possible. Other side-effects include headaches, nausea, drowsiness, joint pain and myalgia.

4. Hepatotoxicity occurs and liver function tests should be carried out regularly to detect early liver damage. Concurrent use of hepatotoxic drugs and alcohol should be discouragred and treatment avoided in the event of existing liver impairment.

5. A further metabolic effect results in an unfavourable shift in the blood lipid profile and hyperlipidaemia. This may have important consequences for patients who have a history of angina or myocardial infarction and other risk factors for coronary heart disease. Care is also required in patients with diabetes in whom altered glucose tolerance may develop.

6. Isotretinoin must not be used in patients with renal failure.

General note

Isotretinoin capsules are stored at room temperature and protected from light.

ISPAGHULA (Fybogel, Isogel)

Presentation

Sachets—3.5 g
Granules—165 g canister

Actions and uses

See the section discussing the actions of laxatives. Ispaghula falls into the bulk forming group, i.e. it is a bulking agent. The ispaghula husk, like bran, is a natural dietary fibre supplement and it is used in those disorders of the bowel thought to be associated with reduced dietary fibre, i.e.:
1. Diverticular disease
2. Spastic or irritable colon
3. Constipation.

Dosage

One sachet (3.5 g) or two 5 ml spoonfuls of granules taken twice daily after meals, stirred into a glass of cold water.

Nurse monitoring

There are no specific problems associated with this drug.

General note

Sachets and granules containing ispaghula husk may be stored at room temperature.

K

KAOLIN

Presentation
Kaolin is included in many anti-diarrhoeal mixtures.

Actions and uses
Kaolin is a highly absorbent powder which absorbs toxic and other substances from the alimentary tract and increases the bulk of the faeces. This has an effect of reducing the frequency and severity of diarrhoea. It is administered in a suspension.

Dosage
1. Adults: 5–25 g as required.
2. Children: 1–5 g as required.

Nurse monitoring
1. Kaolin is not absorbed and therefore has no systemic effects.
2. The only point worthy of note is that as it produces bulk within the gut it is contraindicated in patients with intestinal obstruction.

General note
Preparations containing kaolin may be stored at room temperature. The powder however does not dissolve in water and such mixtures must be thoroughly shaken before each dose is withdrawn.

KETOCONAZOLE (Nizoral)

Presentation
Tablets—200 mg
Oral suspension—100 mg in 5 ml
Cream—2%

Actions and uses
Ketoconazole is an anti-fungal drug. It has a major advantage over other anti-fungal agents in that effective blood levels may be obtained after oral administration. It is used in the treatment of the following disorders:
1. Treatment of fungal infections of skin and hair by dermatophytes and/or yeasts, i.e. dermatomycosis, pityriasis versicolor, chronic mucocutaneous candidosis
2. Treatment of yeast infections of the mouth (*Candida albicans*)
3. For gut sterilization
4. For treatment of systemic mycoses, i.e. systemic candidosis, paracoccidioidomycosis, histoplasmosis, coccidioidomycosis etc.
5. Recurrent vaginal candidosis
6. It may be used prophylactically in 'at risk' groups, i.e. those with reduced immunity due to cytotoxic therapy for malignant disease.

Dosage
1. For the uses described under 1, 2, 3, 4 and 6 above:
   a. Adults: Initially 200 mg once daily is given. The dose may be doubled if a satisfactory response is not achieved. The treatment is continued for at least 1 week after symptoms have cleared and the usual duration of treatment varies widely according to the condition under treatment, i.e. 10 days for oral thrush, 6 months for systemic infections with paracoccidioidomycosis, coccidioidomycosis and histoplasmosis.
   Cream is applied once or twice daily for tinea infection.
   Shampoo is used twice weekly for 2-4 weeks to treat seborrhoeic dermatitis or once daily

for up to 5 days for scalp infection with pityriasis versicolor. It is also used every 1-2 weeks as prophylaxis.
   b. Children: the single daily dose is calculated on the basis of 3 mg per kg.
   See adult use of topical preparations.
2. For the treatment of recurrent vaginal candidosis: 200 mg twice daily for 5 days.

Nurse monitoring

1. The commonest problem associated with administration of this drug is gastrointestinal upset, predominantly nausea.
2. Skin rash and pruritus are also fairly common.
3. Any drug which reduces the acid content of the stomach such as antacids, cimetidine, ranitidine and anticholinergic drugs will impair the absorption of ketoconazole and therefore at least 2 hours should be allowed between administration of ketoconazole and any of these agents.
4. Ketoconazole tablets should be taken with meals when gastric acidity is high.
5. The drug should be avoided in pregnancy.

General note

All preparations may be stored at room temperature.

KETOPROFEN (Alrheumat, Orudis, Oruvail)

Presentation

Capsules—50 mg, 100 mg
Capsules—100 mg, 200 mg sustained release
Injection—100 mg in 2 ml
Suppositories—100 mg

Actions and uses

See the section on non-steroidal anti-inflammatory analgesic drugs.

Dosage

1. Oral: The usual dose is 50–100 mg twice daily although 50 mg three or four times daily is used occasionally. In a few cases some patients achieve adequate control with a single (usually bed-time) dose of 100–200 mg sustained release capsule.
2. Intramuscular: Acute inflammatory pain—100 mg deep i.m. injection 4-hourly up to a maximum dose of 200 mg in one day and no longer than 3 days.
3. Rectal: A single suppository inserted at night to supplement daytime oral dosing.
N.B. No data available in children.

Nurse monitoring

See the section on non-steroidal anti-inflammatory analgesic drugs.

General note

Ketoprofen preparations may be stored at room temperature.

KETOROLAC (Toradol)

Presentation

Tablets—10 mg
Injection—10 mg, 30 mg in 1 ml

Actions and uses

The actions and uses of this potent non-steroidal anti-inflammatory drug (NSAID) are described under the group heading. Ketorolac is however licensed only for short term use (up to 2 days by injection or 7 days orally) and restricted to the treatment of moderate-to-severe post-operative pain. This should be noted in the light of severe adverse reactions to the drug during long term use (see below).

Dosage

1. Adults only:
   a. By intravenous or intramuscular injection, a dose of 10 mg initially with further doses of 10–30 mg 4 to 6-hourly as required up to a total of 90 mg daily. Maximum treatment duration of 2 days.
   b. Orally, 10 mg 4-6 hourly as required for pain up to 40 mg daily in total. Treatment duration should not exceed 7 days.

Nurse monitoring

1. The following dosage restrictions apply in the case of elderly patients: do not exceed 60 mg by injection and do not give oral therapy more frequently than 6-8 hourly.
2. Serious and even fatal reactions have been associated with this drug and long term use is not recommended. Patients especially at risk include those with a history of asthma, haemorrhagic stroke, actively bleeding peptic ulcer, where there is a high risk of haemorrhage associated with surgery, those on current anticoagulant therapy, and patients with renal impairment, hypovolaemia or dehydration.
3. See also the appropriate section under non-steroidal anti-inflammatory analgesic drugs.

General notes

1. Ketorolac preparations are stored at room temperature and protected from light.
2. Though normally administered by bolus i.v. injection, the drug may be diluted in sodium chloride 0.9% or glucose 5% for more prolonged i.v. administration.

KETOTIFEN (Zaditen)

Presentation

Tablets and Capsules—1 mg
Elixir—1mg in 5 ml

Actions and uses

Ketotifen binds to cells present in the airways which under certain conditions would normally release chemicals which would cause an increase in muscle tone in the airways thereby causing bronchospasm manifest as dyspnoea and wheezing. It is, therefore, useful for the prophylactic treatment of conditions associated with bronchospasm.

Dosage

1. The usual adult dosage is 1–2 mg twice daily with food.
2. Children (over 2 years): 1mg twice daily with food.

Nurse monitoring

1. It is important to note that this drug is of prophylactic use only and will not be of any benefit in the treatment of an established attack of bronchospasm.
2. The nurse may play an important role in encouraging patients to persevere with the therapy in the early stages when symptomatic benefit may not be obtained. It has been found in practice that symptomatic benefit is only established after several weeks of treatment.
3. The nurse may also play an important role in encouraging patients to persist with this therapy despite disturbing symptoms in the early treatment period of drowsiness, dizziness and dry mouth, also confidently reassuring them that these symptoms will become far less troublesome as treatment continues.

General note

Ketotifen preparations may be stored at room temperature.

KLEAN-PREP

Klean-Prep is the trade name for a complex mixture of laxative and electrolytes. It is recognised by this title and described as such in the following text.

Presentation

Powder for reconstitution containing polyethylene glycol, sodium sulphate, sodium chloride, sodium bicarbonate, and potassium chloride.

Actions and uses

Once reconstituted, the Klean-Prep mixture is swallowed. It acts as an osmotic laxative designed to completely empty the bowel contents within 4 hours or more, thus facilitating colonoscopy or X-ray or surgery of the lower bowel. The complex formulation should neither remove electrolytes from within nor increase the possibility of potentially harmful absorption of electrolytes.

Dosage

Adults: Quantities of 250 ml are swallowed at 10-minute intervals until the bowel effluent is clear or else the maximum dose of 4 litres has been drunk.

Nurse monitoring

1. Not surprisingly, patients may experience difficulty in swallowing such large volumes of liquid. The following actions may help the patient:
   a. The solution should be reconstituted with warm water.
   b. Fruit juice swallowed at the same time or mixed with Klean-Prep may assist some patients.
   c. If swallowing is not possible, administration via a naso-gastric tube at a rate of 20–30 ml per minute can be tried.
2. Patients should be instructed to fast for at least 4 hours before administration.
3. Nausea, abdominal bloating, cramps and anal irritation are often associated with ingestion of such large volumes of fluid and patients should be reassured accordingly.

General note

Klean-Prep powder (for reconstitution) and ready-prepared liquid may be stored at room temperature.

L

LABETALOL (Trandate)

Presentation

Tablets—50 mg, 100 mg, 200 mg, 400 mg

Injection—100 mg in 20 ml

Actions and uses

Labetalol is a beta-adrenoreceptor blocker and therefore has all the actions of beta-adrenoreceptor blocking drugs (q.v.). However, it also blocks alpha receptor sites in peripheral blood vessels such as arterioles and produces dilation of these vessels. This additional effect adds to its capacity to reduce blood pressure and labetalol's main use is in the treatment of hypertension and co-existing angina pectoris.

Dosage

1. In hypertensive emergencies it may be given by slow intravenous injection (50 mg given over a period of at least 1 minute), or by intravenous infusion of a solution containing 200 mg in 200 ml given at a rate of 2 mg per minute. The maximum intravenous dosage is 300 mg.
2. The usual adult oral maintenance dose is 300–600 mg per day in three divided doses. Up to 2.4 g daily may be given in divided doses to establish control of hypertension.

Nurse monitoring

1. Labetalol has all the side-effects of beta-adrenoreceptor blocking drugs (q.v.).
2. Its additional alpha blocking actions makes it especially likely to produce postural hypotension. Patients must be warned of this and instructed on how to avoid its effects by changing posture slowly.
3. When patients receive intravenous doses of this drug they should be in a supine position to avoid hypotension.
4. Labetalol has a number of side-effects not seen with other beta-blocking drugs and these include difficulty with micturition, epigastric pain, blurred vision, a lichenoid skin rash and tingling sensations in the scalp.

General note

Labetalol tablets and injection may be stored at room temperature. The injection solution is however sensitive to light.

LACTULOSE (Duphalac)

Presentation

Syrup—3.35 g in 5 ml

Actions and uses

Lactulose is a sugar compound which is neither digested in nor absorbed from human gut. When taken it passes into the large bowel where it affects both the bowel bacteria and the amount of water present in the stool. It has two main uses:

1. As a laxative it falls into group 2 in terms of its mode of action (see the section on laxatives).
2. It is used for the treatment of patients with severe liver cell disease and hepatic encephalo-pathy. Its use in this condition is to reduce the amount of protein absorbed from the gut.

Dosage
1. For constipation:
   a. Adults: 15 ml syrup twice per day.
   b. Children: Babies—2.5 ml; Children under 5 years—5 ml; 5-10 years—10 ml.
2. For the treatment of hepatic encephalopathy: doses of 30–50 ml three times daily are given initially and subsequently adjusted to produce two or three soft stools each day.

Nurse monitoring
1. This drug is largely without side-effects, except in two very rare conditions:
   a. Galactosaemia where patients are intolerant of the sugar galactose which is contained in the commercial syrup preparation of this drug.
   b. There is a small group of patients who are actually intolerant to lactulose.

General notes
1. The syrup may be stored at room temperature.
2. It should not be stored in a refrigerator and never be allowed to freeze.
3. For ease of administration it may be diluted with water or with fruit juices etc.

LAMOTRIGINE (Lamictal)

Presentation
Tablets—25 mg, 50 mg, 100 mg
Actions and uses
Lamotrigine is an anticonvulsant which appears to stabilize conducting tissue in the CNS by inhibiting release of certain excitatory neurotransmitter substances, notably glutamate whose presence is thought to be associated with the generation of seizure activity. The drug should not be used as sole anticonvulsant but rather as add-on therapy in refractory epilepsy in which other first line drugs are ineffective when used alone. It is currently indicated in partial and secondary generalized tonic-clonic seizures.

Dosage
Adults: Initially 50 mg bd for 2 weeks, then increased gradually up to a maximum of 200 mg twice daily according to response.

Nurse monitoring
1. This is a relatively new drug and active monitoring and reporting of all suspected adverse reactions should be encouraged.
2. Side-effects so far reported include maculopapular skin rash (up to 10% of patients affected), and rarely angio-oedema and Stevens-Johnson syndrome.
3. Central side-effects include diplopia, blurred vision, dizziness, drowsiness, incoordination, and headache.
4. Gastrointestinal upsets are also reported.
5. The metabolism of lamotrigine is increased by other anticonvulsants which stimulate liver microsomal enzyme production e.g. carbamazepine, phenobarbitone, phenytoin.
6. Lamotrigine has weak antifolate activity and should be avoided in pregnancy.
7. Lamotrigine should be used with caution in patients with renal or hepatic impairment. It is both metabolized by the liver and excreted via the kidney.

General note
Lamotrigine tablets are stored at room temperature in a dry place.

LAXATIVES

Presentation
See individual drugs.
Actions and uses
Laxatives act principally by one of five mechanisms:
1. They may irritate the bowel wall and produce a reflex increased bowel movement, so-called stimulant laxatives.

2. They may increase the amount of water which is taken up and retained by the stool, so-called osmotic laxatives.
3. They may increase the amount of bulk within the stool and promote a more natural colonic action and more regular defaecation i.e. fibre and related bulking agents.
4. They may act as a 'wetting agent' thereby rendering the stool more mobile and easier to pass i.e. stool softeners. Similarly liquid paraffin increases stool mobility by a physical action.
5. Locally acting agents (suppositories and enemas) may stimulate the colon directly or facilitate passage of an impacted formed stool by a local physical effect.

Dosage
See individual drugs.

Nurse monitoring
1. The taking of laxatives is a national pastime. However, the nurse may play an important role in detecting serious disease by noting change in bowel habit manifest by a need for an increase in frequency or dosage of regular laxatives or a failure of their action.
2. In certain situations regular laxative use is totally justified, particularly for all patients receiving regular opioid analgesic therapy in whom constipation can be universally anticipated.
3. Individual side-effects for the various drugs are described under each drug in turn.

General note
See individual drugs.

LEVODOPA (Larodopa)

Presentation
Tablets—500 mg
Actions and uses
In Parkinson's disease it has been shown that certain areas of the brain are depleted of a substance known as dopamine. It has further been shown that treatment with sub-stances which increase concentrations of dopamine in these areas leads to an improvement in symptoms. Levodopa is a precursor of dopamine and is converted in the body to dopamine. It is used, therefore, for the treatment of Parkinson's disease.

Dosage
N.B. This drug is not recommended for administration to children. For adults: an initial dose of 125 mg twice daily immediately after food is recommended. The dose is doubled after a week and thereafter increased at weekly intervals by 375 mg per day, until control is achieved the total daily dose being given in four or five doses.

Nurse monitoring
1. It is important to note that there are new preparations available (madopar and sinemet, q.v.) which combine levodopa with another compound which reduces the rate of metabolism of levodopa in the body and therefore allows low doses to be administered and leads to a reduction in the incidence of side-effects.
2. Side-effects, usually dose-related, occur at some time in most patients. During the initiation of therapy nausea, vomiting, anorexia, weakness and hypotension (commonly postural) may occur. It is important for the nurse to note that nausea and vomiting may be reduced by the administration of the drug immediately after food. Occasionally, however, an anti-emetic drug may be necessary. At any stage in the treatment the following other side-effects may occur.
   a. Psychiatric disturbance including elation, depression, anxiety, agitation, aggression, hallucination and delusion.
   b. Involuntary movements commonly in the form of oral dyskinesia (rhythmic writhing movements of the mouth and tongue) or similar writhing movements of the limbs. These

effects are usually dose-related and may disappear after a reduction in the dose. They are particularly likely to occur in the elderly.

c. Abnormalities in liver function tests and other biochemical blood values may occur.

d. Patients on levodopa may notice a darkening in colour with a reddish tinge of the urine and further darkening if the urine is left to stand. They should be reassured that this is quite normal and does not imply any renal damage.

General note

The drug may be stored at room temperature.

LIGNOCAINE

1. Local anaesthetic—Lignostab, Lidothesin
2. Antidysrhythmic—Xylocard

1. LOCAL ANAESTHETIC

Presentation

Injection—0.5%, 1%, 1.5%, 2% for infiltration anaesthesia and spinal regional nerve block.
Topical solution—4%
Antiseptic gel—2%
Oral gel—2%
Eye drops—4%
Local anaesthetic spray—10%
Ointment—5%
Preparations are also available with adrenaline added (see below).

Actions and uses

Lignocaine is a local anaesthetic with very wide uses and may be applied topically on the cornea, conjunctiva, and mucous surfaces of the mouth, rectum and urethra. It may be injected subcutaneously round specific sites, e.g. before suturing, or into the region of a main nerve branch to block an area of pain receptors prior to dental procedures. It may also be injected around the spinal nerves as they leave the spinal cord to produce regional anaesthesia for obstetric and surgical procedures.

Dosage

Individual doses for infiltration and spinal or regional nerve block vary with the type of procedure—0.5% to 1.5% are generally used for infiltration and 1% to 2% for nerve block and spinal block. Preparations are available with added adrenaline which by its vasoconstrictor effect reduces the rate at which lignocaine leaves the site of injection, and therefore prolongs its effect.

Nurse monitoring

1. By far the most important aspect of nurse monitoring in patients prescribed this drug takes place before the drug is given. Should lignocaine with adrenaline be administered instead of plain lignocaine, especially to the peripheries, severe tissue ischaemia leading perhaps to gangrene and loss of part of a limb may occur. Conversely, administration of plain lignocaine instead of lignocaine and adrenaline may considerably reduce the duration of analgesia, and lead to severe patient discomfort. Thus, the nurse and doctor must check thoroughly in advance that the type and strength of the solution is appropriate.
2. Pain or stinging may occur at the site of application before the onset of local anaesthetic effect.
3. Skin rashes due to local allergy may occur.
4. Excessive dosage may lead to side-effects.

General note

Lignocaine solution may be stored at room temperature.

2. ANTIDYSRHYTHMIC

Presentation

Intravenous—2%
For infusion—20%

Actions and uses

Lignocaine suppresses the conduction of electrical impulses through heart muscle and may be given intravenously to treat serious ventricular dysrhythmias.

Dosage

1. Bolus dosage at onset of treatment: 1 mg/kg given over 5 minutes. This may be repeated once or twice if necessary at 5-10 minute intervals.
2. Maintenance regime: Initially 2 mg per minute, increasing to 3 mg per minute and a maximum of 4 mg per minute if necessary. This regime is usually continued for 48 hours and prior to discontinuation loading doses of oral antidysrhythmic are given.

Nurse monitoring

1. Lignocaine is often given in emergency situations, i.e. at a cardiac arrest and it is imperative in a situation where mistakes can easily be made that the nurse remembers that the 20% solution is never appropriate for bolus injection.
2. Calcium chloride or gluconate cannot be injected into a solution containing lignocaine or the calcium salt will precipitate in a solid form.
3. Too rapid or excessive intravenous dosage may be associated with the following side-effects. nervousness, dizziness, blurred vision, tremor and convulsions; nausea; hypotension and bradycardia; respiratory depression (with very high doses).
4. Patients with impaired liver function are more likely to develop adverse side-effects.

General notes

1. Lignocaine preparation may be stored at room temperature.
2. Lignocaine 20% solution for cardiac use must be added to dextrose 5% or laevulose 5% (1 g added to 500 ml if infusion fluid) to give a final concentration of 0.2%.

LISINOPRIL (Carace, Zestril)

Presentation

Tablets—2.5 mg, 5 mg, 10 mg, 20 mg

Actions and uses

See section on ACE inhibitors.

Dosage

Range: 10–40 mg as a single daily dose.

Nurse monitoring

See section on ACE inhibitors

General note

Lisinopril tablets may be stored at room temperature.

LITHIUM CARBONATE (Camcolit, Phasal, Priadel)

Presentation

Tablets—250 mg, 400 mg
—300 mg, 400 mg (both as slow release tablets)

Actions and uses

Lithium carbonate, by an unknown mechanism, has been found to be useful for the treatment of depression in two particular instances:

1. It has been found to control both the manic and depressive phases of manic depressive psychosis.
2. It has been found that continuing treatment with lithium reduces the recurrence of depressive and manic phases in patients who have already been found to have endogenous depression.

Dosage

For the treatment of depression in adults the precise dosage is that which maintains the plasma lithium level in the range 0.6–1.4 mmol/l. Treatment is usually taken once per day and it is important that all patients receiving the drug have their dosage carefully monitored to keep them within the above range.

Nurse monitoring

1. Side-effects which are usually mainly seen if an excess dose is being taken include anorexia, nausea, vomiting, diarrhoea, thirst, polyuria, fatigue, malaise, dizziness, confusion, hypotension and cardiac dysrhythmias.

2. The drug should not be used in patients with renal failure or cardiac disease.
3. The drug may affect thyroid function rendering the patient clinically hypothyroid. The nurse may aid the detection of this side-effect by noticing the formation of a goitre (thyroid swelling). Most patients on this drug are regularly monitored by clinical and biochemical testing for the development of this effect.
4. Elderly patients require lower doses of this drug if side-effects are to be avoided.

General note
Preparations containing lithium carbonate may be stored at room temperature.

LOFEPRAMINE (Gamanil)

Presentation
Tablets—70 mg
Actions and uses
Lofepramine is a member of the tricyclic antidepressant group and the section under tricyclic anti-depressants should be consulted.
Dosage
Adults: Usually 70 mg twice or three times daily but higher doses are used in severe resistant depression.

Nurse monitoring
The nurse monitoring aspects described under tricyclic anti-depressants apply.

General note
Lofepramine tablets may be stored at room temperature but must be protected from light.

LOMUSTINE (CCNU)

Presentation
Capsules—10 mg, 40 mg
Actions and uses
Lomustine is a cytotoxic drug which inhibits cell growth and division by combining with and rendering useless important substances necessary for cell growth and also by

inhibiting the enzymes responsible for the incorporation of these substances into the cell. It may be used alone, with radiotherapy, or in combination with other cytotoxic drugs in the treatment of the following conditions:
1. Brain tumours
2. Bronchogenic carcinoma
3. Malignant melanoma
4. Hodgkin's disease
5. It has been occasionally given for non-Hodgkin's lymphoma, myeloma, tumours of the gut, kidney, testis, ovary, cervix, uterus and breast.

Dosage
The drug is taken orally. The dose for adults and children is up to 120–130 mg per m^2 as a single dose repeated every 6-8 weeks.

Nurse monitoring
1. Bone marrow suppression is an important side-effect and the resultant leucopenia and thrombocytopenia leaves the patient at risk from severe infection and haemorrhage.
2. Other side-effects include anorexia, nausea, vomiting, alopecia, stomatitis and altered liver function.
3. White blood cell counts, platelet counts and liver function tests are normally monitored during treatment.
4. The nurse should be constantly aware that most cytotoxic drugs are irritant to the skin and mucous surfaces, and are in general very toxic. Great care should therefore be exercised when handling these drugs, and in particular spillage or contamination of personnel or the environment must be avoided. If cytotoxic drugs are handled regularly it is theoretically possible that repeated skin contact or inhalation may produce systemic toxic effects and in nurses who have developed hypersensitivity, severe local and general hypersensitivity reactions

General note
Lomustine capsules may be stored at room temperature. It is important to note that they should be stored in the original container and protected from light and moisture.

LOPERAMIDE (Imodium)

Presentation
Capsules—2 mg
Syrup—1 mg in 5 ml
Actions and uses
Loperamide has a direct action on the nerves which control muscular movement of the intestinal wall. Its overall effect is to slow the passage of substances through the intestine and its use is therefore in the treatment of diarrhoea.
Dosage
1. Adults: 4 mg initially followed by 2 mg after each loose stool. The maximum daily dosage should not exceed 16 mg
2. Children: 4-8 years—1 mg four times per day; 9-12 years—2 mg four times per day.

It is recommended that all the above doses be given until the diarrhoea is controlled.

Nurse monitoring
1. The drug is very poorly absorbed from the gut and therefore produces little in the way of side-effects.
2. Continued use after diarrhoea has been controlled may produce constipation.
3. It should always be remembered that persistent diarrhoea may be indicative of a serious underlying condition and, therefore, the patients should be encouraged to consult their doctors should chronic use of this drug be discovered.

General notes
1. Loperamide preparations may be stored at room temperature.
2. For ease of administration the syrup may be diluted with water.
3. The commercial syrup is sugar-free and is, therefore, suitable for patients who are disaccharide intolerant.

LOPRAZOLAM

Presentation
Tablets—1 mg
Actions and uses
Loprazolam is a benzodiazepine and the section on these drugs should be consulted for a brief general account. It has a marked sedative effect and is taken as a hypnotic to induce sleep. Of particular interest is the short action of this drug in the body which tends to produce a normal length sleep of up to 8 hours without the hang-over effect which occasionally extends into the following day with other hypnotics.
Dosage
Adults: 1–2 mg taken on retiring. Elderly patients should receive the lower dosage.

Nurse monitoring
See the section on benzodiazepines.

General note
Tablets containing loprazolam may be stored at room temperature.

LORAZEPAM

Presentation
Tablets—1 mg, 2.5 mg
Injection—4 mg in 1 ml
Actions and uses
Lorazepam is a benzodiazepine drug (q.v.). It has a short duration of action compared to other drugs of this group. It has two major uses:
1. For the control of anxiety.
2. Because of its short duration of action it is sometimes used as an alternative to diazepam for sedation prior to minor operative or dental procedures.
Dosage
1. For the treatment of anxiety adults receive 1–4 mg daily in divided doses.
2. For sedation prior to minor surgical or dental procedures:

2–4 mg is given as a single dose, 1 or 2 hours before the procedure begins.

3. By intravenous and intramuscular injection: a dose of 0.03–0.05 mg/kg body weight may be given or a single dose of 4 mg (2 mg for children) has been given to control status epilepticus.

Nurse monitoring
See the section on benzodiazepines.

General note
Tablets containing lorazepam may be stored at room temperature.

LOW MOLECULAR WEIGHT HEPARIN/HEPARINOID (LMWH)

Presentation
This new group of injectable anti-coagulants include the following compounds—listed by approved (and trade) name and presentation:
Enoxaparin (Clexane)—2000 i.u. and 4000 i.u. pre-filled syringes
Dalteparin (Fragmin)—2500 i.u. and 10 000 i.u. ampoules; 2500 i.u. and 5000 i.u. pre-filled syringes
Tinzaparin (Innohep, Logiparin)—2500 i.u., 3500 i.u., 4500 i.u. and 5000 i.u. pre-filled syringes
Danaparoid (Orgaron)—Heparinoid—750 i.u. ampoules
Note: Strength of above preparations indicates anti-Factor Xa activity in standard units—see Actions and Uses.

Actions and uses
The LMWHs are a group of specific anticoagulant proteins and heparin-like substances which are derived commercially via a process termed 'fractionation'. They possess certain properties which distinguish them from standard (unfractionated) heparin.

1. They have a much longer duration of action.
2. Their anti-Factor Xa action is more pronounced.
3. They possess less anti-IIa (antithrombin) activity.
4. They have little, if any, inhibitory effect on platelet aggregation or the binding of fibrin to platelets.

It is claimed that, as a result of 1-4 above, LMWHs are more active and persistent than standard heparin on clot formation and less likely to be associated with haemorrhagic consequences. These drugs are used in place of conventional heparin in the prevention of deep-vein thrombosis during and after surgery (various types but particularly if the risk of haemorrhage is high) and in association with haemodialysis.

Dosage
1. Adults only—administered by subcutaneous injection. The usual range is 2000–3500 i.u. (750 i.u. heparinoid) before surgery then once daily for 7-10 days post-operatively (twice daily in the case of heparinoid).
2. Lower doses may be used where the risk of haemorrhage is high (e.g. orthopaedic surgery) or higher doses if the risk of DVT is high.

Nurse monitoring
1. The nurse monitoring aspects of heparin (q.v.) apply to this drug.
2. In surgical patients it is recommended that the first dose be given 2 hours before surgery commences.

General note
Check storage conditions for individual LMWHs with Pharmacy.

M

MADOPAR

Note: This combination now officially known as *co-beneldopa*.

Presentation

Madopar 62.5 capsules containing 50 mg of levodopa and 12.25 mg of benserazide hydrochloride. Madopar 125 capsules containing 100 mg of levodopa and 25 mg benserazide hydrochloride. Madopar 250 capsules containing 200 mg of levodopa and 50 mg of benserazide hydrochloride.

Dispersible tablets containing 50 mg and 100 mg levodopa with respectively 12.5 mg and 25 mg benserazide.

Slow-release capsules containing 100 mg levodopa and 25 mg benserazide.

Actions and uses

This drug contains levodopa and benserazide hydrochloride. (See the section on levodopa for a description of its actions and uses.) The advantage of combining levodopa with benserazide is that the latter drug inhibits conversion of levodopa to dopamine in tissues of the body other than brain, thus allowing more levodopa to reach the brain resulting in an increased clinical effect. It is thought that this drug produces a more rapid response at initiation of therapy, has a simpler dosage regime and is associated with fewer gastrointestinal side-effects.

Dosage

1. Patients not previously treated with levodopa: Initially one capsule of Madopar 125 should be given twice daily and this dose may be increased by one capsule a day every 3rd or 4th day until a full therapeutic effect is obtained or side-effects supervene. The effective dose usually lies within the range of 4–8 capsules of madopar 125 daily in divided doses and most patients require no more than six capsules of madopar 125 daily. Optimal improvement is usually seen in 1 to 3 weeks.

2. Patients previously treated with levodopa: Levodopa should be discontinued 24 hours prior to the first dose of Madopar and the patient may then be initiated on a total of one less Madopar 125 capsule daily than the total number of 500 mg levodopa tablets or capsules previously taken. After a week the initial dose may be increased in the manner described for patients not on previous therapy (see (1) above).

3. Madopar 62.5 capsules are used to gradually tailor individual dosage requirements and are of particular value in the elderly who may readily respond to small dosage increments.

4. The use of slow release capsules, though tailored to the individual patient, may allow less frequent dosage when frequent regular doses are used in patients with 'end of dose' deterioration in their symptoms.

Nurse monitoring

The nurse monitoring aspects of levodopa (q.v.) apply to this drug with two major exceptions:

1. The rate of onset of clinical improvement is faster with this drug.

2. There are fewer gastrointestinal side-effects with this drug compared to levodopa.

General notes

1. The drug should be stored at room temperature.
2. The drug should be protected from moisture.

MAGNESIUM HYDROXIDE (Cream/Milk of Magnesia)

Presentation

Magnesium hydroxide is used alone or more often combined with other antacids in a range of oral liquid and solid dosage forms.

Actions and uses

This drug is an antacid and is often useful for the symptomatic relief of dyspeptic pain. It is also an osmotically active laxative compound (see laxatives).

Dosage

This varies with the type of preparation used.

Nurse monitoring

1. Magnesium hydroxide on its own frequently causes diarrhoea if excessive doses are taken (it is in fact used as a laxative) and therefore as an antacid it is often used in combination with aluminium salts which have a constipating side-effect.
2. In patients with chronic renal failure, increased levels of magnesium in the blood may be produced, leading to signs of magnesium toxicity such as hypotension, flushing and a sensation of heat and thirst, progressing to nausea, vomiting, lethargy and finally coma with weakness and paralysis of all muscles.
3. The absorption and therefore the clinical effect of other drugs such as salicylates, digoxin and antibiotics may be impaired.
4. The dosage of oral anticoagulants may need to be altered if magnesium hydroxide is administered.

General note

Preparations containing magnesium hydroxide may be stored at room temperature. To exert a maximum antacid effect tablets should be thoroughly chewed before swallowing.

MAPROTILINE (Ludiomil)

Presentation

Tablets—10 mg, 25 mg, 50 mg, 75 mg

Actions and uses

Maprotiline is an antidepressant drug which is derived from and is closely related chemically to tricyclic antidepressants. Its actions and uses are similar to those described for tricyclic antidepressants (q.v.).

Dosage

For the treatment of depression in adults: 25–150 mg per day is given either in three divided doses or as a single evening dose taken on retiring.

Nurse monitoring

1. The nurse monitoring notes on tricyclic antidepressants (q.v.) are applicable to this drug.
2. It is worth noting that there is a particularly high incidence of skin rashes with this drug.

General note

Maprotiline tablets may be stored at room temperature.

MAXEPA

Presentation

Capsules and liquid.

Actions and uses

Maxepa is a preparation of fish oils containing two substances called docosahexaenoic acid (DHA) and eicosapentaenoic acid (EPA). DHA and EPA are present in the staple diet of the Eskimo in whom coronary heart disease is almost unknown, possibly as a result of the cholesterol lowering effect of these fatty acids. Maxepa is therefore used as a dietary supplement in order to reduce the blood cholesterol and, mainly, triglyceride and so also the risk of heart disease.

It is of interest that DHA and EPA also inhibit prostaglandin synthesis in a manner similar to the non-steroidal anti-inflammatory analgesics and a future role in the treatment of inflammatory disease, e.g. rheumatoid arthritis, osteoarthritis, etc. is possible.

Dosage

Usually 5 capsules or 5 ml liquid twice daily.

Nurse monitoring

1. Fish oils have a characteristic smell and taste and may cause nausea and 'fishy' breath.
2. They may also increase the risk of bleeding, by platelet stickiness, in patients also receiving anticoagulant therapy.

General note

Maxepa capsules and liquid may be stored at room temperature.

MEBENDAZOLE (Vermox)

Presentation

Tablets—100 mg
Suspension—100 mg in 5 ml

Actions and uses

This drug is effective in the treatment of helminthic infections both in the United Kingdom and the tropics. It is used for the treatment of hookworm, roundworm (Ascaris), threadworm and whipworm.

Dosage

For adults and children aged 2 years and above:

1. Threadworm: A single dose of one tablet or one 5 ml spoonful.
2. Whipworm, roundworm and hookworm: One tablet or one 5 ml spoonful twice daily (morning and evening) for three consecutive days.

Nurse monitoring

1. It is important to note that no special procedures such as purging, use of laxatives, and/or dietary changes are required when using this drug.
2. The drug is not at present recommended for use in children under 2 years.
3. The drug should not be given to pregnant women.
4. Particularly for the treatment of threadworm, it is advisable that all members of a family whether obviously infected or not should be treated at the same time to ensure eradication.
5. Side-effects are mild and consist of transient abdominal pain and occasional diarrhoea.

General note

The drug may be stored at room temperature.

MEBEVERINE (Colofac)

Presentation

Tablets—135 mg

Actions and uses

Mebeverine relieves colonic spasm by a direct action on the smooth muscle of the colon. It is used to relieve abdominal pain, cramps, flatulence, and diarrhoea associated with irritable bowel syndrome and the gastrointestinal spasm associated with diverticular disease, gastritis, duodenitis, oesophagitis, cholecystitis, inflammatory bowel disease, peptic ulceration and hiatus hernia.

Dosage

1. The adult dose is 135 mg three times daily taken 20 minutes before meals.
2. Lower maintenance doses may be used once a therapeutic effect has been achieved.
3. The drug is not recommended for children under 10 years.

Nurse monitoring

No specific problems or side-effects are associated with the administration of this drug.

General note

Mebeverine tablets may be stored at room temperature.

MEBHYDROLIN (Fabahistin)

Presentation

Tablets—50 mg

Actions and uses

Mebhydrolin is an antihistamine. The actions and uses of antihistamines in general are discussed in the section dealing with these drugs. In clinical practice mebhydrolin is used:

1. To suppress generalized minor allergic responses to allergens such as foodstuffs and drugs.
2. To suppress local allergic reactions, i.e. inflammatory skin responses to insect stings and bites, contact allergens, urticaria etc.
3. Orally for allergic ocular inflammatory conditions, e.g. due to hay fever and allergic rhinitis.
4. As a nasal decongestant, e.g. in the treatment of allergic rhinitis and hay fever.

Dosage

Adults only: 50–100 mg three times daily.

Nurse monitoring

See the section on antihistamines.

General note

The drug may be stored at room temperature.

MEDAZEPAM (Nobrium)

Presentation

Capsules—5 mg

Actions and uses

Medazepam is a benzodiazepine drug (q.v.). Its principal use is in the treatment of anxiety.

Dosage

1. Adults. Initial doses of 5 mg two to three times daily increased to a maximum total dosage of 40 mg per day.
2. Children: Dosages are calculated on the basis of 1–1.5 mg/kg body weight in total per day, usually administered in two or three divided doses.

Nurse monitoring

See the section on benzodiazepines.

General note

Medazepam capsules may be stored at room temperature.

MEDROXYPROGESTERONE (Farlutal, Provera, Depo-Provera)

Presentation

Tablets—5 mg, 100 mg, 200 mg, 250 mg, 400 mg, 500 mg
Injection—50 mg/ml
Depot injection—150 mg suspension in 1ml vial, 500 mg suspension in 2.5 ml vial

Actions and uses

1. The actions and uses of progestational hormones in general are discussed in the section on these drugs.
2. In clinical practice this drug is indicated for the treatment of breast cancer, threatened and recurrent abortion, functional uterine bleeding, secondary amenorrhoea, endometrial carcinoma, prostatic cancer, endometriosis, and for prolonged contraception.

Dosage

1. Treatment of breast cancer: Orally 400–800 mg daily (Provera brand) or 1–1.5 g daily (Farlutal brand). The difference in dose reflects differences in bioavailability: check which particular brand is used.
2. Treatment of other malignancies: Orally 100–500 mg daily. By deep intramuscular injection doses vary from 1 g to as little as 250 mg

daily and up to weekly, depending upon the response of the tumour.
3. For the treatment of secondary amenorrhoea and dysfunctional uterine bleeding: 2.5–10 mg per day for 5-10 days of the cycle beginning between days 16-21 repeated for 3 and 2 cycles respectively.
4. For the treatment of threatened abortion: 10–30 mg daily or higher if necessary to be continued 'until fetal viability is evident'.
5. For the treatment of habitual abortion: 10 mg daily during the first trimester, 20 mg daily during second trimester, 40 mg daily during third trimester. Continue therapy to the end of the 8th month.
6. For the treatment of endometriosis: 50 mg intramuscularly once weekly or 100 mg every 2 weeks. Orally, 10 mg three times daily for 90 days, beginning on 1st day of the cycle.
7. For contraception: 150 mg deep intramuscularly during first 5 days of the cycle or within 5 weeks post-partum, repeated every 3 months.

Nurse monitoring
When used as recommended above few problems are encountered with this drug although it remains technically capable of producing the problems described under the nurse monitoring section of progestational hormones (q.v.) in hormones (2).

General note
The drug may be stored at room temperature.

MEFENAMIC ACID (Ponstan)

Presentation
Tablets—500 mg
Capsules—250 mg
Paediatric suspension—50 mg in 5 ml
Actions and uses
See the section on non-steroidal anti-inflammatory analgesic drugs.

Dosage
1. Adults:. The recommended daily dosage is 250 mg to 500 mg three times per day.
2. Children: The recommended total daily doses are as follows:
   a. Infants over 6 months: 25 mg/kg body weight
   b. 1 year plus: 150 mg
   c. 2-4 years: 300 mg
   d. 5-8 years: 450 mg
   e. 9-12 years: 600 mg

Nurse monitoring
1. See the section on non-steroidal anti-inflammatory analgesic drugs.
2. It is worth noting that a particularly troublesome problem with mefenamic acid is the production of diarrhoea which may on occasions be sufficiently severe to require cessation of treatment.

General note
Tablets, capsules and paediatric suspension may be stored at room temperature. For ease of administration the paediatric suspension can be diluted with Syrup B.P. but such dilutions must be used up within a fortnight.

MEFRUSIDE (Baycaron)

Presentation
Tablets—25 mg
Actions and uses
See the section on thiazide and related diuretics.
Dosage
The adult dose is 25–100 mg which is usually taken once daily or occasionally on alternate days.

Nurse monitoring
See the section on thiazide and related diuretics.

General note
Mefruside tablets may be stored at room temperature.

MEGESTROL ACETATE (Megace)

Presentation
Tablets—40 mg, 160 mg

Actions and uses
Megestrol acetate is a progestational hormone and it therefore has the actions of those drugs which are described under hormones (2). In clinical practice it is used to block the growth of oestrogen-dependent neoplasms, such as endometrial and breast carcinoma.

Dosage
1. Breast cancer: 160 mg daily.
2. Endometrial cancer: 40–320 mg daily.

Nurse monitoring
1. Megestrol acetate can theoretically produce all effects described for hormones (2), and the nurse monitoring section for hormones (2) apply to this drug.
2. In practice the drug is generally well tolerated, producing a degree of weight gain, occasional urticaria and nausea.

General note
Tablets may be stored at room temperature.

MELPHALAN (Alkeran)

Presentation
Tablets—2 mg, 5 mg
Injection—100 mg

Actions and uses
Melphalan is a member of the nitrogen mustard group. It prevents cell growth and division by inactivating important constituents of the cell necessary for these activities. Its uses are as follows:
1. It has proved to be of most value in the management of multiple myeloma.
2. It has also been used for the treatment of carcinoma of breast, soft tissue sarcoma, malignant melanoma and seminoma of the testis.

Dosage
1. In multiple myelomatosis a dose schedule of 0.15 mg/kg daily for 4 days in combination with Prednisolone is given. It is repeated at intervals of 6 weeks.
2. For treatment of other tumours regimes are variable:
   a. A single daily dose ranging from 2–35 mg may be given until a total dose of 150–200 mg has been received.
   b. By intravenous injection single doses of 1 mg/kg have been given.
   c. An isolated perfusion technique is used in the treatment of malignant melanoma. By this technique a much higher dose, i.e. up to 100 mg is circulated and confined to a particular part of the body affected by the tumour.

Nurse monitoring
1. Severe bone marrow suppression may occur even at low dose ranges. If these side-effects arise patients may suffer severe and sometimes fatal infection or haemorrhage.
2. Nausea, vomiting and alopecia also occur but are more frequent with higher dosage.
3. The nurse should be constantly aware that cytotoxic drugs are very toxic and must therefore be handled with great care. Spillage and contamination of the skin of the patient or nurse may lead to a degree of absorption of the drug which, if chronically repeated, may cause damage. The skin may also be sensitized to the drug making it, in some cases, impossible for the nurse to continue working with it.

General notes
1. Melphalan is highly irritant and precautions should be taken to avoid contact with skin and eyes.
2. Melphalan tablets may be stored at room temperature.
3. The injection should be stored in a cool place and for this purpose refrigeration may be preferred.

4. The injection must be protected from light.
5. To prepare melphalan injection 1 ml of special solvent is first added to the vial and the mixture shaken before a further 9 ml of diluent is added. Solutions for injection must be used within 15-30 minutes of preparation and unused injection immediately discarded.

MEPROBAMATE (Equanil)

Presentation
Tablets—200 mg, 400 mg
Actions and uses
Meprobamate has sedative and tranquillizing properties and is used in the management of anxiety neuroses, though it has been largely replaced by the newer and more effective benzodiazepines. In addition, the drug produces useful muscle relaxation by an inhibitory action on spinal cord reflexes and it is still widely prescribed in combination with simple analgesics to treat painful muscle injuries associated with muscle spasm.
Dosage
1. Anxiety states:
   a. Adults: 200–800 mg three times daily.
   b. Children: a total daily dose of 50–100 mg per year of age in three divided doses.
2. Muscle injury:
   a. Adults: 300 mg 2-4 times daily.

Nurse monitoring
1. Elderly patients are particularly sensitive to this drug which may produce excessive sedation, confusion and inco-ordination. In general these patients should receive dosages in the lower range.
2. In common with many drugs which act in the CNS, meprobamate may produce dependency in some patients if taken for prolonged periods.
3. CNS depression, and thus the degree of sedation, is more marked in patients who take other sedative drugs and in this context patients should be warned of the danger of taking alcohol in even moderate amounts.
4. Meprobamate should not be taken during pregnancy, by nursing mothers or by epileptic patients in whom seizures may be produced.
5. In patients who have taken the drug for prolonged periods, particularly at high dosage, treatment should never be abruptly withdrawn but rather discontinued gradually. Convulsions may follow if the drug is stopped suddenly.

General note
Tablets should be stored at room temperature. Tablets containing meprobamate and aspirin will deteriorate during storage, particularly if containers are not correctly sealed after use, and this is indicated by the strong 'vinegary' smell produced.

MEPTAZINOL (Meptid)

Presentation
Tablets—200 mg
Injection—100 mg in 1 ml
Presentation
Meptazinol is a strong, non-narcotic analgesic used in the treatment of moderate-to-severe pain, e.g. postoperatively, after myocardial infarction, in obstetrics, etc. It has uses in common with buprenorphine and nalbuphine.
These drugs do not appear to produce significant dependence, respiratory depression or cardiovascular disturbances which are major disadvantages of mor-phine and related analgesics.
Dosage
Adults:
1. Orally: 200 mg every 3-6 hours.
2. Intravenous/intramuscular injection: 50–100 mg repeated every 2-4 hours.

A dose of 100 mg meptazinol produces analgesia comparable to 15 mg morphine or 100 mg pethidine.

Nurse monitoring

1. Though meptazinol is reported to be associated with little, if any, dependence, it is intended for short-term pain relief and the possibility of meptazinol abuse should not be overlooked.
2. In common with opiate analgesics meptazinol may produce nausea and constipation requiring remedial anti-emetic and laxative therapy.
3. There is no evidence that the newborn are adversely affected by meptazinol administered during labour and the respiratory depression associated with pethidine does not occur.

General note

Meptazinol tablets and injection may be stored at room temperature.

MEQUITAZINE (Primalan)

Presentation

Tablets—5 mg

Actions and uses

Mequitazine is an antihistamine. The actions and uses of antihistamines in general are discussed in the section on these drugs. In clinical practice mequitazine is used:

1. To suppress local allergic reactions, i.e. inflammatory skin responses to insect stings and bites, contact allergens, urticaria etc.
2. As a nasal decongestant, e.g. in the treatment of allergic rhinitis and hay fever.

Dosage

Adults: 5 mg twice daily.

Nurse monitoring

See the section on antihistamines.

General note

The drug may be stored at room temperature.

MERCAPTOPURINE (Puri-Nethol)

Presentation

Tablets—50 mg

Actions and uses

Mercaptopurine is an immunosuppressant and cytotoxic drug which inhibits a number of different enzymes involved in the early stages of purine synthesis. Purines are essential for the formation of DNA and subsequent cell division and if their synthesis is blocked cell division is inhibited.

Dosage

The oral daily dose for adults is usually 2.5–5 mg/kg body weight. Children's doses are as for adults.

Nurse monitoring

1. Bone marrow suppression is an important side-effect and may produce anaemia, bleeding due to thrombocytopenia and infection due to suppression of white cell production. Regular blood tests are frequently carried out during treatment to detect the onset of these side-effects.
2. This drug commonly causes gastrointestinal side-effects including anorexia, nausea, vomiting, diarrhoea and oral ulceration.
3. This drug may also damage the liver and therefore blood tests of liver function should be carried out regularly.
4. The drug allopurinol (q.v.) which is used in the treatment of hyperuricaemia may alter the body metabolism in such a way that the effect of a particular dose of mercaptopurine may be markedly increased in patients who are given both drugs. The dose of mercaptopurine should be reduced to approximately one-quarter of that intended if patients are already on allopurinol.
5. The nurse should be constantly aware that most cytotoxic drugs are irritant to the skin and mucous surfaces, and are in general very toxic. Great care

should therefore be exercised
when handling these drugs, and
in particular spillage or
contamination of personnel or the
environment must be avoided. If
cytotoxic drugs are handled
regularly it is theoretically
possible that repeated skin
contact or inhalation may
produce systemic toxic effects
and in nurses who have
developed hypersensitivity,
severe local and general
hypersensitivity reactions.

General notes
1. Mercaptopurine tablets may be
   stored at room temperature.
2. They should be protected from
   light and kept dry.

MESALAZINE (Asacol)

Presentation
Tablets—400 mg resin coated,
positioned release
Suppositories—250 mg, 500 mg

Actions and uses
Mesalazine is chemically
aminosalicylic acid, a component of
sulphasalazine (q.v.) which is formed
after administration of
sulphasalazine. Mesalazine
possesses an anti-inflammatory
action and is used in the
maintenance of remission of
ulcerative colitis for patients who are
intolerant of sulphasalazine.

Dosage
Adults only
1. Orally: 2.4 g (6 tablets) in 3
   divided doses in acute disease.
   1.2–2.4 g daily in 3-4 divided
   doses as maintenance therapy.
2. Rectal: 750–1500 mg daily in
   divided doses with the last dose at
   night on retiring.
Note that 400 mg mesalazine is
theoretically the dose available
from a 1 g dose of sulphasalazine.

Nurse monitoring
1. Tablets are specially formulated
   to release the active ingredient in
   the terminal ileum and colon and

it is most important that patients
swallow these whole and that
they are not crushed for ease of
administration.
2. Since mesalazine is chemically
   related to aspirin, it should be
   avoided in patients with a history
   of aspirin sensitivity.
3. Side-effects are mainly
   gastrointestinal and include
   nausea, diarrhoea and
   abdominal pain.
4. Mesalazine appears to be a
   safe alternative to sulphasalazine
   in pregnancy. It is also of
   value in males who develop
   low sperm counts and
   infertility during sulphasalazine
   therapy.

General note
Mesalazine preparations may be
stored at room temperature. They
should be protected from direct
sunlight.

M

MESTEROLONE (Pro-Viron)

Presentation
Tablets—25 mg

Actions and uses
1. The actions and uses of
   androgenic hormones and
   anabolic steroids are
   discussed in the sections
   dealing with these drugs under
   hormones (4).
2. In clinical practice this drug is
   used primarily for the treatment of
   hypogonadism in males.

Dosage
The dosage is adjusted according to
individual response but is usually in
the range of 25 mg two to four times
daily.

Nurse monitoring
See the section on androgenic
hormones and anabolic steroids in
hormones (4).

General note
The drug may be stored at room
temperature.

MESTRANOL (Menophase)

Presentation
   The above preparation combines
   mestranol with a progestational
   hormone.
Actions and uses
   1. The actions and uses of
      oestrogenic hormones in general
      are discussed in the section on
      these drugs in hormones (1).
   2. The actions and uses of
      the proprietary preparations
      in which this hormone is
      included are:
      a. For the treatment of functional
         uterine bleeding.
      b. For the treatment of
         endometriosis.
Dosage
   The doses vary considerably
   with the indications for use
   and the individual proprietary
   preparation.

Nurse monitoring
   See the section on combined
   oestrogen and progestrogenic
   hormones in hormones (3).

General note
   All the above preparations
   may be stored at room
   temperature.

METFORMIN (Glucophage)

Presentation
   Tablets—500 mg, 850 mg
Actions and uses
   The actions and uses of biguanide
   drugs are described in the section
   on these drugs.
Dosage
   For adults: 3 x 500 mg or 2 x 850 mg
   tablets in three or two divided doses
   respectively with meals.

Nurse monitoring
   See the section on biguanide drugs.

General note
   The drug may be stored at room
   temperature.

METHADONE (Physeptone)

Presentation
   Tablets—5 mg
   Mixture—1mg in 1ml (for methadone
   maintenance)
   Injection—10 mg in 1 ml
Actions and uses
   1. Methadone is a narcotic analgesic
      with a long duration of action and
      its general actions and uses are
      described in the section dealing
      with these drugs.
   2. Methadone has an additional
      specific use in that it is less
      addictive than other narcotic
      analgesics such as morphine and
      diamorphine and if used when
      patients are being weaned off
      these drugs it may lead to a
      reduction in the severity of
      withdrawal symptoms.
Dosage
   1. For analgesia: Adults should
      receive 5–10 mg 6-8 hourly
      initially increasing if necessary to
      30 mg 6 hourly.
   2. For methadone maintenance in
      addicts: the dose is widely
      variable.
   3. Avoid in children.

Nurse monitoring
   See the section on narcotic
   analgesics.

General notes
   1. The drug should be stored in a
      locked (controlled drug) cupboard.
   2. The drug should be stored at
      room temperature.

METHICILLIN (Celbenin)

(See Note 3, p. 362)
Presentation
   Injection—1 g vials
Actions and uses
   Methicillin is a member of the
   penicillin group of drugs with actions
   and uses similar to those described
   for benzylpenicillin (q.v.). Methicillin,
   however, has an important advantage over benzylpenicillin in that it is
   more likely to be effective against

infections caused by Staphylococcus aureus than benzylpenicillin. In addition therefore to the general recommendations in that section it is specifically indicated for the treatment of infections due to Staphylococcus aureus.

Dosage
1. Adult:
   a. Intramuscular: 1 g every 4-6 hours.
   b. Intravenous: 1 g every 4-6 hours.
   c. Intra-articular: 500 mg–1 g once daily.
   d. Intrapleural: 500 mg–1 g once daily.
   e. Subconjunctival: 500 mg once daily.
2. Children:
   a. Under 2 years: one-quarter of the adult dose.
   b. Over 2 years: one-half of the adult dose.

Nurse monitoring
See the section on benzylpenicillin.

General notes
1. Methicillin injection may be stored at room temperature.
2. Once reconstituted, solutions for injection should be used immediately and any unused solution discarded.
3. Solutions should be prepared as follows:
   a. For intramuscular dosage: 1.5 ml water for injection should be added to each 1 g vial.
   b. For intravenous administration: The vial should be diluted to 20 ml which can then either be given slowly over 3-4 minutes or added to normal saline, 5% dextrose or dextrose/saline mixtures and infused over 4-6 hours.
   c. Intra-arterial injections should be prepared in 5 ml of water for injection.
   d. Intrapleural injections should be prepared in 10 ml of water for injection.
   e. Subconjunctival injections should be prepared in 0.5–0.75 ml of sterile water.

METHIXENE (Tremonil)

Presentation
Tablets—5 mg

Actions and uses
The actions and uses of this drug are identical to those described for benzhexol (q.v.).

Dosage
Adults: 15–30 mg in total daily given in three divided doses.

Nurse monitoring
The nurse monitoring aspects of benzhexol (q.v.) apply to this drug.

General note
The drug may be stored at room temperature.

METHOHEXITONE (Brietal)

Presentation
Injection—100 mg, 500 mg, 2.5 g, 5 g

Actions and uses
Methohexitone sodium is a potent barbiturate (q.v.) with a rapid onset and short duration of action. Its main use therefore is by intravenous injection for the induction of anaesthesia.

Dosage
Methohexitone sodium is administered intravenously as a 1% solution (10 mg/ml) and is given at a rate of 1 ml in 5 seconds until anaesthesia is induced. If given alone the patient will remain unconscious for 5-7 minutes during which time prolonged anaesthesia using inhalation therapy may be induced if required.

Nurse monitoring
See the section on barbiturates.

General notes
1. Once prepared solutions of methohexitone sodium should be used immediately. If they are not discarded they rapidly turn cloudy and precipitate free drug rendering them useless.
2. Methohexitone solution for injection should not be mixed with other drugs in the same syringe.

METHOTREXATE

Presentation
Tablets—2.5 mg
Injection—2.5 mg/ml, 5 mg/2 ml,
25 mg/ml, 50 mg/2 ml, 250 mg/10 ml
Powder—50 mg/vial

Actions and uses
The mode of action of methotrexate is as follows:

All cells require for growth a vitamin known as folic acid. Folic acid is converted by a number of enzymatic steps in the cell to its biologically active form, folinic acid. Methotrexate blocks this conversion and therefore reduces cell growth and multiplication by depriving the cell of folinic acid. It is used in the treatment of the following conditions:

1. It is used in the treatment of acute lymphoblastic leukaemia. Initial treatment is usually with other drugs but once the leukaemia is under control, methotrexate is used as maintenance therapy. It is also used for the prevention and treatment of meningeal leukaemia.
2. Other malignancies which have been reported to respond to treatment with methotrexate include:
   a. Choriocarcinoma and related trophoblastic diseases
   b. Lymphosarcoma
   c. Burkitt's lymphoma
   d. Tumours of the head and neck.
3. Methotrexate is occasionally used in the treatment of severe cases of psoriasis and rheumatoid arthritis which do not respond to conventional therapy.

Dosage
The drug may be given by oral, intramuscular, intravenous, intra-arterial, intra-articular and intrathecal routes. The doses vary widely according to the route of administration, type of malignant disease under treatment and with the variety of other cytotoxic or immunosuppressant drugs which are used in combination. Because of the wide variety of dosage regimes, none are specifically stated here. However, it should be noted that intrathecal doses are very much smaller than doses given by other routes.

Courses of treatment with methotrexate are very often followed by the administration of calcium folinate which is a methotrexate antagonist. This has been found to reduce the incidence of associated toxic effects.

Nurse monitoring
1. The principal toxic effects are suppression of the bone marrow and gastrointestinal disturbance. The former effect leads to leucopenia and thrombocytopenia and a resultant increased risk of severe infection or haemorrhage.
2. One of the earliest manifestations of toxicity is oral soreness frequently progressing to ulceration in the mouth. Other gastrointestinal effects include nausea, vomiting and diarrhoea.
3. Megaloblastic anaemia, skin rashes, alopecia, altered ovarian and testicular function, enteritis with bleeding episodes and intestinal perforation may occur.
4. Damage to specific tissues such as the kidneys, liver, lungs and nervous system have been reported. Liver damage is thought to occur more commonly with long-term oral therapy and renal damage is thought to be more common in intermittent high dose regimes. Intrathecal therapy is the commonest cause of neurotoxicity.
5. The drug has produced abortion and a wide range of fetal abnormalities and must not be taken during pregnancy.
6. The nurse should be constantly aware that most cytotoxic drugs are irritant to the skin and mucous surfaces, and are in general very toxic. Great care should therefore be exercised when handling these drugs, and in particular spillage or contamination of personnel or the environment must be avoided. If cytotoxic drugs are handled regularly it is theoretically possible that repeated skin

contact or inhalation may produce systemic toxic effects and in nurses who have developed hypersensitivity, severe local and general hypersensitivity reactions.

General notes

1. Methotrexate should only be diluted with 0.9% sodium chloride injection and should not be mixed with other drugs before administration.
2. Preparations of methotrexate may be stored at room temperature. Vials containing powder may similarly be stored for up to 2 weeks after reconstitution.

METHOTRIMEPRAZINE (Nozinan)

Presentation
Tablets—25 mg
Injection—25 mg in 1 ml

Actions and uses
Methotrimeprazine is a member of the phenothiazine group. It is therefore a neuroleptic or major tranquilliser and has a limited role in the treatment of severe anxiety, schizophrenia and manic depressive psychosis. In practice, however, the main role for this drug is as an anxiolytic and anti-emetic when used in combination with diamorphine (or a related opioid analgesic) in pain control. In particular it is widely used in the control of pain in terminal cancer when it is often mixed with diamorphine in the same syringe and delivered by continuous subcutaneous infusion via a syringe driver.

Dosage

1. Oral: Doses vary from as low as 25 mg to as high as 200 mg three times daily with a maximum of 40 mg for children under 10 years. In pain control, the injectable route is most often used.
2. Injection: Usually 12.5–50 mg by i.m. injection administered every 6-8 hours. Doses of 2–3 g may be administered by continuous s.c. infusion over 24 hours in combination with diamorphine.

Nurse monitoring

1. The nurse monitoring aspects for phenothiazines apply to this drug.
2. In particular methotrimeprazine may produce severe postural hypotension and close monitoring of ambulant patients is necessary.
3. Methotrimeprazine should not be administered by the i.v. route.

General note
Methotrimeprazine tablets and ampoules may be stored at room temperature. They must however be protected from light; note that on exposure to light the injection solution will develop a pink or yellow discolouration in which case it should be discarded.

METHYLCELLULOSE (Celevac)

Presentation
Tablet—500 mg

Actions and uses
The actions of laxatives are discussed in the section dealing with these drugs. Methylcellulose is a member of the bulk forming group i.e. it swells the volume of faeces and induces a more natural bowel action and increase in frequency of defaecation.

Dosage
Adults: 3–6 tablets taken night and morning. Children should receive an appropriate dose in proportion to this.

Nurse monitoring

1. There are no specific problems with this drug.
2. It is worth noting that ingestion of this drug may be associated with a feeling of fullness and it is therefore also used as an aid to dieting.
3. Doses should be taken with at least one half pint of liquid.

General notes

1. Methylcellulose tablets may be stored at room temperature.

M

2. They can be physically broken up for ease of administration.

METHYLDOPA (Aldomet)

Presentation
Tablets—125 mg, 250 mg, 500 mg
Injection—250 mg in 5 ml

Actions and uses
Methyldopa reduces the blood pressure through a direct action on the centres controlling blood pressure in the brain. It is available for use orally on a regular basis but may be given intravenously in hypertensive emergencies. It has been used for many years safely in obstetrics and is therefore often used for control of hypertension in pregnancy.

Dosage
1. Adult dose: 250 mg two to three times daily, rising to a maximum of 3 g per day in three divided doses.
2. Adult emergency intravenous dose: 250–500 mg 6-hourly as required.
3. Children's dosage: Up to 1 year— 6 mg/kg; 1-6 years—62.5 mg; 7 years plus—125 mg. All these doses should be taken three times per day. The maximum dosage in each age range is four times the dose stated, three times per day. Similar doses are given by intravenous injection if necessary.

Nurse monitoring
Although methyldopa is a very .
effective drug in the treatment of hypertension, the major problem with its use is the large number of potentially serious side-effects which may occur, and it is in the early detection of these side-effects that the nurse can make a major contribution.
1. Neurological side-effects: Depression is by far the most important, but paraesthesia, Parkinsonism, involuntary muscle twitching, nightmares, confusion, light-headedness and dizziness may also occur.

2. Cardiovascular: Postural hypotension, fluid retention, worsening of existing angina and bradycardia.
3. Gastrointestinal: Nausea, vomiting, distension, excess flatus, constipation, dry mouth, black tongue and very rarely pancreatitis.
4. Blood: Haemolytic anaemia, leucopenia, granulocytopenia, thrombocytopenia.
5. Other side-effects include nasal stuffiness, a raised blood urea, gynaecomastia/galactorrhoea, impotence in males, loss of libido, skin rashes, drug fever and abnormal liver function tests.

General note
Methyldopa tablets and injection may be stored at room temperature. The injection is diluted with 100 ml 5% dextrose injection and infused over a period of 30-60 minutes.

METHYLPHENOBARBITONE (Prominal)

Presentation
Tablets—30 mg, 60 mg, 200 mg

Actions and uses
See the section on barbiturates. Methylphenobarbitone has a specific anticonvulsant action and it is used in the treatment of all forms of epilepsy.

Dosage
100–600 mg daily in divided doses.

Nurse monitoring
See the section on barbiturates.

General note
Tablets containing Methylphenobarbitone may be stored at room temperature.

METHYLPREDNISOLONE (Medrone, Depo-Medrone, Solu-Medrone)

Presentation
Tablets—2 mg, 4 mg, 16 mg
Intravenous or intramuscular injection—40 mg, 125 mg, 500 mg in 1 g

Long-acting intramuscular and intra-articular injection—40 mg in 1 ml, 80 mg in 2 ml, 200 mg in 5 ml
Acne lotion and cream—0.25%

Actions and uses

Methylprednisolone is a corticosteroid drug (q.v.). Its rapid onset of action following intravenous injection makes it particularly useful in the management of severe shock.

Dosage

1. Oral: This varies widely with the nature and severity of the condition being treated.
2. Intravenous injection: For the treatment of severe shock doses of up to 30 mg/kg body weight daily may be given.
3. Intra-articular injection: Dosages vary between 4 and 80 mg according to the size of the joint under treatment.
4. The lotion is applied sparingly once or twice daily and the cream once to three times daily.

Nurse monitoring

See the section on corticosteroid drugs. It must be remembered that even topical applications may lead to sufficient of the drug being absorbed to produce the systemic effects described in this section.

General note

Preparations containing methyl-prednisolone may be stored at room temperature.

METHYLTESTOSTERONE

Presentation

Tablets—5 mg, 10 mg, 25 mg and 50 mg

Actions and uses

Methyltestosterone is an androgenic hormone. Its actions and uses are discussed in the section on these drugs.

Dosage

The dosage varies according to the indication for its use.

Nurse monitoring

See the section on androgenic hormones in hormones (4).

General note

The drug may be stored at room temperature.

METHYSERGIDE (Deseril)

Presentation

Tablets-1 mg

Actions and uses

Methysergide has two actions:
1. It constricts blood vessels.
2. It is an antagonist of 5-hydroxytryptamine, a chemical which is released in tissues involved in acute inflammation.

In clinical practice Methysergide has two major uses:
1. For the treatment of the rare carcinoid syndrome where excess production of 5-hydroxytryptamine leads to attacks of flushing and diarrhoea.
2. It is effective for the prophylactic treatment of migraine but it is now rarely used for this because of toxicity.

Dosage

1. For the treatment of carcinoid syndrome: Up to 20 mg per day may be required according to individual patient response.
2. For the prophylaxis of migraine: 1 or 2 mg three times a day with meals.

Nurse monitoring

1. This drug on rare occasions may cause extensive fibrosis involving the heart, pleura, lung and retroperitoneal tissues. It should, therefore, be given in short courses only and should not be administered for long periods.
2. Common side-effects include nausea, epigastric pain, dizziness, drowsiness, restless-ness, muscle cramps and psychological effects. Vomiting, muscle weakness, ataxia, weight increase, oedema, tachycardia

and postural hypotension may also occur.
3. The vasoconstrictor effect may lead to cold extremities.
4. The drug should be used with great caution in patients with peripheral vascular disease, coronary heart disease, peptic ulceration and reduced kidney or liver function.

General note
The drug should be stored at room temperature.

METIPRANOLOL (Glauline)

Presentation
Eye drops—0. 1%, 0.3%, 0.6%

Actions and uses
Metipranolol is a beta-blocking drug and it has the actions and uses of other drugs described in the section on beta-adrenoreceptor blocking drugs. In practice, however, metipranolol is only used in the form of eye drops for the treatment of ocular hypertension and chronic open-angle glaucoma: topical beta-blockers lower raised intra-ocular pressure by an unknown mechanism which is associated with a reduction in aqueous humour production.

Dosage
Glaucoma: One drop is instilled in the affected eye twice daily, therapy being initiated with 0.1% strength drops and increased in time as necessary.

Nurse monitoring
1. Despite the fact that this drug is administered externally, sufficient may be absorbed from the cornea to produce systemic side-effects in susceptible patients (see beta-adrenoreceptor drugs). Thus patients with obstructive airways disease (particularly asthmatics) and those with uncontrolled heart failure should not be treated with beta-blocker eye drops.
2. Other patients in whom metipranolol must be used with

caution include those with sinus bradycardia and 2nd or 3rd degree heart block.
3. Metipranolol eye drops may cause stinging of the eye on application and should be avoided if the patient uses soft contact lenses.

General note
Metipranolol eye drops may be stored at room temperature. They have a relatively short life during use when a risk of bacterial contamination after opening exists and normally eye drops of any kind should not be used after 1 week for a hospitalized patient or after 4 weeks for others.

METOCLOPRAMIDE (Maxolon)

Presentation
Tablets—10 mg
Syrup—5 mg in 5 ml
Paediatric liquid—1 mg in 1 ml
Injection—10 mg in 2 ml, 100 mg in 20 ml

Actions and uses
Metoclopramide has two major modes of action:
1. It has a direct action on the gut increasing normal gut motility (peristalsis) and increasing gastric emptying time.
2. It has an anti-emetic effect via an action on the central nervous system.

It has the following uses:
1. It can be used to control vomiting associated with gastrointestinal disease, drug therapy (particularly cytotoxic drugs), radiotherapy and postoperative period.
2. In diagnostic radiology metoclopramide is used to speed the passage of barium through the stomach and also as an aid to duodenal intubation.

Dosage
1. Adults:
   a. Oral: 10 mg three times a day.
   b. Parenteral: 10 mg three times a day.

2. Children:
   a. Oral: Under 1 year—1 mg b.d.; 5-15 years—2.5–5 mg three times daily. The total daily dose for children should not exceed 0.5 mg/kg body weight.
   b. Parenteral: As for oral dosage regimes. High dose intravenous infusion using doses of up to 2 mg/kg body weight or more have been administered prior to cytotoxic chemotherapy. This may be repeated every 2 hours up to a maximum dose of 10 mg/kg in 24 hours. Infusions are administered over 15 minutes.
3. For diagnostic procedures a single dose of metoclopramide is given 9-10 minutes before the examination. Dosage is as follows:
   a. Adults: 10–20 mg.
   b. Children under 3 years: 1 mg.
   c. Children 5-14 years: 2.5–5 mg.

Nurse monitoring
1. It is important to note that metoclopramide is of little benefit in the prevention or treatment of motion sickness or in the treatment of nausea and vertigo due to Menière's disease or other labyrinthine disturbances.
2. Metoclopramide blocks the action of dopamine in the central nervous system and produces a range of symptoms and signs similar to those seen in Parkinson's disease. This effect is particularly likely to occur in children and young adults and where higher dosages are used. The effects include facial muscle spasm, trismus, a rhythmic protrusion of the tongue, bulbar speech, muscle spasm around the eyes, rolling of the eyeballs and an unnatural positioning of the head and shoulders.
3. Because drugs of the phenothiazine group (q.v.) also produce similar effects, metoclopramide and phenothiazines should only be given together with great caution.

4. Metoclopramide stimulates the production of prolactin by the pituitary. This may lead to an increase in breast size in males and galactorrhoea in females.
5. Metoclopramide and anticholinergic drugs (see the section on poldine and other related compounds) should be avoided as the latter drugs antagonize the effects of metoclopramide on the gut.

General note
Preparations containing metoclopramide may be stored at room temperature. Liquid preparations are sensitive to light and ampoules containing injection solution which show a yellow discolouration should be discarded.

METOLAZONE (Metenix, Xuret)

Presentation
Tablets—500 microgram, 5 mg
Actions and uses
See the section on thiazide and related diuretics. Metolazone has additional diuretic properties because of its further action on the proximal renal tubule where some reabsorption of sodium takes place. This makes it an extremely potent diuretic so that it is generally reserved for the treatment of heart failure which is refractory to first line thiazide diuretics.
Very low dose metolazone may be used in the control of hypertension.
Dosage
1. Heart failure: The usual adult dose is 5–20 mg once daily; the duration of action is approximately 18-24 hours.
2. Hypertension: 500 microgram or 1 mg daily.

Nurse monitoring
See the section on thiazide and related diuretics.
Note that low dose (Xuret) and high dose (Metenix) have very different indications and are not interchangeable.

General note
> Metolazone tablets may be stored at room temperature.

METOPROLOL (Betaloc, Lopresor)

Presentation
> Tablets—50 mg, 100 mg, 200 mg (sustained release)

Actions and uses
> Metoprolol is a cardioselective beta-blocker and its actions are described in the section dealing with these drugs.

Dosage
> The adult dose range is 100–400 mg per day which is usually given in two equal doses. Sustained release tablets of metoprolol may be given as a single daily dose.

> **Nurse monitoring**
> See the section on beta-adrenoreceptor blocking drugs.

General note
> Metoprolol tablets may be stored at room temperature.

METRONIDAZOLE (Flagyl)

(See Note 3, p. 362)

Presentation
> Tablets—200 mg and 400 mg
> Suppositories—500 mg and 1 g (for vaginal and rectal administration)
> Injection—0.5% for intravenous infusion

Actions and uses
> Metronidazole has been found to be effective in the treatment of both bacterial and parasitic infections in man. Its main uses are as follows:
> 1. Trichomonal vaginitis.
> 2. Amoebiasis.
> 3. Giardiasis.
> 4. Vincent's angina.
> 5. Infections due to anaerobic organisms such as bacteroides species and clostridia.
> 6. Metronidazole is now being used more commonly for the prevention of wound infection and peritonitis after abdominal surgery.

Dosage
> 1. For the treatment of trichomonal vaginitis:
>   a. Adults and children greater than 10 years: 200–400 mg three times a day for 7-10 days or a single dose of 2 g.
>   b. Children: Less than 3 years— 150 mg per day for 7-10 days; 3-7 years—200 mg per day for 7-10 days; 7-10 years old—300 mg per day for 7-10 days.
> This condition may also be treated with 10-20 days' treatment with 500 mg or 1 g as pessaries once per day.
> 2. Acute and chronic hepatic or intestinal amoebiasis:
>   a. Adults: 2–2.4 g for 3 days or 400–800 mg three times a day for 5-10 days.
>   b. Children: 7.5 mg/kg three times a day for 10 days.
>   c. For cyst eradication in symptomless carriers of amoebiasis the same doses apply although shorter courses of treatment are usually effective.
> 3. For the treatment of giardiasis:
>   a. Adults: 2 g for 3 days.
>   b. Children: Less than 3 years old—400 mg for 3 days; 3-7 years—600 mg for 3 days; 7-10 years—1 g for 3 days.
> 4. For the treatment of Vincent's angina: Adult doses are 200 mg three times per day or 400 mg twice a day for a week.
> 5. For the treatment of serious bacterial infections due to bacteroides or clostridia:
>   a. Oral therapy is as follows:
>   i. Adult doses vary from 200–400 mg three times a day.
>   ii. Children and infants should receive 7.5 mg/kg body weight three times daily.
>   b. Rectal administration:
>   i. Adults and children over 12 years: 1 g suppository 8-hourly.
>   ii. Children 5-12 years: 500 mg 8-hourly.
>   iii. Children 1-5 years: One-half of a 500 mg suppository 8-hourly.

M

iv. Children less than 1 year: one-quarter of a 500 mg suppository 8-hourly.
   c. For parenteral treatment:
      i. Adults receive 500 mg 8-hourly by i.v. infusion.
      ii. Children under 12 years receive 7.5 mg/kg 8-hourly.
6. For the prevention of wound infection and peritonitis after abdominal surgery the recommended dose for adults is:
   a. 500 mg 8-hourly by i.v. infusion over 20 minutes or
   b. 400 mg three times a day orally or
   c. 1 g three times a day rectally.

Nurse monitoring
1. It is important to note that this drug may cause darkening of the urine and urethral discomfort. The patient should be warned of this possibility to prevent anxiety.
2. Gastrointestinal effects are common. These include anorexia, nausea, an abnormal taste in the mouth and dryness of the tongue.
3. Neurological side-effects such as headache are common. More serious neurological side-effects such as vertigo, depression, insomnia and drowsiness are less common.
4. Patients with disorders of the blood and disease of the central nervous system should not be given this drug.
5. It is recommended that the drug be avoided in pregnant women.
6. It is noteworthy that some patients may become profoundly sick if they take alcohol when on this drug and they should therefore be warned of this possible effect.
7. It is very important to note that the drug has no effect on diseases caused by *Candida albicans* (thrush).

General notes
1. The drug may be stored at room temperature.

2. Care should be taken to ensure that suppositories are not stored in a warm place, e.g. above a radiator, as they might melt.

METYRAPONE (Metopirone)

Presentation
Capsules—250 mg

Actions and uses
Metyrapone acts on the adrenal cortex to inhibit production of hydrocortisone (cortisol) by a specific effect on the chemical process called 11 -P-hydroxylation. Its use is therefore associated with an increase in the urinary excretion of precursors of cortisol which, if not detected, indicates either failure of the adrenal cortex or hypopituitarism, or both.
Metyrapone, since it inhibits cortisol production, has also been used in the treatment of Cushing's syndrome.

Dosage
Test for adrenal insufficiency or hypopituitarism: six doses, each of 750 mg (or 15 mg/kg for children) are given at intervals of 4 hours.

Nurse monitoring
1. Metyrapone may produce nausea and vomiting and doses should be taken with food.
2. Special care is necessary if major impairment of pituitary function exists.
3. The measurement of urinary steroid output, which is the basis for the metyrapone test, may be affected by the steroid-like drugs which the patient might be taking concurrently.

General note
Metyrapone capsules may be stored at room temperature.

MEXILETINE (Mexitil)

Presentation
Capsules—50 mg, 200 mg, 360 mg (slow release)
Injection—250 mg in 10 ml

Actions and uses

Mexiletine is an antidysrhythmic drug which is used to abolish or prevent serious ventricular dysrhythmias in patients who have had a myocardial infarction. It is given by intravenous injection initially and subsequently orally for the long-term prophylaxis of these rhythm disturbances.

Dosage

The adult intravenous loading dose is 100–250 mg by bolus injection at a rate of 25 mg/minute. This is followed by intravenous infusion containing 500 mg in 500 ml. The first 250 ml is given over 1 hour, the second 250 ml is given more slowly over 2 hours. Further maintenance infusions may be given using 250 mg in 500 ml at a rate of 0.5 mg/ minute. For oral maintenance therapy an initial loading dose of 400 mg is followed by 200–250 mg three or four times a day.

Alternatively 360 mg twice daily as slow release capsules may be administered.

Nurse monitoring

This drug requires careful monitoring for adverse effects which tend to be dose-related. When the drug is being administered intravenously the patient should be observed for lightheadedness, confusion, drowsiness, dizziness, diplopia, blurred vision, nystagmus, dysarthria, ataxia, paraesthesias, convulsions, hypotension, bradycardia, atrial fibrillation, nausea, vomiting, dyspepsia, an unpleasant taste and hiccoughs. Such effects are both less frequent and milder with oral therapy.

General note

Mexiletine capsules and injection may be stored at room temperature. The injection may be added to several infusion solutions including 0.9% sodium chloride injection, 5% dextrose injection, 5% laevulose injection, 1.4% sodium bicarbonate injection and sodium lactate injection.

MIANSERIN (Bolvidon, Norval)

Presentation

Tablets—10 mg, 20 mg, 30 mg

Actions and uses

Mianserin is an antidepressant drug derived from and chemically related to tricyclic antidepressants. Its actions and uses are similar to those described for tricyclic antidepressants (q.v.).

Dosage

For the treatment of depression in adults 30–200 mg is given daily either in divided doses or as a single evening dose taken on retiring.

Nurse monitoring

The nurse monitoring notes for tricyclic antidepressants (q.v.) are applicable to mianserin with two possible exceptions:
1. Following acute overdosage there has been a lower incidence of cardiac side-effects, principally tachycardias.
2. Mianserin has less 'anti-cholinergic' side-effects, such as dry mouth, blurred vision, urinary retention, constipation and tachycardia. It is therefore preferable for use in three groups:
   a. Patients with glaucoma.
   b. Patients with prostatism.
   c. Patients in whom the above side-effects are intolerable.

General note

Tablets containing mianserin may be stored at room temperature.

MICONAZOLE (Daktarin)

Presentation

Tablets—250 mg
Oral gel, cream and powder—2%
Injection—200 mg in 20 ml
Pessaries and tampons—100 mg

Actions and uses

1. In oral or topical preparation this drug is an effective antifungal agent used in clinical practice for the treatment of disease caused by pathogenic fungi (mainly

yeasts and dermatophytes) such as candidiasis.
2. An intravenous solution is available and intravenous infusions of the drug are used to treat systemic infection:
   a. Candida albicans
   b. Candida tropicalis
   c. Candida parapsilosis
   d. Aspergillus fumigatus
   e. Cryptococcus neoformans
   f. Coccidioides immites
   g. Paracoccidioides brasiliensis

Dosage
1. Oral gel:
   a. Adults: 5-10 ml of gel four times daily.
   b. Children aged over 6: 5 ml four times daily.
   c. Children aged 2-6: 5 ml twice daily.
   d. Children less than 2 years: 2.5 ml twice daily.
2. Miconazole tablets: Adults: 250 mg four times a day.
3. Pessaries and tampons: One should be inserted into the vagina at night.
4. Topical miconazole should be applied once or twice daily.
5. Intravenous infusion:
   a. The usual adult dose is 600 mg three times daily as an infusion in 200-500 ml infusion fluid. As a guide clinically effective daily doses have ranged from as low as 600 mg per day to, in a few patients, as high as 3600 mg per day.
   b. In children a daily dose of 40 mg/kg in total is recommended. A dose of 15 mg/kg per infusion should not be exceeded.

Nurse monitoring
1. Miconazole intravenous solution must be diluted with either normal saline or 5% dextrose and administered by slow infusion over at least 30 minutes. Usually a dose of 600 mg would be diluted in 200–500 ml of infusion fluid and lower doses in proportionately lower volumes of fluid.

2. The intravenous infusion can be associated with phlebitis, pruritus, nausea, vomiting, fever, skin rash, drowsiness, diarrhoea, anorexia and flushing.
3. Oral preparations are associated with mild gastrointestinal upset.
4. Topical applications have no side-effects.

General notes
1. Topical and oral miconazole preparations may be stored at room temperature.
2. The injection solution should be refrigerated.

MINOCYCLINE (Minocin)

(See Note 3, p. 362)
Presentation
Tablets—50 mg, 100 mg
Actions and uses
General notes on the actions and uses of tetracyclines (q.v.) apply to minocycline. In addition the drug has been found to be of particular use for the prevention of meningitis due to *Neisseria meningitidis* in the families of carriers of the disease.
Perhaps the most common use for this drug is in the treatment of acne vulgaris.
Dosage
The adult dose is 50–100 mg every 12 hours. It is worth noting that food appears to have less effect on the absorption of minocycline than tetracyclines in general and there-fore the drug may be taken with food. For acne: 50 mg twice daily for 6 weeks or longer.

Nurse monitoring
1. For general nurse monitoring notes see the section on tetracyclines.
2. It is worth noting that neuro-logical side-effects are particularly prominent with this drug as compared to other tetracyclines. These effects cause light-headedness, dizziness and vertigo.

M

3. Tetracyclines should be avoided in children under 12 years.

General note
The drug may be stored at room temperature.

MITOBRONITOL (Myelobromol)

(Also known as Dibromomannitol)
Presentation
Tablets—125 mg
Actions and uses
Mitobronitol is a cytotoxic drug which is an alkylating agent and has a similar mode of action to busulphan (q.v.). It is used mainly in the treatment of chronic myeloid leukaemia and occasionally to achieve and maintain remission in the treatment of polycythaemia rubra vera.
Dosage
Adults: Initially 250 mg per day is given until the white cell count is reduced to less than 20 000/mm³. Thereafter maintenance doses of 125 mg per day or on alternate days are given to maintain the white cell count at an appropriate level.

Nurse monitoring
1. Suppression of bone marrow function may be produced leading to anaemia, haemorrhage due to thrombocytopenia and infection due to suppression of white cell function.
2. Gastrointestinal disturbances, alopecia, skin pigmentation, skin rash and menstrual abnormalities may also occur.
3. The nurse should be constantly aware that most cytotoxic drugs are irritant to the skin and mucous surfaces, and are in general very toxic. Great care should therefore be exercised when handling these drugs, and in particular spillage or contamination of personnel or the environment must be avoided. If cytotoxic drugs are handled regularly it is theoretically

possible that repeated skin contact or inhalation may produce systemic toxic effects and in nurses who have developed hypersensitivity, severe local and general hypersensitivity reactions.

General note
Mitobronitol tablets may be stored at room temperature.

MOCLOBEMIDE (Manerix)

Presentation
Tablets—150 mg
Action and uses
This drug is a reversible inhibitor of the enzyme monoamine oxidase type A (hence RIMA). Its action in the brain results in accumulation of high levels of the monoamine neurotransmitters, noradrenaline and 5-hydroxytryptamine (serotonin) which is associated with mood elevation and the reversal of depression. Moclobemide is therefore used in the treatment of major depressive illness unresponsive to tricyclic and related antidepressants as an alternative to the traditional monoamine oxidase inhibitors (MAOIs). Because of its specific and reversible action on type A receptors it is much less likely to produce the serious hypertensive episodes which occur with other MAOIs when certain well known foodstuffs containing tyramine (e.g. cheeses, yeast extracts, soya based products, etc) are eaten. Similarly the drug is much less likely to interact with monoamine decongestants present in various cough and cold remedies.
Dosage
Initially 150 mg twice daily increased according to response up to a maximum dose of 600 mg daily.

Nurse monitoring
1. This drug is preferably taken with or immediately after food to limit possible gastrointestinal upsets.

2. As noted above the various well known interactions involving traditional MAOIs appear to be much less likely to occur with this drug. Caution is nevertheless advised and excessive ingestion of foods rich in tyramine should be avoided. Similarly patients should avoid cough and cold remedies containing monoamines such as ephedrine, pseudoephedrine and phenylpro-panolamine, which can generally be purchased over-the-counter.

3. In common with traditional MAOIs, this drug should be used with caution in agitated or excited patients (unless additional sedation is used) and in patients with severe liver disease and thyrotoxicosis.

4. Moclobemide is likely to exacerbate an existing acute confusional state and increase the risk of dangerously elevated BP in patients with phaeochromocytoma. It is therefore contraindicated in such cases.

5. Common side-effects include sleep disturbances, agitation, restlessness, dizziness, nausea, headaches, confusion, and a rise in liver enzymes.

General note
Moclobemide tablets are stored at room temperature.

MONOAMINE OXIDASE INHIBITORS

Isocarboxazid   Phenelzine
Tranylcypromine
Actions and uses
When the enzyme monoamine oxidase, which is present in many tissues in the body, is inhibited by the group of drugs known as monoamine oxidase inhibitors there is a resultant increase in the concentration of 5-hydroxytryp-tamine and catecholamines in the central nervous system. This leads to marked effects on mental function ranging from feelings of well-being and increased energy to, in some patients, psychosis. This group of drugs is therefore used for the treatment of depression. However, they have many serious side-effects and for this reason are usually only used when other drugs, such as tricyclic antidepressants, have been found to be ineffective.

Dosage
See specific drugs.

Nurse monitoring
1. Severe headache and dangerous hypertensive crisis may be precipitated in patients taking monoamine oxidase inhibiting drugs by the ingestion of certain foodstuffs. These include cheese, yoghurt, pickled herrings, broad beans, yeast extracts, meat extracts (Bovril, Marmite, etc.) wines and beers. The nurse may play an important role in both educating patients about food intake and monitoring their diets.

2. The nurse may also play an important role in warning patients that they must never indulge in self-medication of any kind particularly those sold for coughs and colds, as these contain chemicals which may lead to serious hypertension and headache if they are taken at the same time as monoamine oxidase inhibiting drugs.

3. A number of other drugs are extremely dangerous if they are given at the same time as monoamine oxidase inhibitors. The nurse may play an important role in identifying such potential combinations. The major group of drugs contraindicated for concurrent administration with monoamine oxidase inhibitors are as follows:
   a. Other antidepressants: If tricyclic and monoamine oxidase inhibiting drugs are given together mental excitement and hyperpyrexia may occur.

b. Antihypertensives: Hypertension and excitement may occur with methyldopa.

c. Narcotic analgesics: The coincident administration of pethidine and monoamine oxidase inhibiting drugs may lead to respiratory depression, restlessness, coma and hypotension.

d. Central nervous system depressants: Barbiturates, tranquillizers, antihistamines, alcohol and anti-Parkinsonian drugs are contraindicated for concurrent administration with monoamine oxidase inhibitor drugs.

e. Insulin and tolbutamide are contraindicated for concurrent administration with monoamine oxidase inhibiting drugs.

f. Drugs which stimulate the sympathetic nervous system, e.g. ephedrine, phenylephrine and the amphetamines may produce serious (and even fatal) rises in blood pressure which result in brain haemorrhage.

4. A common side-effect produced by monoamine oxidase inhibiting drugs is hypotension. Symptoms of dizziness on standing, indicating postural hypotension, may occur. It is important to remember that hypertensive crises can still occur in patients who have been rendered hypotensive by the drug.

5. Other side-effects include cardiac dysrhythmias, dizziness, headache, anxiety, tremor, convulsions and liver toxicity.

6. It is advisable that all patients receiving monoamine oxidase inhibiting drugs be issued with a warning card which provides a complete list of substances which they may accidentally take and which may lead to the effects described above.

MORPHINE (As Hydrochloride, Sulphate or Tartrate)

Presentation
Morphine sulphate is available in numerous preparations, often in combination with other drugs and in varying strengths. The following are only examples of the many preparations in common use:
Tablets—MST Continus, 10 mg, 30 mg, 60 mg and 100 mg as slow release
Injection—15 mg and 30 mg in 1 ml
Suppositories—15 mg and 30 mg
Mixtures—containing 10, 20, 30 mg in 10 ml

Actions and uses
See the section on narcotic analgesics.

Dosage
N.B. The following doses are given as a guideline only and both initial dosage and maintenance dosage may vary considerably depending on the condition under treatment and the development of tolerance to the drug in the patient.

1. Adults:.
   a. Orally:
      i. Standard preparations: 10–20 mg 4 to 6-hourly as required.
      ii. Slow release tablets (MST Continus) 30–100 mg twice daily.
   b. By subcutaneous or intramuscular injection: 15–30 mg 4 to 6-hourly as required for pain.
   c. Intravenous injections may cause a rapid fall in blood pressure. They should be administered slowly and the dosage recommended is 10–20 mg 4 to 6-hourly as required.
2. Children: For oral, subcutaneous or intramuscular administration: Less than 1 year—0.15–0.2 mg/kg 8-hourly; 1-7 years—2–5 mg 8-hourly.

Nurse monitoring
See the section on narcotic analgesics.

General notes
1. Preparations may be stored at room temperature.
2. By law this drug must be kept in a locked (controlled drug) cupboard.

MULTIVITAMINS (Pabrinex)

Presentation
1. There are numerous oral vitamin and multivitamin preparations available either by prescription or direct over-the-counter sales.
2. Parenteral multivitamins are available as Pabrinex, either IMM (intramuscular maintenance), IMHP (intramuscular high potency) or IVHP (intravenous high potency).

Actions and uses
1. Oral preparations: Vitamins and multivitamin supplements are frequently prescribed and even more frequently purchased directly for use as tonics. There is no real evidence that they are of any benefit for this purpose.
2. In patients who have a documented history and clinical signs of inadequate diet, oral or parenteral preparations may be usefully prescribed to aid physical recovery.
3. In patients with impaired absorption of foodstuffs due either to disease of the gall bladder, pancreas or gut, parenteral vitamin preparations are an essential component of therapy.
4. Parenteral multivitamins have been shown to be useful in the management of delirium tremens, a state of agitated confusion caused by acute cessation of prolonged heavy drinking.
   It should be noted that Pabrinex contains primarily a number of the vitamin B complex compounds and vitamin C.

Dosage
1. The dosage of oral preparations varies according to the proprietary brand and nurses are advised to consult manufacturers' literature.
2. Parenteral therapy:
   a. For the treatment of adults with acute psychotic disturbances: Initially 2–4 pairs of intravenous high potency ampoules 4-8 hourly for 48 hours followed by one pair of intravenous or intramuscular high potency ampoules daily for 5–7 days. Maintenance therapy should consist of 1–2 pairs of intramuscular maintenance ampoules given daily until full health is restored.
   b. Children: Parenteral therapy is rarely necessary but when it is indicated doses are:
      i. 6–10 years: one-third of the adult dose.
      ii. 10–14 years: one-third to one-half of the adult dose.
      iii. 14 years and over: should receive adult doses.

Nurse monitoring
1. The ill-effects caused by administration of an excess of vitamins are discussed more fully under the individual headings (see the sections covering vitamin A, vitamin B complex, vitamin C, vitamin D and vitamin E).
2. Parenteral administration of Pabrinex has a number of problems which are:
   a. With repeated injections anaphylactic shock may occur and appropriate measures such as the injection of adrenaline and soluble glucocorticoids or antihistamines should be readily available during administration of this therapy.
   b. Pabrinex contains pyridoxine and this may antagonize levodopa therapy for Parkinson's disease.
   c. Flushing of the face may rarely occur.
   d. Perhaps the most important point for the nurse to note is that the intramuscular (IMM) preparation should never be given intravenously.

General note
Ampoules of Pabrinex should be stored in a cool, dry place.

M

MUSTINE

Presentation
Injection—10 mg

Actions and uses
Mustine is a cytotoxic drug of the nitrogen mustard group which arrests cell growth by a chemical binding (alkylating) action on substances which are essential for cell division to proceed. Its uses are as follows:

1. In combination with other cytotoxics in the treatment of Hodgkin's disease and other lymphomas.
2. In the treatment of carcinoma of the lung and other solid tumours.
3. By intracavitary injection in the treatment of malignant effusions, particularly pleural effusions.
4. Topically to skin lesions in mycosis fungoides.

Dosage
This varies considerably according to the nature of the malignant disease and the route of administration, and the following is a rough guide only.

1. Intravenous: 400 microgram/kg body weight as a single dose or in 4 divided daily doses by slow injection into the tubing of a running sodium chloride 0.9% infusion.
2. Intracavitary: 200–400 microgram/kg body weight in 20–50 ml sodium chloride 0.9%.
3. Topical: A solution of 0.02% has been applied to skin lesions.

Nurse monitoring

1. Severe nausea and vomiting are commonly produced within 1 hour of intravenous therapy and last for several hours thereafter.
2. Bone marrow suppression with anaemia, neutropenia and thrombocytopenia is a serious dose-related side-effect.
3. Tinnitus, vertigo and deafness may occur.
4. Patients may display hyper-sensitivity, particularly following topical use, varying from urticaria and other skin reactions to anaphylaxis.
5. The nurse should be constantly aware that most cytotoxic drugs are irritant to the skin and mucous surfaces and are in general very toxic. Great care should therefore be exercised when handling these drugs and in particular spillage or contamination of personnel or the environment must be avoided. If cytotoxic drugs are handled regularly it is theoretically possible that repeated skin contact or inhalation may produce systemic toxic effects and in nurses who have developed hypersensitivity, severe local and general hypersensitivity reactions.

General notes

1. Mustine injection should be stored under refrigeration and attention is drawn to the provision of an expiry date on labelled vials.
2. After reconstitution, the drug should be used immediately and any remaining drug discarded.

N

NABILONE (Cesamet)

Presentation
Capsules—1 mg

Actions and uses
Nabilone is an anti-emetic drug which is chemically related to substances called cannabinoids which are found in cannabis resin. It is used in the management of vomiting associated with anti-cancer therapy.

Dosage
Adults: 1–2 mg taken the night before anti-cancer therapy and repeated 1–3 hours prior to the first dose of anti-cancer drug administered.

Nurse monitoring
1. The major problem with this drug is that it will be liable to misuse since it resembles cannabis and for this reason it is restricted to prescription in hospitals only. The nurse may therefore play a valuable role in ensuring that dosages are taken and that tablets are not allowed to accumulate in the home.
2. Alertness may be impaired and patients should be aware of the risks of impairment of driving skills. This is particularly true if other sedative drugs are taken, particularly alcohol.
3. Patients with a history of psychotic illness may react adversely and should be carefully monitored.

General note
Nabilone capsules may be stored at room temperature.

NABUMETONE (Relifex)

Presentation
Tablets—500 mg
Suspension—500 mg in 5 ml

Actions and uses
This drug is converted after absorption to its active metabolite which is a non-steroidal anti-inflammatory drug (see under this section). It has anti-inflammatory and analgesic properties and is used in the treatment of chronic arthritic disease.

Dosage
Adults: Usually 1 g taken as a single dose at bedtime. This may be supplemented by an additional 500 mg to 1 g dose in the morning.

Nurse monitoring
See non-steroidal anti-inflammatory drugs.

General note
Nabumetone tablets and suspension may be stored at room temperature and should be protected from light.

NADOLOL (Corgard)

Presentation
Tablets—40 mg, 80 mg

Actions and uses
Nadolol is a non-selective beta-adrenoreceptor blocking drug and its actions and uses are described in the section dealing with these drugs.

Dosage
The usual daily adult dose is in the range 40 mg to 240 mg daily as a single dose or in two divided doses, depending upon the range of indications for this drug.

Nurse monitoring

See the section on beta-adrenoreceptor blocking drugs.

General note

Nadolol tablets may be stored at room temperature.

NAFTIDROFURYL (Praxilene)

Presentation

Capsules—100 mg
Injection—200 mg in 10 ml

Actions and uses

This drug acts on the cardiovascular system to produce vasodilation. It is used in clinical practice for the following disorders:

1. For the treatment of peripheral vascular insufficiency including Raynaud's phenomenon, intermittent claudication, night cramps and frostbite.
2. It is also used to improve blood supply to the brain in cerebrovascular insufficiency.

Dosage

1. Orally: 100 mg three times per day.
2. Parenterally: By intravenous or intra-arterial infusion: in sodium chloride 0.9%, dextrose 5% or dextran injection: 200 mg twice daily.

Nurse monitoring

1. It is important to note that this drug must never be administered by intravenous bolus injection.
2. Nausea, epigastric pain, flushing of the skin of the head and neck, tachycardia, postural hypotension, headache and dizziness may occur.

General notes

1. The drug may be stored at room temperature.
2. Solutions should be protected from light.

NALBUPHINE (Nubain)

Presentation

Injection—20 mg in 2 ml

Actions and uses

Nalbuphine is a strong, non-narcotic analgesic used in the treatment of moderate-to-severe pain, e.g. postoperatively, after myocardial infarction, etc. It has uses in common with buprenorphine and meptazinol. These drugs do not appear to produce significant dependence, respiratory depression or cardiovascular disturbances which are major disadvantages of morphine and related analgesics.

Dosage

Adults: 10–20 mg by intravenous, intramuscular or subcutaneous injection.

Nurse monitoring

1. Though nalbuphine is reported to be associated with little if any dependence, it is intended for short term pain relief and the possibility of abuse should not be overlooked.
2. In common with opiate analgesics nalbuphine may produce nausea and constipation requiring remedial anti-emetic and laxative therapy.

General note

Nalbuphine injection may be stored at room temperature but ampoules should be protected from light.

NALIDIXIC ACID (Negram)

Presentation

Tablets—500 mg
Suspension—300 mg in 5 ml

Actions and uses

This drug has a bactericidal action, i.e. it kills the bacteria present in the body. It has been found to be particularly effective against the Gram-negative organisms which commonly cause urinary tract infections. These are *E. coli*, Klebsiella, Enterobacter and Proteus species. It is important to remember that infections due to *Pseudomonas aeruginosa* are rarely, if ever, effectively treated by nalidixic acid.

Dosage
1. Adults:
   a. For acute urinary tract infections: 1 g four times a day.
   b. For prolonged treatment of chronic infections: 500 mg four times a day.
2. Children: Children under 3 months of age should rarely, if ever, be given this drug as their livers are incapable of metabolizing it. Older children should receive 50 mg/kg body weight in total daily, given in divided doses.

Nurse monitoring
1. As noted above the drug should rarely, if ever, be given to children under the age of 3 months.
2. If given to infants, raised intracranial pressure manifest by drowsiness, convulsions and papilloedema may occur.
3. Side-effects in older patients may include skin rash, visual disturbance, headache and gastrointestinal symptoms such as nausea, vomiting and abdominal pain.
4. Photosensitivity reactions, urticaria, pruritus, fever and blood disorders may occur in patients who prove to be hypersensitive to the drug.
5. The drug enhances the effect of two other major groups of drugs
   a. Warfarin, leading to a danger of bleeding unless the dosage is carefully monitored and reduced appropriately.
   b. Oral anti-diabetic drugs where hypoglycaemia may be induced.
6. Nalidixic acid may cause positive reactions to urinary tests with Benidix solution and Clinitest.

General note
The drug may be stored at room temperature.

NANDROLONE (Durabolin, Deca-Durabolin)

Presentation
Injection—25 mg, 50 mg in 1 ml (as the decanoate salt)
—50 mg in 1 ml (as the phenyl-propionate salt)

Actions and uses
The actions and uses of anabolic steroids are described in the section dealing with these drugs in hormones (5). In its decanoate form this drug has a duration of action of 3 weeks while in the phenylpropionate form it has a duration of action of 1 week.

Dosage
By deep intramuscular injection:
1. Adults.
   a. As the phenylpropionate salt: 25 mg to 50 mg once weekly.
   b. As the decanoate salt: 25 mg to 50 mg every 3 weeks.
2. Children:
   a. Up to 1 mg/kg per month as the phenylpropionate form.
   b. 0.75–1.5 mg/kg every week as the decanoate form.

Nurse monitoring
See the sections on androgenic hormones and anabolic steroids in hormones (5).

General notes
1. The drug may be stored at room temperature.
2. Injection solution should be protected from direct sunlight.

NAPROXEN (Naprosyn, Synflex)

Note: Also combined with misoprostol in Napratec
Presentation
Tablets—250 mg, 275 mg, 375 mg, 500 mg
Tablets (enteric-coated)—250 mg, 375 mg, 500 mg
Tablets (sustained release)—500 mg
Suspension—250 mg in 10 ml
Granules—500 mg sachets
Suppositories—500 mg

Actions and uses
See the section on non-steroidal anti-inflammatory analgesic drugs.

Dosage
1. Adults:
   a. The initial dosage is usually 250 mg twice per day.
   b. Maintenance dosage is usually adjusted to within the range of 370 mg to 1 g in total daily
   c. As an alternative to oral therapy, one suppository (500 mg) may be inserted at night.
2. Children: In the treatment of rheumatoid disease a dose of 10 mg/kg per day has been used but only in children over the age of 5 years.
3. In the treatment of acute gout 750 mg is given initially followed by 250 mg 8-hourly until the attack has clinically resolved.

Nurse monitoring
See the section on non-steroidal anti-inflammatory analgesic drugs.

General note
Naproxen preparations may be stored at room temperature.

NARCOTIC ANALGESICS

Note: Such drugs are usually collectively termed opioids (opium-like). They comprise a group of drugs derived from opium and termed opium alkaloids, and synthetic compounds based on the opium alkaloids. They include the following preparations:

Buprenorphine
Codeine
Dextromoramide
Dextropropoxyphene
Diamorphine
Dihydrocodeine
Dipipanone
Meptazinol
Methadone
Morphine
Nalbuphine
Papaveretum
Pentazocine
Pethidine
Phenazocine

Actions and uses
1. Narcotic analgesic drugs have a powerful analgesic action mediated by their direct effect on the central nervous system. They are used for the treatment of conditions associated with acute or chronic severe pain such as myocardial infarction, childbirth, postoperative pain and the pain associated with malignant disease. They are also used regularly for pre-operative medication.
2. One of the weaker members of the group, codeine, is used both as an analgesic and for its cough suppressant and constipating action.

Nurse monitoring
1. The most important point for the nurse to note is that the use of many of the drugs in this group is strictly controlled by law and the legal aspects of prescribing these drugs is further discussed in Appendix 1.
2. The most serious problem encountered with patients who receive these drugs is the production of physical dependence and addiction. Nurses play an important role in giving patients support when such drugs are being withdrawn after short-term use, in identifying patients who may be becoming dependent on these drugs and in providing support to patients who are being weaned off prolonged use of these drugs.
3. Narcotic analgesics produce a dose-related depression of neurological function resulting in sedation, drowsiness, sleepiness. They may eventually produce profound depression of respiratory function and therefore must be used with great caution in patients who already have poor respiratory function or in those in whom the sedative effect may be enhanced, such as patients with liver cirrhosis.

4. Many analgesics in this group produce severe nausea and vomiting and for this reason they are commonly used in combinations containing anti-emetics.

5. Narcotic analgesics influence the motility of the gut and cause constipation. This may be a major problem which may give rise to great discomfort especially in elderly and bedridden patients.

6. Narcotic analgesics must be used with extreme caution in patients who are also receiving monoamine oxidase inhibitors (q.v.) as the combination of these two types of drug may produce serious cardiovascular reactions.

7. In addition to physical dependence, the phenomenon of tolerance may arise in patients receiving prolonged treatment with these analgesics. The term 'tolerance' basically means that with prolonged treatment patients receive less benefit from doses which were previously effective. This may mean that the frequency of administration and dosage may have to be increased as duration of therapy progresses. As many patients receiving prolonged narcotic analgesia are suffering from chronic pain due to malignant conditions the nurse may play an important role in observing such patients and identifying the relative efficacy of their treatment regimes so that the need for change in therapy may be brought to the attention of the medical staff.

General note
   See specific drugs.

NATAMYCIN (Pimafucin)

Presentation
   Pessaries—25 mg
   Cream—2%
   Oral suspension—1%
Actions and uses
   This anti-fungal drug is used most commonly in clinical practice for the treatment of infections due to *Candida albicans.*
Dosage
   1. Pessaries: One at night.
   2. Cream: Apply twice daily.
   3. 4 drops after feeds in infants.

Nurse monitoring
   No problems are associated with the administration of this drug.

General note
   The drug may be stored at room temperature.

NEDOCROMIL (Tilade)

Presentation
   Pressurized inhaler—2 mg per metered dose.
Actions and uses
   Nedocromil is a specific anti-inflammatory drug with an action in the lung. In asthma there is a tendency for a variety of cells present within the bronchial mucosa to break down on exposure to certain environmental trigger factors (animal dander, cigarette smoke, house dust mite, etc.) resulting in the release of chemicals which provoke bronchospasm. Nedocromil inhibits the release of such substances; it is administered by inhalation for the prevention of asthmatic attacks.
Dosage
   Adults and older children: 4 mg by inhalation 2–4 times daily.

Nurse monitoring
   1. It is important to recognize that this is a prophylactic drug. It must be taken regularly and never to treat an asthmatic attack.
   2. The action of nedocromil is somewhat similar to that of sodium cromoglycate (intal) which is the drug of choice for young children.
   3. Occasionally headaches and nausea have been reported and some patients may complain of an unpleasant bitter taste.

General note

Nedocromil aerosol inhalers may be stored at room temperature. Each unit contains 112 individual doses: when finished it should not be disposed of by incineration.

NEFOPAM (Acupan)

Presentation

Tablets—30 mg

Injection—20 mg in 1 ml

Actions and uses

Nefopam is an analgesic drug which acts by a direct effect on the central nervous system. It is chemically unrelated to the narcotic analgesic drugs and it is indicated for the management of moderate to severe pain which is not amenable to treatment with mild analgesics but is not felt to be of sufficient severity to require narcotic analgesia.

Dosage

1. Orally: 30–90 mg three times per day.
2. By intramuscular or intravenous injection: 20 mg four times per day (see nurse monitoring section for administration procedure).

Nurse monitoring

1. When this drug is given by intramuscular injection care must be taken to ensure that accidental intravenous injection is avoided. If intravenous injection is contemplated, the drug should be administered slowly, the maximum rate of administration recommended being 5 mg/minute. Too rapid intravenous injection may cause syncope.
2. Common side-effects include nausea, vomiting, blurred vision, nervousness, light-headedness, dry mouth, drowsiness, sweating, insomnia, headache and tachycardia.
3. Patients with a history of fits should not receive this drug.
4. The metabolism and excretion of nefopam may be impaired in patients with liver or kidney disease.

General notes

1. The drug may be stored at room temperature.
2. Notes on intramuscular and intravenous administration are included in the nurse monitoring section.

NEOMYCIN

(See Note 3, p. 362)

Presentation

Tablets—500 mg

N.B. Neomycin is included in a vast range of preparations for topical use including ointments, creams, eye drops and ear drops. It is usually combined with other medicaments particularly other antibiotics and corticosteroids.

Actions and uses

Neomycin is an antibiotic of the aminoglycoside group which resembles gentamicin (q.v.). It is not absorbed orally and is too toxic for systemic use. It is therefore only useful in the following situations:

1. It may be given in an attempt to sterilize the gut. This is useful before bowel surgery and also may lead to a decrease in protein absorption from the bowel which is useful in patients with cirrhosis of the liver when they develop encephalopathy.
2. It is an effective antibiotic for the treatment of superficial infections of the skin, eye and ear.

Dosage

1. To attempt bowel sterilization:
   a. Adults receive 500 mg–1 g four times per day.
   b. Children: Less than 1 year—2 mg/kg four times a day; More than 1 year—125–250 mg four times a day.

Nurse monitoring

1. Systemic adverse effects are unlikely as very little of the drug is absorbed.
2. Despite the fact that the drug is very poorly absorbed, a large number of patients develop skin rashes due to hypersensitivity.

3. Nurses who are sensitive to the drug develop severe skin rashes if they handle it. Therefore the wearing of protective gloves is advised.

General note
Neomycin tablets may be stored at room temperature.

NEOSTIGMINE (Prostigmin)

Presentation
Tablets—15 mg neostigmine bromide
Ampoules—0.5 mg and 2.5 mg neostigmine methylsulphate in 1 ml

Actions and uses
Neostigmine prevents the action of the enzyme that destroys acetylcholine in the body. This in effect leads to a prolongation of acetylcholine action which is to stimulate the parasympathetic component of the autonomic nervous system. It has the following uses in clinical practice:
1. For the treatment of myasthenia gravis.
2. As an antidote to non-depolarizing or competitive (curariform) muscle relaxants used in surgery.

Dosage
1. For the treatment of myasthenia gravis:
   a. Adults: A daily dose of 5–20 tablets by mouth or 1–2.5 mg by injection is commonly given but doses higher than these may be needed in some patients.
   b. Children: The doses should be decided by the attending physician. A guideline is as follows:
      i. Neonates: 0.05–0.25 mg by injection or 1–5 mg orally every 4 hours.
      ii. Older children: 0.2–0.5 mg daily by injection or 15–60 mg daily orally.
2. As an antidote to curariform drugs: 1–5 mg intravenously. Atropine 0.4–1.25 mg should normally be given some minutes before this injection.

Nurse monitoring
1. Side-effects include excess salivation, anorexia, nausea, vomiting, abdominal cramp and diarrhoea. Bradycardia and hypotension may occur along with bronchoconstriction and increase in bronchial secretions. Rarely weakness, paralysis, convulsion and coma may occur.
2. It is important to note that the major symptom of overdosage with this drug is increased muscular weakness. When used for the treatment of myasthenia gravis, the patient may become weak and it is then difficult to differentiate whether this is due to inadequate or excessive treatment. In this situation the intravenous administration of edrophonium chloride (Tensilon) will produce a rapid and short-lived improvement in muscle power if inadequate dosage is the cause of weakness but will not have this effect if overdosage is the cause of weakness.
3. The drug should never be given to patients who are known to suffer from intestinal or urinary obstruction.
4. Patients with bradycardia, bronchial asthma, heart disease, epilepsy, hypotension and Parkinsonism should not receive this drug.

General notes
1. All preparations should be protected from light.
2. Tablets should be stored in well closed containers.

NETILMICIN (Netillin)

(See Note 3, p. 362)

Presentation
Injection—10 mg in 1.5 ml, 50 mg in 1 ml, 100 mg in 1 ml

Actions and uses
Netilmicin is a member of the aminoglycoside group of antibiotics. Its actions and uses are identical to those of gentamicin. It is administ-

ered only by injection and is
frequently favoured since it produces
a lower incidence of adverse effects
than do other aminoglycosides.

Dosage
As for gentamicin, though slightly
higher doses may be used.

Nurse monitoring
See the section on aminoglycoside
antibiotics.

General notes
1. Netilmicin injections may be
   stored at room temperature.
2. The drug should never be mixed
   with other antibiotics prior to
   administration.
3. Intravenous infusions are
   prepared in 100 ml sodium
   chloride 0.9%, dextrose 5% or
   dextrose/saline mixtures and
   infused over 30 minutes to 2
   hours.

NICARDIPINE (Cardene)

Presentation
Capsules—20 mg, 30 mg
Capsules—30 mg, 45 mg (sustained
release)

Actions and uses
Nicardipine has the actions and uses
described for nifedipine.

Dosage
1. Hypertension: 20–40 mg three
   times daily or 30–60 mg sustained
   release capsules twice daily.
2. Angina pectoris: maintenance
   therapy only, dosages as for
   hypertension.

Nurse monitoring
The nurse monitoring section for
nifedipine also applies to this drug.

General note
Nicardipine capsules may be stored
at room temperature.

NICLOSAMIDE (Yomesan)

Presentation
Tablets—500 mg

Actions and uses
This antihelminthic drug is used for
the treatment of the following
tapeworm infections:
1. Beef tapeworm (*Taenia saginata*)
2. Pork tapeworm (*Taenia solium*)
3. Fish tapeworm (*Diphyllobothrium
   latum*)
4. Dwarf tapeworm (*Hymenolepis
   nana*)

Dosage
1. For the treatment of beef, pork
   and fish tapeworm:
   a. Adults and children over 6
      years: 2 g
   b. Children 2–6 years: 1 g
   c. Children under 2 years: 500
      mg
2. For the treatment of dwarf
   tapeworm:
   a. On the first day adults and
      children over 6—2 g; Children
      2–6 years—1 g; Children
      under 2 years—500 mg
   b. For the subsequent 6 days:
      adults and children over 6—1
      g daily; Children 2–6 years—
      500 mg daily; Children under 2
      years—250 mg daily.

Nurse monitoring
1. A laxative given 2 hours after
   treatment with this drug ensures
   a rapid and complete expulsion
   of the worm which would
   otherwise be excreted in pieces
   during the next few days. It is felt
   that in the treatment of *Taenia
   solium* a laxative is essential.
2. The drug may be given without
   danger to patients with liver,
   biliary or kidney disease.

General note
The drug may be stored at room
temperature.

NICOFURANOSE (Bradilan)

Presentation
Tablets—250 mg enteric-coated

Actions and uses
This drug dilates peripheral blood
vessels and is therefore used in
clinical practice to treat the following
disorders:

1. Raynaud's syndrome
2. Intermittent claudication
3. Night cramps and chilblains.

Dosage
For adults 500 mg–1 g three times daily.

Nurse monitoring
1. The side-effects of all drugs which have vasodilator effect include flushing of the skin of the face and the neck, hypotension, dizziness, faintness (especially on standing up). These side-effects may make a reduction in dosage necessary.
2. Gastrointestinal symptoms encountered with this drug include nausea and vomiting.

General note
The drug may be stored at room temperature.

NICOTINYL ALCOHOL (Ronicol)

Presentation
Tablets—25 mg and 150 mg (slow release)

Actions and uses
The actions and uses of this drug are identical to those described for nicofuranose (q.v.).

Dosage
Adults: 25–50 mg four times a day or 150–300 mg twice daily as slow release tablets.

Nurse monitoring
The nurse monitoring section on nicofuranose (q.v.) applies to this drug.

General note
The drug may be stored at room temperature.

NICOUMALONE (Sinthrome)

Presentation
Tablets—1 mg

Actions and uses
A number of substances present in blood which play an important part in preventing bleeding by forming clots are produced by the liver from vitamin K. Nicoumalone inhibits the synthesis of these substances (known as clotting factors) and therefore reduces the ability of the blood to clot. Its principal uses are for the prevention and treatment of thromboembolic states such as deep venous thrombosis and pulmonary embolus. They are also used to prevent the formation of clot in cardiovascular disease either on artificial heart valves or in the atria of patients who have atrial dysrhythmias.

Dosage
1. Adults:.
   a. Loading dose: Day 1: 8–16 mg; Day 2: 4–12 mg; Day 3: Dosage should be adjusted according to result of blood clotting test.
   b. Maintenance dose: Varies according to individual response and should be decided after reference to the results of blood clotting test.

Nurse monitoring
1. The daily maintenance dose of nicoumalone is, as noted above, determined by the results of clotting studies. As the effects of bleeding due to overcoagulation or thrombosis due to undercoagulation can be so rapidly catastrophic, strict adherence to the recommended dose is mandatory and the nurse may play an important role in ensuring that patients are aware of this.
2. The effects of nicoumalone may be influenced by a number of factors listed below and the nurse may play an important role by identifying their occurrence and alerting both the patient and medical staff. The following circumstances may lead to a requirement for alteration in dosage:
   a. Acute illness such as chest infection or viral infection.
   b. Sudden weight loss.

N

c. The concurrent administration of other drugs: A number of drugs may affect the patient's dosage requirements. Where drugs are known to interfere with anticoagulant control this has been noted in the nurse monitoring sections of the drugs in this book.

3. The occurrence of haemorrhage in a patient on nicoumalone is an indication for immediate withdrawal of the drug and if the haemorrhage is at all serious or repetitive the patient should be referred immediately to hospital for further assessment and, if necessary, they may be given vitamin K which accelerates a return to normal clotting function.

4. Nicoumalone is relatively contraindicated in patients with severe liver or kidney disease, haemorrhagic conditions or uncontrolled hypertension. It should also be used with great caution immediately after surgery or labour.

5. Nausea, loss of appetite, headache and dizziness may occur.

General note

The tablets may be stored at room temperature

NIFEDIPINE (Adalat, Coracten, Nifensar XL))

Presentation

Capsules—5 mg and 10 mg
Tablets—10 mg, 20 mg (Retard)
Tablets —20 mg, 30 mg, 60 mg (sustained release)
Capsules—10 mg, 20 mg (sustained release)

Actions and uses

Nifedipine has three main actions

1. It decreases the work done by the heart in two ways:
   a. It directly affects heart muscle, depressing its activity.
   b. It dilates peripheral vessels, reducing the pressure against which the heart has to work.

2. It lowers raised blood pressure by its action on peripheral blood vessels which results in vasodilation.

3. It improves peripheral perfusion in patients with vascular insufficiency.

These properties make it useful for the treatment of angina pectoris, hypertension and Raynaud's phenomenon.

Dosage

1. Angina pectoris:
   a. Prophylaxis: 10 mg three times a day initially increasing to a maximum of 20 mg three times a day if necessary. 5 mg capsules may be useful when carefully tailoring doses to individual need.
   b. Treatment of acute attack: a capsule may be bitten and placed under the tongue to produce a more rapid onset of effect.

2. Hypertension: 20–40 mg as 'Retard' tablets or 'Coracten' taken twice a day. Slow release capsules may be taken once daily in a dose of 30 mg and up to 90–100 mg if necessary.

Nurse monitoring

1. Note that different modified release preparations exist and that these are not necessarily interchangeable.

2. Headaches and flushing may be expected in patients on this drug. Lethargy or tiredness may also occur.

3. There is some evidence that occasionally the drug, after an acute myocardial infarction, may divert blood to healthy rather than damaged muscle and so increase the extent of damage.

4. Sometimes angina may be paradoxically exacerbated and require the drug to be stopped.

General note

The drug may be stored at room temperature. It is light-sensitive.

NITRAZEPAM (Mogadon)

Presentation
Tablets—5 mg
Capsules—5 mg
Suspension—2.5 mg in 5 ml.

Actions and uses
Nitrazepam is a member of the benzodiazepine group (q.v.) which has a pronounced sedative effect and is taken at night as an hypnotic.

Dosage
5–10 mg on retiring.

Nurse monitoring
1. See the section on benzodiazepines.
2. It is essential to re-emphasize that nitrazepam is particularly likely to cause a hang-over effect with drowsiness and headache the following day. This may be particularly severe when high dosage is used in elderly patients and may lead to frank confusion. It is recommended that the elderly should only very rarely receive a dose exceeding 5 mg of this drug if side-effects are to be avoided.

General note
Preparations containing nitrazepam may be stored at room temperature.

NITROFURANTOIN (Macrodantin, Furadantin)

Presentation
Tablets—50 mg and 100 mg
Capsules—50 mg and 100 mg
Suspension—25 mg in 5 ml

Actions and uses
Nitrofurantoin is bactericidal, i.e. it kills organisms in the body if the concentration of the drug obtained is sufficiently high. At lower concentrations it is bacteriostatic, i.e. it inhibits growth and further multiplication of bacterial cells. It is so rapidly excreted from the body that it is only of use in bacterial infections of the bladder. It is debatable whether sufficient concentration is obtained in the kidney for it to be useful in pyelonephritis and it is certainly not useful for infections of other organs of the body. It is usually effective against *E. coli*, Klebsiella and Enterobacter but resistance is a greater problem with Proteus and *Pseudomonas aeruginosa*. It is used both in the treatment of urinary tract infections and for prophylaxis against urinary tract infections.

Dosage
1. For the treatment of urinary tract infections:
   a. Adults: 100 mg four times a day with meals.
   b. Children: Less than 1 year— 2.5 mg/kg body weight four times a day; 1–7 years—25– 50 mg four times a day; Over 7 years—adult doses are administered.
2. For the prophylaxis of urinary tract infection half of the dose recommended for treatment of acute infections is given.

Nurse monitoring
1. Nausea, vomiting and diarrhoea occur commonly. The incidence and severity of these effects may be reduced if the drug is taken with meals or milk.
2. An uncommon but important side-effect is peripheral neuropathy. Patients should be continually asked to report symptoms of numbness or tingling of the feet and if such symptoms occur the drug should be immediately withdrawn before irreversible and more severe changes occur.
3. Other neurological side-effects include headache, vertigo, drowsiness, nystagmus and muscle pain.
4. Megaloblastic anaemia is a rare adverse effect.
5. Hypersensitivity reactions including chills, fever, jaundice, liver damage, leucopenia, granulocytopenia and haemolytic anaemia may occur.
6. The drug may rarely damage the lungs especially in elderly patients producing pneumonitis and pulmonary fibrosis.

N

> 7. The drug should not be given to patients who have severe renal damage as it may accumulate in the body and produce severe toxic effects.

General note
The drug may be stored at room temperature.

NIZATIDINE (Axid)

Presentation
Capsules—150 mg, 300 mg
Actions and uses
See histamine H_2-receptor antagonists.
Dosage
1. Treatment of peptic ulcer: 150 mg twice daily or 300 mg at bed-time for up to 8 weeks.
2. Prevention of relapse: usually a single bed-time dose of 150 mg since it appears that overnight acid output is important in determining ulcer relapse rates.

> ### Nurse monitoring
> The nurse monitoring aspects described for histamine H_2-receptor antagonists apply.

General note
Nizatidine tablets may be stored at room temperature.

NON-STEROIDAL ANTI-INFLAMMA-TORY ANALGESIC DRUGS

Actions and uses
This group of drugs relieves pain and reduces inflammation in a variety of diseases affecting the joints, tendons, cartilage and muscle. Thus they are useful in such disorders as rheumatoid arthritis, osteoarthritis, ankylosing spondylitis and gouty arthritis. If given in lower doses for minor painful conditions they are effective analgesics but this practice is to be discouraged as simple analgesics such as paraceta-mol are equally effective and do not have the potentially serious side-

effects of this group of drugs. For convenience the drugs may be classified according to their chemical structure.
1. Anthranilic acid derivatives
   Mefenamic acid
2. Indole acetic acid derivatives
   Etodolac
   Indomethacin
   Sulindac
3. Salicylates
   Aspirin.
   Benorylate, converted to aspirin in blood.
   Diflunisal, a long-acting aspirin-like drug which is less irritant to the gastric mucosa than is aspirin.
   Salsalate, converted to aspirin in the blood.
4. Phenylacetic acid derivatives
   Diclofenac
5. Pyrazoles
   Azapropazone
6. Propionic acid derivatives
   Fenbufen
   Fenoprofen
   Flurbiprofen
   Ibuprofen
   Ketoprofen
   Naproxen
   Tiaprofenic acid.
7. Others
   Acemetacin
   Ketorolac
   Nambumetone
   Piroxicam

Dosage
See individual drugs.

> ### Nurse monitoring
> 1. As mentioned above this group of drugs are very effective analgesics but they have potentially serious side-effects and perhaps the major role to be played by the nurse in the management of patients who are in possession of these drugs is to ensure that they are taken in the correct dosage and only for the problems for which they are prescribed.
> 2. These drugs frequently have gastrointestinal side-effects which may range from loss of appetite, nausea, vomiting and

diarrhoea to gastric bleeding which may be either chronic and go unnoticed or be acute and result in haematemesis or melaena. In patients with chronic painful disorders, adequate nutrition is absolutely essential and it is important that the nurse monitors the nutrition of patients on these drugs and where necessary encourages patients to try to overcome any associated anorexia. As a substantial number of patients on these drugs will gradually develop an anaemia, it is important that the nurse observes all patients on these drugs for the clinical signs of anaemia such as pallor, tiredness and dyspnoea on exertion.

3. These drugs are relatively contraindicated in patients with peptic ulceration and they may exacerbate the symptoms of this problem.

4. Asthma may be precipitated in a few patients who are hypersensitive to drugs of this type. This occurs most commonly in the salicylate group but it may also rarely occur with the other groups. An important point to note is that patients who suffer from salicylate-induced asthma may not have their symptoms relieved by changing to one of the other chemical groups.

5. All drugs in this group may cause salt and water retention. This may exacerbate or produce hypertension or cardiac failure. This effect is rarely seen in salicylates except when high dosage is given for the treatment of rheumatic fever.

6. Most anti-inflammatory drugs are metabolized to some extent by the liver and/or are excreted as metabolites or unmetabolized drugs by the kidney.
They will therefore tend to accumulate in patients who have impaired liver or kidney function and be more likely to produce toxic effects.

7. Non-steroidal anti-inflammatory drugs are carried in the blood attached to sites on proteins which circulate in the blood. They have the capacity to displace other drugs from these proteins as the actual active component of any drug is that part which lies free in the plasma rather than that part which is bound to the protein. Any displacement of a drug from the protein will lead to an increased effect. This is especially important with two groups of drugs:
   a. Anticoagulants such as warfarin. If non-steroidal anti-inflammatory drugs are given to patients who are receiving warfarin or other anticoagulants, the anticoagulant may be displaced from the proteins and therefore be proportionately more active. This may lead to bleeding and may be especially dangerous if non-steroidal anti-inflammatory drugs' other side-effects such as peptic ulceration or gastrointestinal bleeding occur coincidentally.
   b. Oral hypoglycaemics such as chlorpropamide may also be displaced with resultant increase in effect and this may cause hypoglycaemia.

General note
See specific drugs.

NORFLOXACIN (Noroxin, Utinor)

Presentation
Tablets—400 mg
Eye drops—0.3%

Actions and uses
Norfloxacin is an aminoquinolone antibiotic chemically related to nalidixic acid, ciprofloxacin and ofloxacin. Its spectrum of activity is similar to that of other drugs but norfloxacin is used mainly in the treatment of urinary tract and ophthalmic infections.

Dosage

1. Urinary tract and other systemic infection:
   a. Adults: A dose of 400 mg twice daily is given for 3 days in uncomplicated lower urinary tract infections, for 7-10 days in more resistant cases, and for up to 12 weeks in chronic relapsing cases.
2. Ophthalmic infections.
   a. 1–2 drops instilled in the affected eye 4 times a day.

Nurse monitoring

1. In common with other broad spectrum antibiotics, disturbances of gastrointestinal function are possible.
2. A few patients may develop allergy to norfloxacin. This usually presents as skin rashes but in more severe cases breathlessness, tachycardia, angioedema, and even anaphylaxis may occur.
3. Central nervous system side-effects include restlessness, agitation, hallucinations and confusion. Seizures have been reported in a few cases and treatment in epileptics should be avoided.
4. Since norfloxacin has been shown to impair development of joint tissue in immature animals, it should be avoided in infants and young children if possible.
5. Eye drops once opened should be retained for 7 days in hospitalized patients or 4 weeks if in the community.

General note

Norfloxacin tablets and eye drops are stored at room temperature.

NORTRIPTYLINE (Aventyl, Allegron)

Presentation

Tablets—10 mg, 25 mg
Capsules—10 mg, 25 mg
Syrup—10 mg in 5 ml

Actions and uses

Nortriptyline is a tricyclic antidepressant drug. Its actions and uses are described in the section on these drugs.

Dosage

For the treatment of depression:
1. Adult dose ranges vary from 10–25 mg three to four times daily.
2. Children over the age of 12 may be given 10–25 mg three times daily.
3. Children under the age of 12 and the elderly may be given 10 mg three or four times daily.

Nurse monitoring

See the section on tricyclic antidepressant drugs.

General note

Preparations containing nortriptyline may be stored at room temperature.

NYSTATIN (Nystan, Mycostatin)

Presentation

Tablets—500 000 units
Suspension—100 000 units in 1 ml
Pessaries—100 000 units
Gel—100 000 units in 1 g
Vaginal cream—100 000 units in 4 g
Cream and ointment—100 000 units in 1 g

Actions and uses

This anti-fungal drug is used most commonly in clinical practice to eradicate infection due to *Candida albicans* either in the gut or the genital tract.

Dosage

1. Orally: one tablet or 1 ml of suspension three or four times daily.
2. Vaginally: One or two pessaries at night.
3. Topical applications should be administered two to four times daily.
4. Nystatin solutions have been used in a variety of strengths for e.g. bladder/wound irrigation, inhalation via nebulizer, soaks for dentures, etc. Advice on special mixtures of this type should be sought from Pharmacy Departments.

Nurse monitoring
1. It is important to note that the drug is not absorbed after oral administration and is not used for systemic infections.
2. The drug does not produce any known side-effects.

General note
The drug may be stored at room temperature.

N

O

OESTRADIOL (Estraderm TTS)

Presentation

Transdermal patch—25, 50 and 100 microgram released from a reservoir of 2, 4 and 8 mg respectively.

Actions and uses

The Estraderm TTS (Transdermal Therapeutic System) provides a means of achieving gradually, and at a relatively constant rate, blood levels of the natural oestrogen, 17 beta-oestradiol via the trans-dermal route from application of an impregnated patch to the skin. This obviates the need for frequent oral administration and mimics to some extent the natural release of oestrogen from the functioning ovary. Skin patches of oestradiol are used as a method of hormone replacement after ovarian failure, i.e. in menopausal women or younger women after hysterectomy and oophorectomy. This route is associated with more natural control, less risk of cardiovascular complications and improvement in associated symptoms such as hot flushing, mood disturbances, loss of libido and vaginal dryness, and infection. See also an account of oestrogens under hormones (1).

Dosage

A single patch is applied to the skin twice weekly at 3–4 day intervals, starting with an average dose of 50 mg (Estraderm 50) and increasing up to 100 mg as required according to the response. The patch should produce oestradiol levels similar to those seen during early follicular release.

Nurse monitoring

1. Patients require careful instruc-tions in application of Estraderm patches. Each patch is applied to an area of dry, smooth skin below the waist. Patches must never be applied to the breast since high local concentrations may predispose to malignancy. Patches are of course contraindicated in oestrogen-dependent cancer.
2. Each patch is applied to the skin and pressed firmly to the site using the warm palm of the hand for at least 10 seconds.
3. If applied correctly Estraderm patches will remain in situ despite normal mechanical friction, and hot and cold bathing. It should never be necessary to stick patches with adhesive tape.
4. See also notes on hormones (1). This form of therapy however provides relatively very low systemic levels of oestradiol and is much less likely than oral oestrogen therapy to increase cardiovascular risk. It can therefore be used when other risk factors exist, including cigarette smoking and hypertension.
5. Occasionally an allergic contact skin rash occurs in sensitive patients for which an inactive component of the patch may be responsible.

General note

Estraderm skin patches may be stored at room temperature. Each patch is enclosed in a protective pouch which is removed immediately before application.

OESTRADIOL VALERATE (Progynova)

Also combined with norgestrel in Cyclo-Progynova

Presentation
Tablets—1 mg, 2 mg

Actions and uses
Oestradiol valerate is an oestrogenic substance. The general actions and uses of oestrogens are described in the section on these drugs. Oestradiol valerate in clinical practice is used for the alleviation of menopausal symptoms and the prophylaxis and treatment of post-menopausal sequelae of oestrogen withdrawal such as osteoporosis and senile vaginitis.

Dosage
For the treatment of menopausal symptoms: 21-day cycles of 1 or 2 mg are administered.

Nurse monitoring
1. See the section on oestrogenic hormones under hormones (1).
2. When used as hormone replacement therapy in women with an intact uterus (i.e. who have not undergone hysterectomy) it is necessary to counter uterine hyperplasia and an increased risk of cancer by combining this drug with a progestogen, hence the use of Cyclo-Progynova.

General note
The drug may be stored at room temperature.

OESTRIOL (Ortho-Gynest, Ovestin)

Presentation
Tablets—250 microgram
Vaginal cream—0.01%
Vaginal pessary—0.5 mg

Actions and uses
Oestriol is an oestrogenic substance. The general actions and uses of oestrogens are described in the section on contraceptives (oral).

Dosage
1. For the treatment of functional dysmenorrhoea: 1 mg daily for 14 days prior to the expected onset of pain.
2. For the treatment of senile vaginitis: 250–500 microgram per day.
3. Topical therapy for senile vaginitis: One pessary as one metered dose inserted into the vagina each evening.

Nurse monitoring
See the section on oestrogens in hormones (1).

General note
The drug may be stored at room temperature.

OESTROGENS, CONJUGATED (Premarin)

Also combined with norgestrel in Prempak C

Presentation
Tablets—0.625 mg, 1.25 mg, 2.5 mg
Injection—25 mg in 5 ml
Vaginal cream—0.625 mg/g

Actions and uses
1. The actions and uses of oestrogenic hormones in general are described in the section on contraceptives (oral).
2. The oral preparation of this drug has a number of recommended uses:
   a. For the treatment of symptoms due to post-menopausal oestrogen deficiency.
   b. For the treatment of senile vaginitis.
   c. For the treatment of post-menopausal osteoporosis.
   d. For the suppression of lactation.
   e. For the treatment of amenorrhoea.
   f. For the treatment of prostatic carcinoma.
   g. For the regulation of abnormal uterine bleeding.
3. The parenteral (intravenous) preparation is used to achieve haemostasis due to capillary bleeding such as in epistaxis or abnormal uterine bleeding.
4. The vaginal cream is used for the treatment of atrophic vaginitis.

Dosage

1. Orally:
   a. For the treatment of post-menopausal oestrogen deficiency: 0. 625–1.25 mg daily administered cyclically for 21 days every 28 days.
   b. For the treatment of senile vaginitis: Cyclical administration for 21 days every 28 days of 1.25–3.75 mg per day.
   c. For the treatment of post-menopausal osteoporosis: Cyclical administration for 21 days every 28 days of 1.25–3.75 mg per day.
   d. For the suppression of lactation: 3.75 mg every 4 hours for five doses, or 1.25 mg every 4 hours for 5 days.
   e. For the treatment of amenorrhoea: 3.75 mg daily in divided doses for 20 days (for the last 5 days progesterone therapy should be added).
   f. For the treatment of prostatic carcinoma: 4.5–7.5 mg daily in divided doses.
   g. For the treatment of abnormal uterine bleeding:
      i. To achieve haemostasis: 3.75–75 mg daily in divided doses (Haemostasis can usually be expected within 2–4 days).
      ii. For cycle regulation: The daily dose required to produce haemostasis is continued without interruption for 20 days. During each of the last 5–10 days of oestrogen therapy an oral progesterone is given and within 2–5 days of cessation of drugs bleeding should commence.
2. Parenteral administration: To achieve haemostasis:
   a. For adults 25 mg intramuscularly or intravenously.
   b. For children 5–10 mg intramuscularly or intravenously.
3. Topical application: 2–4 g daily.

Nurse monitoring
1. See the section on oestrogenic hormones in hormones (1).
2. When used as hormone replacement therapy in women with an intact uterus (i.e. who have not undergone hysterectomy) it is necessary to counter uterine hyperplasia and an increased risk of cancer by combining this drug with a progestogen, hence the use of Prempak C.

General notes
1. Tablets and vaginal cream may be stored at room temperature.
2. Injection vials should be stored in a refrigerator.
3. Once reconstituted with the diluent provided, injections may be kept for up to 2 months.

OFLOXACIN (Tarivid)

Presentation
Tablets—200 mg, 400 mg

Actions and uses
Ofloxacin is an aminoquinolone antibiotic chemically related to nalidixic acid, ciprofloxacin and enoxacin.
Its spectrum of activity includes Staphylococcus spp., Neisseria spp., Gram-negative microorganisms (including *Pseudomonas auruginosa*), *Haemophillus influenzae,* Chlamydia, Mycoplasma, and Legionella. As a result, ofloxacin may be used in the treatment of upper and lower infections of the urinary tract and respiratory tract, and in various forms of venereal disease.

Dosage
Adults: 200–400 mg once daily and up to 400 mg twice daily in severe infections. Lower urinary tract infections, e.g. cystitis, are generally treated with doses in the lower range. A single dose of 400 mg may be sufficient in uncomplicated urethral and cervical gonorrhoea. For other indications, courses of

between 5 and 10 days are normally required.

Nurse monitoring

1. In common with other broad spectrum antibiotics disturbances of gastrointestinal function are possible.
2. A few patients may develop allergy to ofloxacin. This usually presents as skin rashes but in more severe cases breathlessness, tachycardia, angioedema, and even anaphylaxis may occur.
3. Side-effects on the central nervous system may appear as sleep disturbances, headaches, dizziness, unsteady gait, restlessness, anxiety or confusion. Acute psychotic reactions have been reported after the initial doses, in which case treatment should be promptly discontinued.
4. Rarely, bone marrow suppression leading to anaemia, neutropenia, and thrombocyto-penia has occurred. This may be suspected if patients complain of increasing tiredness or lethargy, infection, or bleeding tendency.
5. Administration of ofloxacin with antacids should be avoided. If possible, a dose of ofloxacin should not be taken within 4 hours of an antacid dose.

General note

Ofloxacin tablets may be stored at room temperature.

OMEPRAZOLE (Losec)

Presentation

Capsules—20 mg and 40 mg, containing enteric-coated granules

Actions and uses

Omeprazole is described as an inhibitor of the 'proton pump', an intracellular mechanism located in acid-secreting cells of the gastric mucosa which is essential for production of gastric acid. It therefore inhibits acid output and, if given in sufficiently high dosage, can actually 'switch off' gastric acid output completely. Omeprazole is currently used in the treatment of peptic ulcer disease and reflux oesophagitis which has proved resistant to more conventional treatment with drugs such as cimetidine or ranitidine. Most recently it has also been licensed for long term maintenance therapy. It is of particular value in Zollinger-Ellison syndrome, a serious condition associated with a gastrinoma which gives rise to excessive gastric acid production.

Dosage

Adults:

1. Duodenal ulcer: 20 mg daily for 4 weeks.
2. Gastric ulcer: 20 mg daily for 8 weeks.

Maintenance therapy is given at above doses.

Double the above dosage in severe disease.

3. Zollinger-Ellison syndrome: doses up to 60 mg once, or even twice, daily are required.
4. Reflux oesophagitis: 20 mg daily for 4 weeks and up to 8 weeks if not adequately healed. 40 mg may be required in refractory cases. Thereafter 20 mg daily maintenance therapy can be used.

Nurse monitoring

1. Long-term suppression of gastric acid is not recommended, and continuous (maintenance) therapy, as seen with drugs such as cimetidine, should not normally occur with omeprazole. An exception arises in the case of reflux oesophagitis when long term low dose therapy may be necessary.
2. Headaches, nausea, diarrhoea, and skin rashes have been reported.
3. Omeprazole should not be administered to pregnant or breast feeding women.
4. Interactions with diazepam, phenytoin, and warfarin have resulted in increased sedation, phenytoin toxicity, and haemorrhage, respectively.

General note

Omeprazole capsules may be stored at room temperature.

ONDANSETRON (Zofran)

Presentation

Tablets—4 mg, 8 mg
Injection—4 mg in 2 ml; 8 mg in 4 ml

Actions and uses

Ondansetron is a member of the group of drugs including granisetron and tropisetron which selectively inhibit the effects of 5-hydroxytryptamine (5-HT, serotonin) at specific binding sites called $5-HT_3$ receptors. Stimulation of these receptors in the gastrointestinal tract and chemoreceptor trigger zone induces nausea and triggers the vomiting reflex. Drugs of this type are therefore used to prevent and treat nausea and vomiting in patients who are exposed to various emetogenic stimuli including anti-cancer drugs and radiotherapy. More recently they have been shown to be similarly effective in the control of post-operative nausea and vomiting.

Dosage

Adults: For therapy associated with moderate nausea and vomiting, an oral dose of 8 mg 8–hourly starting 1–2 hours before therapy is given and continued for up to 5 days is usually sufficient. The initial dose may be given by slow intravenous injection or rapid intravenous infusion immediately before therapy.

Where therapy is likely to produce severe nausea and vomiting, an initial 8 mg dose is usually given by the intravenous route and followed by continuous intravenous infusion at a rate of 1 mg/h for 24 hours, or by two further intravenous bolus doses of 8 mg 4-hourly.

Children: An initial intravenous dose of $5 mg/m^2$ body surface area given as above and followed by oral doses of 2–4 mg 8-hourly for up to 5 days.

Nurse monitoring

1. Cytotoxic therapy which is most likely to cause severe nausea and vomiting consists of regimes containing cisplatin. Less emetogenic drugs include cyclophosphamide, carboplatin, doxorubicin, and daunorubicin. Radiotherapy, too, is usually associated with moderate nausea and vomiting. Ondansetron may be of benefit in all these situations.

2. Since 5-HT also increases gut motility, ondansetron, as might be expected, slows gut transit and produces constipation. As many cancer patients are also treated with strong morphine-like analgesics which also cause constipation, laxative therapy is generally required (if not already given).

3. Other side-effects of ondansetron include headache, facial flushing, and a feeling of warmth in the head and epigastrium which can be explained by the effect on 5-HT at these sites.

4. When given by intravenous infusion, ondansetron may be added to sodium chloride or glucose solutions, or mixtures of these. It is also compatible with mannitol, compound sodium lactate (Ringer's) solution, and solutions to which potassium chloride has been added. Ondansetron should not however be mixed with any other drugs either in the syringe or the infusion fluid.

General note

Ondansetron tablets and injection should be stored at room temperature and solutions must be protected from light during storage. Prepared infusions are, however, stable for 24 hours even in the presence of direct light.

ORCIPRENALINE (Alupent)

Presentation
Tablets—20 mg
Syrup—10 mg in 5 ml
Metered aerosol—750 microgram
per dose
Injection—0.5 mg in 1 ml, 5 mg in
10 ml

Actions and uses
This drug stimulates the beta
component of the sympathetic
nervous system. Its useful effects
are:
1. It causes relaxation of the smooth
   muscle in the walls of the large
   airways (bronchi) and therefore
   may be used to treat reversible
   airways obstruction
   (bronchospasm) due to asthma or
   other diseases such as bronchitis
   and emphysema.
2. It inhibits uterine contraction and
   therefore may be used in obstetric
   practice for the treatment of
   premature labour.

Dosage
1. For the treatment of
   bronchospasm:
   a. Orally:
      i. Adults: 20 mg four times a
         day.
      ii. Children: 3–12 years—10
          mg four times a day to 20
          mg three times a day; 1–3
          years—5–10 mg four times
          a day; 0–1 year—5–10 mg
          three times a day.
   b. Metered aerosol:
      i. Adults: 1–2 puffs, a
         maximum number of 12
         puffs in 24 hours with at
         least 30 minutes between
         each dosage.
      ii. Children: 6–12 years—1–2
          puffs, a maximum of four
          doses in 24 hours with at
          least 30 minutes between
          each dosage.
   Children under 6 years—1 puff, a
   maximum of four puffs in 24 hours
   with at least 30 minutes between
   each dosage.
   c. By intramuscular injection:
      i. Adults: 0.5 mg repeated
         after 30 minutes if
         necessary.

ii. Children: 6–12 years—0.5
    mg repeated after 30
    minutes if necessary;
    Children under 6 years—
    0.25 mg repeated after 30
    minutes if necessary.

Nurse monitoring
1. Patients, as well as being
   instructed in the correct use of
   the metered aerosol, must be
   warned never to exceed the
   prescribed dosage of this drug.
2. It is worth noting that the beta-
   blocking drugs (q.v.) antagonize
   the action of Alupent and,
   therefore, their concurrent
   administration is undesirable.
3. Transient side-effects after
   administration include palpitation,
   tachycardia, headache, nausea
   and abdominal discomfort.
4. The drug should never be given
   to patients already receiving
   monoamine oxidase inhibitors.
5. The drug should be used with
   great care in patients with heart
   disease, hypertension or
   thyrotoxicosis.

General notes
1. Preparations containing
   orciprenaline may be stored at
   room temperature.
2. Injection solution and syrup
   should be protected from light.
3. The pressurized aerosols should
   never be punctured or incinerated
   after use.

ORPHENADRINE (Disipal)

Presentation
Tablets—50 mg
Injection—40 mg in 2 ml

Actions and uses
The actions and uses of this drug are
identical to those described for
benzhexol (q.v.).

Dosage
In adults:
a. Orally: 150–300 mg in total given
   in three divided doses.
b. Parenterally: 20–40 mg as a
   single dose by intramuscular
   injection.

Nurse monitoring
The nurse monitoring aspects of benzhexol (q.v.) apply to this drug.

General note
This drug may be stored at room temperature.

OXAZEPAM

Presentation
Tablets—10 mg, 15 mg, 30 mg
Actions and uses
Oxazepam is a member of the benzodiazepine group (q.v.). Its principal use is in the treatment of anxiety.
Dosage
10–30 mg three times daily with occasionally an additional 10 or 30 mg dose at night.

Nurse monitoring
See the section on benzodiazepines.

General note
Tablets containing oxazepam may be stored at room temperature.

OXETHAZAINE (Mucaine)

Presentation
Suspension—10 mg in 5 ml
Actions and uses
Oxethazaine is a local anaesthetic drug which is taken in an antacid mixture to anaesthetize the lower oesophagus. It is used in the management of oesophagitis, heartburn and hiatus hernia.
Dosage
5–10 ml of suspension four times daily before meals and at bedtime.

Nurse monitoring
The drug is not absorbed and therefore produces no systemic toxic effects.

General note
Oxethazaine suspension may be stored at room temperature.

OXPENTIFYLLINE (Trental)

Presentation
Tablets—400 mg (slow release)
Actions and uses
Oxpentifylline is a vasodilator which is also said to make red blood cells more able to alter their shape and therefore to penetrate narrowed and damaged vessels improving oxygen supply. It is recommended for use in:
1. Peripheral vascular disease including Raynaud's disease, intermittent claudication, chilblains and night cramps.
2. Cerebrovascular insufficiency.
Dosage
Adults: 400 mg two or three times a day (slow-release tablets).

Nurse monitoring
1. Symptoms which may be experienced during administration of this drug include nausea, gastric upset, dizziness, flushing and malaise.
2. The drug should be used with great caution in patients who already have hypotension or who are receiving antihypertensive drugs or have heart disease.

General note
The drug may be stored at room temperature.

OXPRENOLOL (Trasicor)

Presentation
Tablets—20 mg, 40 mg, 80 mg, 160 mg (slow release)
Injection—2 mg powder in 2 ml ampoule
Actions and uses
See the section on beta-adrenoreceptor blocking drugs. Oxprenolol is a 'non-selective' drug.
Dosage
1. Intravenous dosage for the management of serious cardiac dysrhythmias is 1–2 mg given over a period of 5 minutes and repeated as necessary every 10–20 minutes to a maximum dosage of 5 mg. The patient's pulse and

blood pressure should be carefully monitored during administration and also a continuous ECG monitor must be maintained and injection must be stopped if there is widening of the QRS complex.
2. Intramuscular drug treatment may be given as an alternative to intravenous treatment and the dosage and monitoring is as described for the intravenous administration.
3. Adult oral dosage ranges from 80–480 mg per day usually in three divided doses. For the treatment of hypertension a twice-daily or once-daily dosage regime may be used. A sustained release preparation is available and may be given once per day.
4. For the control of cardiac dysrhythmias in children the drug is given in a dosage of 1 mg/kg body weight usually divided into three doses.

Nurse monitoring
See the section on beta-adrenoreceptor blocking drugs.

General note
Oxprenolol tablets and powder for injection may be stored at room temperature. Powder for injection should be dissolved in water for injection immediately before use.

OXYMETHOLONE (Anapolon)

Presentation
Tablets—50 mg
Actions and uses
1. The actions and uses of anabolic steroids and androgenic hormones in general are discussed in the sections on these drugs in hormones (4).
2. In clinical practice this drug is used for:
   a. The treatment of aplastic and refractory anaemia.
   b. As adjunctive therapy in patients with malignant disease where treatment with cytotoxic agents and/or radiotherapy is

likely to cause bone marrow depression.
Dosage
For the treatment of aplastic anaemia: 2–5 mg/kg body weight daily for adults and 2–4 mg/kg body weight daily for children in divided doses. The dose should be adjusted within this range according to individual response. Therapy must be maintained for at least 3 months before a response can be expected and minimum duration of therapy should be 6 months. After response is obtained it is recommended that that dose be continued for 3 months and then halved and maintained for at least a further 3 months. Therapy should be withdrawn gradually.

Nurse monitoring
See the sections on anabolic steroids and androgenic hormones in hormones (4).

General note
The drug should be stored at room temperature.

OXYTETRACYCLINE (Terramycin, Imperacin)

(See Note 3, p. 362)
Presentation
Tablets—250 mg
Capsules—250 mg
Syrup—125 mg in 5 ml
Injection—100 mg (intramuscular); 250 mg (intravenous)
Ointment—3%
Oxytetracycline is also included in compound eye ointments and drops.
Actions and uses
See the section on tetracycline.
Dosage
See the section on tetracycline.

Nurse monitoring
See the section on tetracycline.

General notes
1. The drug may be stored at room temperature.
2. The syrup should be used within 1 week of preparation.

OXYTOCIN (Syntocinon)

Presentation

Injection—2 units in 2 ml; 5 units in 1 ml; 10 units in 1 ml; 50 units in 5 ml
Nasal spray—40 units in 1 ml

Actions and uses

Oxytocin, of which Syntocinon is a synthetic derivative, is a hormone normally found in the posterior lobe of the pituitary gland in the brain. It has two actions which make it useful in clinical practice:

1. It stimulates the milk ejection reflex, i.e. the mechanism by which breast milk passes from its site of production to reach the suckling infant.
2. It stimulates the contraction of the pregnant uterus.

It has the following uses:

1. It may be administered by nasal spray to facilitate breast feeding.
2. It may be administered by intra-venous infusion to induce labour.
3. It may be administered by intravenous infusion (often in combination with ergometrine as 'Syntometrine') for the treatment of missed abortion or postpartum haemorrhage.

Dosage

1. Intranasally for the facilitation of breast feeding: The nasal spray should be administered 2–5 minutes before feeds.
2. Intravenously to induce labour: Most maternity units have a documented procedure for the administration of this drug to induce labour and therefore no specific doses are given here.
3. For the treatment of postpartum haemorrhage or missed abortion: Again the nurse is recommended to acquaint herself with the treatment schedule of the centre to which she is attached.

Nurse monitoring

1. High doses may cause excessive uterine contraction and dosage should therefore be carefully monitored to prevent the potentially disastrous occurrence of a ruptured uterus.
2. When high doses of Syntocinon are given with large volumes of electrolyte free fluid, water intoxication may occur. Initially headache, anorexia, nausea, vomiting and abdominal pain may be the presenting features and this progresses to lethargy, drowsiness, unconsciousness and grand mal type seizures. The concentration of blood electro-lytes may be markedly disturbed.

General notes

1. The drug should be stored in a refrigerator.
2. Infusions are generally administ-ered in 5% dextrose solution.

P

PACLITAXEL (Taxol)

Presentation
Injection—30 mg in 5 ml vial

Actions and uses
This drug is a novel cytotoxic which blocks the mitotic phase of the cell cycle by impairing microtubular assembly and reorganization during interphase. The result is that normal cell division cannot take place. The current licensed indication for paclitaxel is in the treatment of metastatic ovarian carcinoma in which cisplatin and carboplatin regimens have proved ineffective. It is likely however that its uses will eventually extend to lung cancer and other solid tumours.

Dosage
A single dose of 175 mg/m² body surface area is administered by intravenous infusion. Repeat doses may be given at 3 weekly intervals but only once the neutrophil count has returned to above a reference value—1.5×10^9/litre.

Nurse monitoring
1. The occurrence of severe hypersensitivity reactions (hypotension, dyspnoea, rash, angioedema, etc) to this drug is such that steroid and complete antihistamine (H_1 and H_2) cover is essential. Thus single doses of oral dexamethasone 20 mg and chlorpheniramine 10 mg i.v. plus cimetidine 300 mg i.v. are administered at 6–12 hours and 30–60 minutes respectively prior to paclitaxel.
2. Bone marrow suppression (mainly neutropenia but also anaemia and thrombocytopenia) is a life-threatening and hence dose-limiting adverse event.
3. Peripheral neuropathy (commonly paraesthesia) generally occurs but more severe neurotoxicity is a signal that dosage reduction of as much as 20% is required with future doses.
4. Gastrointestinal side-effects including mucositis, nausea and vomiting, and diarrhoea are very common. Alopecia occurs in almost all patients.
5. A rise in liver enzymes (transaminases, alkaline phosphatase and bilirubin) has been noted and this drug should be used with caution in patients with pre-existing liver impairment.
6. Cardiac arrhythmias (ventricular tachycardia, A-V block) are uncommon side-effects.
7. The nurse should be constantly aware that most cytotoxic drugs are irritant to the skin and mucous surfaces, and are in general very toxic. Great care should therefore be exercised when handling these drugs, and in particular, spillage or contamination of personnel or the environment must be avoided. If cytotoxic drugs are regularly handled it is theoretically possible that repeated skin contact or inhalation may produce systemic toxic effects and in nurses who have developed hypersensitivity, severe local and general allergic reactions.

General notes

1. Paclitaxel vials are stored at 'cool' room temperature and protected from light.
2. If refrigerated a precipitate may form but the drug should redissolve when gently shaken on returning to room temperature.
3. Infusions are prepared in 250 ml or 500 ml sodium chloride 0.9%, glucose 5% or glucose/saline injection and administered over 3 hours.
4. Prepared infusions are stable for up to 27 hours at room temperature. Do not refrigerate.
5. A hazy appearance is quite normal and due to the solubilizing agent which is present in the vial. Solutions must be filtered via a 0.22 micron filter during administration.
6. A reaction with PVC is possible and this material must be avoided when preparing and mixing the injection.

PAMIDRONATE (Aredia)

Presentation

Injection—15 mg, 30 mg powder vials.

Actions and uses

Pamidronate is chemically a bis(di-)phosphonate compound which is used in the management of hypercalcaemia due to malignant disease, notably associated with myeloma, lymphoma, and solid tumours which have spread to bone (bone metastases). It appears to act by inhibiting loss of bone density with subsequent release of calcium into the circulation (bone resorption). The serum calcium usually starts to fall within 48 hours of administration of pamidronate, and levels may remain within the normal range for several weeks thereafter.

Other uses for pamidronate, e.g. in Paget's disease and osteoporosis in menopausal women, are currently under investigation, but are not approved indications for its use.

Dosage

Adults: Usually a single dose of 30–90 mg is given by intravenous infusion in sodium chloride 0.9% or glucose 5%, 500 ml over at least 2 hours.

Nurse monitoring

1. Intravenous injections of pamidronate are irritant and must be administered slowly.
2. Patients may develop transient pyrexia during drug administration.
3. Pamidronate produces oliguria in some patients and should be used with extreme caution if renal impairment exists.
4. Use in pregnancy and epilepsy should be avoided.

General note

Pamidronate injection should be stored in the refrigerator. It must never be administered in solutions containing calcium, e.g. compound sodium lactate (Ringer's) injection.

PANCREATIN

Presentation

See dosage table

Actions and uses

This preparation is a mixture of enzymes normally produced by the pancreas. In pancreatic disease, where insufficient enzymes are being produced, food cannot be absorbed. Pancreatin, therefore, is used in cases of malabsorption due to pancreatic deficiency.

Dosage

Preparation	Usual Dosage
Creon caps	2 with meals swallowed whole or sprinkled over food
Nutrizym tabs	1–2 capsules with meals
Pancrease caps	2 with meals swallowed whole or sprinkled over food
Pancrex	5–10 g as powder four times daily before meals

Pancrex V powder	500 mg–2 g as powder four times daily before, or mixed with meals
Pancrex V caps	Contents of 1–3 capsules sprinkled over food four times per day
Pancrex V tabs	5–15 tablets four times per day before meals
Pancrex V Forte tabs	2–6 tablets four times per day before meals.
Panzyrat caps	1–2 capsules with meals

Note that a variety of strengths for each of the above exists and the true dose is widely variable. It is that which is sufficient generally to prevent steatorrhoea.

Nurse monitoring
1. When used in very young babies irritation of the skin may occur around the mouth and the anus. Barrier creams will effectively prevent this.
2. Rarely hypersensitivity reactions such as sneezing and skin rash may occur.
3. These preparations are, to say the least, unpleasant. The nurse may play an important supportive role in encouraging the patient to persevere with this treatment.

General note
Preparations should be stored in a well-closed container in a cool place.

PAPAVERETUM (Omnopon)

Presentation
Injection—contains 13.44 mg morphine, 1.2 mg papaverine, 1.04 mg codeine per 1 ml ampoule
Paediatric injection—contains 6.72 mg morphine, 0.6 mg papaverine, 0.52 mg codeine per 1 ml ampoule

Actions and uses
Papaveretum is a mixture of narcotic substances derived from natural opium which has been suitably refined to remove noxious sub-stances and standardized on the above strengths. In practice its analgesic activity is due to the morphine content. The actions and uses discussed under the narcotic analgesic drugs apply to papaveretum.

Dosage
1. Adults: Intramuscular, subcutaneous or intravenous routes: 1–2 ml repeated 4–6 hourly as required.
2. Children: As above. Up to 1 month—0.015 ml/kg; 1 month to 1 year—0.015–0.02 ml/kg; older children—0.02–0.03 ml/kg.

Nurse monitoring
See the section on narcotic analgesic drugs.

General notes
1. The drug should be stored in a locked (controlled drug) cupboard.
2. The drug should be stored at room temperature.

PARACETAMOL (Calpol, Disprol, Panadol)

Presentation
Tablets—500 mg (plain and soluble)
Syrup—120 mg in 5 ml: 250 mg in 5 ml

Actions and uses
Paracetamol has both analgesic (pain relieving) and anti-pyretic (temperature reducing) properties. It is used where mild analgesia is indicated for such common complaints as headache and musculoskeletal pain. It is particularly useful for the treatment of mild pain or pyrexia in groups of patients for whom salicylate therapy is contraindicated, such as those with previous gastrointestinal bleeding and also for the treatment of children under 8 years, who should not normally be given salicylates.

Dosage
1. Adults: 500 mg–1 g 4 to 6-hourly as required for pain.
2. Children: Less than 1 year—120 mg four times a day; 1–5 years—240 mg four times a day; 5 years and over—up to 480 mg four times a day.

P

Nurse monitoring
1. Few if any side-effects are associated with the administration of this drug.
2. This drug is widely available for sale without prescription in Great Britain and although it is associated with negligible side-effects when taken in normal dosage, it is extremely dangerous if taken as an overdose when severe and fatal liver damage may occur. A specific intravenous treatment regime with N-acetylcysteine is available but its efficacy depends on how quickly the patient receives it after taking the overdose. Thus any patient who has taken such an overdose must be referred to hospital with the utmost speed.
3. As well as liver damage after overdosage, renal and cardiac damage may occur.

General note
The drug may be stored at room temperature.

PENICILLAMINE (Distamine)

Presentation
Tablets—50 mg, 125 mg and 250 mg

Actions and uses
Penicillamine has two main actions:
1. It binds heavy metal ions by a process called 'chelation' and therefore may be used in the treatment of the following disorders:
   a. Lead poisoning where it is thought to reduce the absorption of lead.
   b. Wilson's disease (hepatolenticular degeneration) where it increases the excretion of copper.
   c. Mercury poisoning.
   d. Cystinuria where it promotes the excretion of the more soluble form of cystine.
2. It also reduces the inflammatory response in patients with severe rheumatoid arthritis. The reduction in the inflammatory response leads to a subsequent relief of symptoms.

Dosage
1. Lead poisoning and Wilson's disease:
   a. Adults: 1–2 g daily in divided doses.
   b. Children: up to 20 mg/kg daily in divided doses.
2. Rheumatoid arthritis:
   a. Adults: Initially 125–250 mg per day is given and gradually increased until a response is obtained. Usually the required dose is in the range of 500–750 mg per day although the response may take several weeks to develop. After maintaining patients on these high doses for several months it is often possible to reduce the maintenance dose without loss of effect.
   b. Children: Up to 2 years—25–50 mg twice a day; 2–4 years—50–100 mg twice a day; 4–10 years—100 mg twice or three times per day.

Nurse monitoring
1. This drug should never be given to patients who are already receiving gold salts or anti-malarial treatment such as chloroquine or hydroxychloroquine.
2. Routine checks of white cell counts, platelet counts and urine tests for albumin should be performed at weekly intervals in patients on this treatment.
3. Patients may be allergic to penicillamine. Patients who have already been found to be allergic to penicillin are particularly at risk from this.
4. Adverse effects include headaches, sore throat, fever, skin rash, nausea, pruritus, muscle and joint pain, altered taste sensitivity, eosinophilia, lymphadenopathy, leucopenia, agranulocytosis, thrombocytopenia, proteinuria and nephrotic syndrome.
5. Patients who have already been found to be allergic to gold injections should never be given penicillamine.

General note

Penicillamine tablets may be stored at room temperature.

PENICILLIN V

(See Note 3, p. 362)
N.B. Also referred to as phenoxymethylpenicillin. Several proprietary brands are available.

Presentation

Tablets—125 mg, 250 mg
Syrup, suspension and elixir—62.5 mg in 5 ml; 125 mg in 5 ml; 250 mg in 5 ml.

Actions and uses

Phenoxymethylpenicillin has a mode of action similar to that described for benzylpenicillin (q.v.). It is usually effective against streptococcus, pneumococcus, meningococcus and gonococcus and rarely effective against staphylococcus. It is therefore indicated for the treatment of diseases caused by these organisms as outlined in Note 3. Phenoxymethylpenicillin has an advantage over benzylpenicillin in that it is better absorbed and therefore is the drug of choice for oral penicillin treatment.

Dosage

1. Adults and older children: 500 mg four times a day.
2. Children aged 1–7 years: 125–250 mg four times a day.
3. Children less than one year 62.5 mg four times a day

It is important to note that the drug should preferably be given 30 minutes to 1 hour before meals.

Nurse monitoring

See the section on benzylpenicillin.

General notes

1. Tablets and powder for preparing oral liquid preparations may be stored at room temperature.
2. Syrup, suspension and elixir should be discarded 7 days after reconstitution or 14 days after reconstitution if refrigerated.

PENTAZOCINE (Fortral)

Presentation

Tablets—25 mg
Capsules—50 mg
Injection—30 mg in 1 ml; 60 mg in 2 ml
Suppositories—50 mg

Actions and uses

Pentazocine is a derivative of the narcotic analgesic group of drugs but it has a much less potent analgesic effect when compared with morphine. It is, therefore, used in the management of moderate to severe pain.

Dosage

1. Adults.
   a. Orally: 25–100 mg 4 to 6-hourly as required.
   b. By intramuscular, intravenous or subcutaneous injection: 30–60 mg 4 to 6-hourly as required.
   c. Rectally: 50 mg 4 to 6-hourly as required.
2. Children:
   a. Orally:
      i. Less than 1 year: there are no dosage recommend-ations for this age group.
      ii. 1–12 years: It is recom-mended that if this drug is required in this age group, parenteral therapy be used.
   b. Parenterally:
      i. By intramuscular or subcutaneous injection: 1 mg/kg body weight is the maximum single dose recommended. This should be repeated 3 to 4-hourly as required.
      ii. By intravenous injection: 0.5 mg/kg body weight is the maximum single dose recommended, repeated every 3 to 4-hours as required.
   c. By suppository: Suppositories are not recommended as being suitable for administration to children under the age of 12.

Nurse monitoring

1. See the section on narcotic analgesic drugs.

2. Hallucinations and other behavioural abnormalities have been found to be a particular problem with this drug and occur in 10% of patients. The reason they have been reported only rarely is that they tend to be of a pleasant nature.
3. Pentazocine is not subject to the legal requirements associated with 'controlled drugs'.

General notes
1. The drug may be stored at room temperature.
2. Note that high dose (30 mg) capsules and injection are controlled drugs and are therefore subject to the storage conditions which apply to such drugs.

PERINDOPRIL (Coversyl)

Presentation
Tablets—2 mg, 4 mg
Actions and uses
See section on ACE inhibitors.
Dosage
Range: 4–8 mg as a single daily dose.

Nurse monitoring
See section on ACE inhibitors

General note
Perindopril tablets may be stored at room temperature.

PERPHENAZINE (Fentazin)

Presentation
Tablets—2 mg, 4 mg
Actions and uses
Perphenazine is a phenothiazine drug and its actions and uses are described in the section on these drugs. It is used predominantly for the treatment of severe anxiety and agitation associated with psychotic disorders but it is occasionally, in addition, used for the treatment of nausea and vomiting.

Dosage
1. The usual oral adult dose is 4 mg three times daily increasing to a maximum of 24 mg per day if required.
2. Not recommended for children.

Nurse monitoring
See the section on phenothiazine drugs.

General note
Perphenazine tablets may be stored at room temperature.

PERICYAZINE (Neulactil)

Presentation
Tablets—2.5 mg, 10 mg, 25 mg
Syrup—10 mg in 5 ml
Actions and uses
Pericyazine is a neuroleptic drug of the phenothiazine group which is used for its tranquillizing or calming effect in severely agitated patients with behavioural disorders such as schizophrenia, senile dementia and mental subnormality. When compared to other major tranquillizers such as chlorpromazine, pericyazine produces a marked sedative effect, thus it is of particular use in disorders characterized by aggressive or impulsive tendencies.
Dosage
1. Adults: Initially 15–75 mg daily in divided doses increased gradually until control of symptoms is achieved. Thereafter the dosage is reduced to the lowest possible daily dose to maintain control in the individual patient.
2. Elderly adults: Smaller initial doses are used, e.g. 10 mg daily increased gradually.
3. Children: Daily dosages have been calculated on the basis of 0.5 mg for each year of age.

Nurse monitoring
1. The nurse monitoring section on phenothiazines apply to pericyazine.

2. It is important to note that pericyazine has a strong sedative action and may produce marked postural hypotension. It is for this reason that correspondingly low initial doses should be used for elderly subjects who are particularly susceptible to sudden falls in blood pressure and in whom fainting attacks and palpitation may occur.

3. Children are similarly susceptible to the sedative and hypotensive actions of the drug.

4. The unwanted effects of pericyazine may be less troublesome if the dosage is divided in such a way that the larger portion is administered at night.

General note
Tablets and syrup preparations of pericyazide should be stored at room temperature.

PETHIDINE

Presentation
Tablets—25 mg and 50 mg
Injection—50 mg in 1 ml; 100 mg in 2 ml

Actions and uses
The actions and uses of this narcotic analgesic drug are described in the section on narcotic analgesic drugs.

Dosage
1. Adults:
    a. Orally: 50–100 mg 3 to 4-hourly as required.
    b. By subcutaneous, intramuscular or intravenous injection: 50–100 mg 4-hourly as required.
2. Children: By oral, intramuscular, subcutaneous or intravenous injection:
    a. Less than 1 year: 1 mg/kg up to three times daily.
    b. 1-7 years: 12.5 mg up to three times daily.
    c. Over 7 years: 25 mg three times daily.

Nurse monitoring
1. The nurse monitoring aspects of narcotic analgesic drugs in general are described in the section on these drugs.
2. It is worth noting that the side-effects experienced with pethidine are particularly severe in the elderly.

General notes
1. The drug should be stored in a locked (controlled drug) cupboard.
2. The drug should be stored at room temperature.

PHENAZOCINE (Narphen)

Presentation
Tablets—5 mg

Actions and uses
Phenazocine is a narcotic analgesic and its actions and uses are described in the section on these drugs.

Dosage
For adults: 5–20 mg every 4-6 hours as required.

Nurse monitoring
1. See the section on narcotic analgesic drugs.
2. This drug may also be taken by the sublingual route in patients with swallowing difficulty.

General notes
1. The drug should be stored in a locked (controlled drugs) cupboard.
2. The drug should be stored at room temperature.

PHENELZINE (Nardil)

Presentation
Tablets—15 mg

Actions and uses
Phenelzine is a monoamine oxidase inhibiting drug. Its actions and uses are described in the section on these drugs.

P

Dosage
15 mg three times daily.

Nurse monitoring
See the section on monoamine oxidase inhibitors.

General note
Phenelzine tablets may be stored at room temperature.

PHENINDAMINE (Thephorin)

Presentation
Tablets—25 mg

Actions and uses
Phenindamine is an antihistamine. The actions and uses of antihistamines in general are described in the section on these drugs. In clinical practice phenindamine is used:
1. To suppress generalized minor allergic responses to allergens such as foodstuffs and drugs.
2. To suppress local allergic reactions, i.e. inflammatory skin responses to insect stings and bites, contact allergens, urticaria, etc.

Dosage
Adults: 25–50 mg one to three times per day.

Nurse monitoring
1. See the section on antihistamines.
2. It is particularly interesting to note that this drug tends to produce symptoms of CNS stimulation rather than the drowsiness produced by other antihistamines.

General note
The drug may be stored at room temperature.

PHENINDIONE (Dindevan)

Presentation
Tablets—10 mg, 25 mg and 50 mg

Actions and uses
A number of the substances present in blood which play an important part in preventing bleeding by forming clots are produced by the liver from vitamin K. Phenindione inhibits the synthesis of these substances (known as clotting factors) and therefore reduces the ability of the blood to clot. Its principal uses are for the prevention and treatment of thromboembolic states such as deep venous thrombosis and pulmonary embolus. It is also used to prevent the formation of clot in cardio-vascular disease either on artificial heart valves or in the atria of patients who have atrial dysrhythmias.

Dosage
1. Adults:
   a. Loading dose: 200 mg on day 1; 100 mg on day 2. The dosage on day 3 should depend on the result of clotting studies.
   b. Maintenance dosage: depends on the results of blood clotting studies but usually lies within the range of 50–150 mg per day.

Nurse monitoring
1. The daily maintenance dose of phenindione is, as noted above, determined by the results of clotting studies. As the effects of bleeding due to overcoagulation or thrombosis due to undercoagulation can be so rapidly catastrophic, strict adherence to the recommended dose is mandatory and the nurse may play an important role in ensuring that patients are aware of this.
2. The effects of phenindione may be influenced by a number of factors listed below and the nurse may play an important role by identifying their occurrence and alerting both the patient and medical staff. The following circumstances may lead to a requirement for alteration in dosage:
   a. Acute illness such as chest infection or viral infection.
   b. Sudden weight loss.

c. The concurrent administration
of other drugs: A number of
drugs may affect the patient's
dosage requirements. Where
drugs are known to interfere
with anticoagulant control this
has been noted in the nurse
monitoring sections of the
drugs in this book.

3. The occurrence of haemorrhage
in a patient on phenindione is an
indication for immediate withdrawal of the drug and if the
haemorrhage is at all serious or
repetitive the patient should be
immediately referred to hospital
for further assessment and, if
necessary, they may be given
vitamin K which accelerates a
return to normal clotting function.

4. Phenindione is relatively
contraindicated in patients with
severe liver or kidney disease,
haemorrhagic conditions or
uncontrolled hypertension. It
should also be used with great
caution immediately after surgery
or labour.

5. Skin rash, fever, blood dyscrasia,
diarrhoea, liver and kidney
damage may all occur with this
drug and because of these
effects it is now less commonly
used than warfarin.

6. It is important for the nurse to
note that metabolites of this drug
may impart a pink or orange
colour to the urine and this may
be mistaken for haematuria. This
is particularly important as
haematuria is an indication for
stopping drug therapy and
urgently reassessing blood
clotting status.

General note
The drug may be stored at room
temperature.

PHENOBARBITONE

Presentation
Tablets—15 mg, 30 mg, 60 mg,
100 mg
Tablets—30 mg, 60 mg (as sodium
salt)

Capsules—60 mg and 100 mg (as
slow release)
Elixir—15 mg in 5 ml
Injection—15 mg, 30 mg, 60 mg and
200 mg in 1 ml

Actions and uses
Phenobarbitone is a member
of the barbiturate group. Full
information is contained in the
sections on anticonvulsants and
barbiturates. Its major use in
clinical practice is in the management of epilepsy, particularly
grand mal, petit mal and
psychomotor seizures. It is
additionally occasionally used
as a sedative and hypnotic
though this is a declining role for
barbiturate drugs since safer
alternatives exist.

Dosage
1. As an anticonvulsant:
   a. Orally:
      i. Adults: 90–375 mg
      (maximum 600 mg) daily
      taken as a single dose or in
      divided doses.
      ii. Children: 5–10 mg/kg body
      weight daily as a single
      dose or in two divided
      doses.
   b. By intramuscular injection:
      i. Adults: 50–200 mg single
      dose.
      ii. Children: 3–6 mg/kg
      body weight as a single
      dose.
N.B. The subcutaneous and
intravenous routes may also be used
though the strong irritant nature of
phenobarbitone injection should be
noted.
2. As a sedative or hypnotic: Adults:
15–30 mg 3 or 4 times a day or up
to 200 mg at night as a single
dose.

Nurse monitoring
See the sections on anticonvulsants
and barbiturates.

General note
Preparations containing
phenobarbitone may be stored at
room temperature.

PHENOTHIAZINES

Chlorpromazine
Clopenthixol
Flupenthixol
Fluphenazine
Methotrimeprazine
Perphenazine
Prochlorperazine
Promazine
Promethazine
Thioridazine
Trifluoperazine
Trimeprazine

Actions and uses

The phenothiazine group of drugs possesses a wide range of actions. They are used in clinical practice for three main reasons:

1. They have been found to be useful as major tranquillizers (neuroleptics) and are used for the treatment of severely anxious patients and to control the marked behavioural abnormality in schizophrenia.
2. A few of this group of drugs possess potent anti-emetic activity and are used in the treatment of conditions associated with vomiting.
3. This group of drugs is used commonly in the routine management of patients with senile dementia, to control behavioural abnormalities.

Dosage

See individual drugs.

Nurse monitoring

1. Contact dermatitis can occur in people handling these drugs regularly. Precautions should therefore be taken against repeated direct contact between the nurse's skin and formulations of these drugs.
2. Solutions of Chlorpromazine cause irritation at injection sites. Injection sites should therefore be varied and discomfort may be relieved by the addition of a local anaesthetic to the injection solution.

3. A common side-effect of this group of drugs is postural hypotension. This is especially important in patients who are receiving other anti-hypertensive drugs and should always be borne in mind as a cause of symptoms of dizziness or faintness.
4. Other common side-effects include excessive sedation, gastrointestinal upset, photosensitivity and variation in body temperature—more often hypothermia but rarely hyperthermia may occur.
5. Endocrine side-effects of this drug include amenorrhoea, failure of ovulation, galactorrhoea and gynaecomastia.
6. Various troublesome neurological side-effects may occur in patients, especially those receiving the drug for a prolonged period of time. These are:
   a. A clinical picture similar to Parkinson's disease with a slow shuffling gait, a tremor and a dull, expressionless face.
   b. Tardive dyskinesia which is manifest as writhing movements of the muscles of the head and neck may occur and may be irreversible.
7. Phenothiazines may produce cholestatic jaundice and should be used with extreme caution in patients with liver disease.
8. Occasionally phenothiazines may affect the production of white blood cells. This makes the patient more susceptible to infection. Any patient presenting with even simple symptoms such as a sore throat should have their white blood cell count checked.

General note

See individual drugs.

PHENOXYBENZAMINE (Dibenyline)

Presentation

Capsules—10 mg
Injection—100 mg in 2 ml

Actions and uses

Phenoxybenzamine affects the sympathetic nervous system and produces peripheral vascular dilation. It is therefore used for the treatment of diseases where improvement in peripheral blood flow is desired. These include:

1. Raynaud's disease.
2. Intermittent claudication.
3. Chilblains.
4. Frostbite.

It has two further uses in clinical practice:

1. Its ability to block the alpha-receptors of the sympathetic nervous system make it useful in the treatment of phaeochromocytoma (an adrenaline-secreting tumour).
2. The drug has been given by intravenous infusion to attempt to increase tissue perfusion in states of severe shock.

Dosage

1. For the treatment of peripheral vascular disease:
   a. Orally: 20–60 mg per day in 2–4 divided doses.
   b. By intravenous infusion: 0.5 mg–1 mg/kg in 500 ml of sodium chloride 0.9% infused over 1 hour.
2. In the treatment of phaeochromocytoma: Up to 200 mg in total per day in divided doses may be necessary.
3. In the treatment of severe shock: An infusion of 0.5 mg–1 mg/kg in 500 ml of 200–500 ml of sodium chloride injection is given over a period of at least 1 hour.

Nurse monitoring

1. The drug's vasodilator action may produce flushing of the skin of the head and neck, headache, dizziness, tachycardia and postural hypotension.
2. The drug may occasionally cause slight gastrointestinal upset.
3. Inhibition of ejaculation may occur.
4. Other side-effects include nasal congestion, dryness of the mouth, constricted pupils, drowsiness and sedation.

General note

The drug should be stored at room temperature.

PHENTERMINE (Duromine, Ionamin)

Presentation

Capsules–15 mg and 30 mg (both sustained-release)

Actions and uses

Anorexogenic drugs abolish hunger by a direct action on the central nervous system. They are thought to have a supplementary effect in that they increase the ability to perform mental and physical work without the need for increased food intake.

Dosage

For adults only: 15 or 30 mg daily at breakfast.

Nurse monitoring

1. The nurse monitoring aspects of this drug are identical to those described for diethylpropion (q.v.).
2. Note that this is now classified as a 'controlled drug' as a result of recognition of its abuse potential.

General note

The drug is subject to the storage conditions of other drugs controlled by the Misuse of Drugs Act.

PHENTOLAMINE (Rogitine)

Presentation

Injection—10 mg in 1 ml

Actions and uses

This drug causes a reduction in blood pressure by dilating peripheral vessels via an inhibitory effect on alpha-receptors of the sympathetic nervous system (i.e. it is an alpha-blocker). It is no longer used to treat hypertension but may still rarely be seen in use during the surgical removal of phaeochromocytomata which are tumours associated with the production of excess catecholamines.

P

Dosage
1. Adults: 2–5 mg by intravenous injection.
2. Children: 1 mg by intravenous injection.

Nurse monitoring
Parenteral phentolamine frequently produces flushing, dizziness, weakness and tachycardia.

General notes
1. Solutions should be protected from light and stored in a cool place.
2. The drug is diluted in 50–100 ml sodium chloride 0.9% or glucose 5% and administered over 20–30 minutes.

PHENYTOIN (Epanutin)

Presentation
Tablets and capsules—25 mg, 50 mg, 100 mg
Suspension—30 mg in 5 ml
Injection—250 mg in 5 ml

Actions and uses
Phenytoin inhibits the spread of abnormal electrical activity through both the brain and the heart. It therefore has two major uses.
1. It may be given intravenously (or more rarely intramuscularly) to control status epilepticus, and orally to prevent seizures particularly of the grand mal and temporal lobe types.
2. Phenytoin may be given intravenously or more rarely orally to control certain ventricular dysrhythmias, especially when these dysrhythmias are associated with digoxin overdosage.

Dosage
1. For the treatment of epilepsy:
  a. When given intravenously for status epilepticus the usual adult dose is 150–250 mg. Maximum infusion rate should be 50 mg per minute. Children's dosages are lower than for adults and calculated in proportion to the body weight.
  b. Regular maintenance dose should be between 25–50 mg two or three times daily. It is now accepted that the dosage should be adjusted according to measured blood levels.
2. In the treatment of cardiac arrhythmias, 3.5–5 mg/kg by slow intravenous injection is administered. A second dose may be given if necessary, oral maintenance therapy thereafter would be between 25–50 mg two to three times a day.

Nurse monitoring
The nurse's principal role in the management of patients on these drugs is to contribute to the early detection of either effects of excess dosage or side-effects of the drug.
1. The effects of overdosage can be seen:
  a. With too rapid intravenous injection when cardiac arrhythmias may arise. Patients receiving this drug should therefore have pulse, blood pressure and ECG monitoring.
  b. The clinical signs of excess dosage are ataxia, nystagmus, dysarthria and confusion.
2. Side-effects include tenderness and hyperplasia of the gums, hirsutism, blood disorders, i.e. megaloblastic anaemia, low white cell counts, low platelet counts, pancytopenia and aplastic anaemia. Skin rashes, joint pains, fever and hepatitis can also occur. Finally the nurse should be aware that patients receiving phenytoin may experience problems if other drugs are added to their regime if these drugs alter liver metabolism. One example of this is chloramphenicol, which reduces the metabolism of phenytoin in the liver and may produce toxicity with doses of phenytoin which previously had produced no unwanted effects.

General notes

1. All preparations containing phenytoin may be stored at room temperature.
2. The solution for injection must be given undiluted and never mixed with other drugs.
3. Solutions of phenytoin should be protected from light.

PIMOZIDE (Orap)

Presentation
Tablets—2 mg, 4 mg, 10 mg

Actions and uses
Pimozide is a neuroleptic drug which is used for its tranquillizing or calming effect in severely agitated patients with a range of behavioural disorders including schizophrenia, hyperactivity and aggressive behavioural disorders. In this respect pimozide possesses many of the properties of the phenothiazine tranquillizers discussed in the section on phenothiazines.

Dosage
1. Adults: The dosage varies widely according to the nature and severity of the disorder under treatment. Initially 4–10 mg (increasing to up to 20 mg for acutely agitated patients) is administered. Thereafter the dose is gradually reduced to that which maintains the individual symptom-free.
2. Children: In children over 12 years of age a dose of 1–3 mg daily has been used.

Nurse monitoring
1. Adverse effects which are associated with the phenothiazine tranquillizers may also occur in patients treated with pimozide. The nurse monitoring section on phenothiazines thus applies to this drug.
2. Extrapyramidal (Parkinsonian) symptoms and tardive dyskinesia appear to be more common with pimozide than with the phenothiazines though the occurrence of unwanted sedation is less likely.

3. Other common side-effects include skin rashes, glycosuria and altered liver function.

General note
Pimozide tablets may be stored at room temperature.

PINDOLOL (Visken)

Presentation
Tablets—5 mg, 15 mg

Actions and uses
Pindolol is a non-selective beta-adrenoreceptor blocking drug. Its actions and uses are described under beta-adrenoreceptor blocking drugs (q.v.).

Dosage
The adult dosage regime is usually a daily dose of 15 mg. Alternatively up to 45 mg may be given in two or three divided doses per day.

Nurse monitoring
See the section on beta-adrenoreceptor blocking drugs.

General note
Pindolol tablets may be stored at room temperature.

PIPERAZINE (Pripsen)

Presentation
Sachets–4 g (each sachet contains 4 g of piperazine phosphate and standardized senna equivalent to 15.3 mg; total sennoside calculated as sennoside B)

Actions and uses
This antihelminthic drug is effective in the treatment of threadworm (enterobiasis) and roundworm (ascariasis).

Dosage
1. Enterobiasis: The dose should be calculated according to age or weight and is given once daily for 7 days.
   a. Adults (approximate weight over 55 kg): 2 g

b. Children over 13 (approximate weight over 40 kg): 2 g
c. Children 5–12 (approximate weight 17–40 kg): 1.5 g
d. Children 2–4 (approximate weight 13–16 kg): 750 mg
e. Children less than 2 (approximate weight below 13 kg): Dose to be recommended by a physician.
2. For the treatment of roundworm:
a. Adults (approximate weight over 55 kg): 4 g
b. Children 13–16 years (approximate weight 41–55 kg): 3.75 g
c. Children 9–12 years (approximate weight 26–40 kg): 3 g
d. Children 2–8 years (approximate weight 13–25 kg): 2.5 g
e. Children less than 2 (approximate weight below 13 kg): Dose to be recommended by a physician.

Nurse monitoring
1. When more than one member of the family is affected all affected members should be treated simultaneously.
2. Occasional neurological abnormalities including visual disturbance, dizziness and vertigo may occur.

General note
The drug may be stored at room temperature.

PIPERAZINE OESTRONE SULPHATE (Harmogen)

Presentation
Tablets—1.5 mg
Actions and uses
1. The actions and uses of oestrogenic substances in general are described in the section on these drugs.
2. In clinical practice this drug is used for oestrogen replacement therapy and the relief of oestrogen deficiency symptoms at or after the menopause and following surgical or radio-therapeutic oophorectomy.

Dosage
The drug is administered in 21–28 day cycles with 5–7 days between each cycle. The dosage varies according to individual response between 1.5 and 4.5 mg per day.

Nurse monitoring
See the section on oestrogenic hormones.

General note
The drug may be stored at room temperature.

PIRBUTEROL (Exirel)

Presentation
Capsules—10 mg, 15 mg
Inhaler—200 microgram per metered dose
Actions and uses
This drug has the actions and uses described for fenoterol (q.v.)
Dosage
1. Oral:
a. Adults and children over 12 years: 10–15 mg three or four times daily.
b. Children 6–12 years: 7.5 mg four times daily.
2. Inhaler: Adults and children over 12 years: 200-400 microgram (1–2 metered doses) three or four times a day up to a maximum of 12 inhalations per 24 hours.

Nurse monitoring
See the section on fenoterol.

General note
See the section on fenoterol.

PIRENZEPINE (Gastrozepin)

Presentation
Tablets—50 mg
Actions and uses
Pirenzepine is an anticholinergic (parasympathetic blocking) drug which resembles atropine but has some specificity for the gastrointestinal tract. Its

anti-secretory effect in the stomach, as a result of vagal inhibition of gastric acid output, promotes healing of gastric and duodenal ulcers.

Dosage

Adults: Usually 50 mg twice daily but in the treatment of resistant ulcers this may be increased to three times daily.

Nurse monitoring

1. Most ulcers should heal within 6 weeks and alternative medical treatments (or surgery) exist for those which fail to respond.
2. The anticholinergic action of pirenzepine elsewhere on the gut and in the eye may result in troublesome dry mouth and blurring of vision, despite the relative specificity of this drug.
3. For maximum effect, patients should be instructed to take pirenzepine about 30 minutes before meals.

General note

Pirenzepine tablets may be stored at room temperature.

PIROXICAM (Feldene)

Presentation

Capsules—10 mg, 20 mg
Injection—20 mg in 1 ml
Suppositories—20 mg
Topical gel—0.5%

Actions and uses

See the section on non-steroidal anti-inflammatory analgesic drugs.

Dosage

1. The adult oral dose is 20 mg once per day. Double this dose may be taken for 48 hours following an acute skeletal muscle injury.
2. For acute gout 40 mg per day may be prescribed.
3. Gel: Apply to the affected area 3–4 times daily.
4. Oral doses, above, may be administered by deep intramuscular injection in acute musculoskeletal injury or exacerbation of arthritis.
5. The rectal dose is as for the oral route when compromised.

Nurse monitoring

1. See the section on non-steroidal anti-inflammatory analgesic drugs.
2. Note that dispersible tablets and 'Melt' tablets (which very rapidly dissolve in the mouth) are oral alternatives for patients with swallowing difficulty, especially the elderly with dysphagia.

General note

Piroxicam preparations may be stored at room temperature.

PIZOTIFEN (Sanomigran)

Presentation

Tablets—0.5 mg, 1.5 mg

Actions and uses

Pizotifen inhibits the action of substances which are released within the blood vessels and which cause the vascular changes which lead to the symptoms of severe headache and migraine. In clinical practice it is used for the prophylaxis of migraine.

Dosage

The dose ranges from 0.5–6 mg per day depending on individual patient response.

Nurse monitoring

1. The nurse may play an important role in cautioning patients about the dangers of drowsiness associated with taking this drug, especially in relation to driving vehicles and operating machinery.
2. The drug should never be given to patients who have glaucoma or a predisposition to urinary retention.
3. Apart from drowsiness, common side-effects include weight gain and increased appetite. Less frequently, dizziness and nausea have occurred.

General note

The drug may be stored at room temperature.

POLDINE SULPHATE (Nacton)

Presentation
Tablets—2 mg, 4 mg

Actions and uses
Poldine sulphate is an anticholinergic drug which acts by reducing the amount of acid produced by the cells of the stomach. A reduction in gastric acid secretion in patients with peptic ulcer may produce symptomatic relief and may aid ulcer healing.

Dosage
For adults the initial dose of 2 mg three times daily and at bedtime may be increased gradually up to a maximum of 4 mg four times a day. The optimum dose is that which provides adequate pain relief without producing troublesome side-effects.

Nurse monitoring
Poldine has anticholinergic side-effects similar to those described under hyoscine-N-butylbromide (Buscopan) (q.v.).

General note
Preparations containing poldine may be stored at room temperature.

POLYTHIAZIDE (Nephril)

Presentation
Tablets—1 mg

Actions and uses
See the section on thiazide and related diuretics.

Dosage
The adult dose is 0.5–4 mg taken as a single daily dose. The diuretic action may last up to 48 hours.

Nurse monitoring
See the section on thiazide and related diuretics.

General note
Polythiazide tablets may be stored at room temperature.

POTASSIUM CLORAZEPATE (Tranxene)

Presentation
Capsules—7.5 mg, 15 mg

Actions and uses
Potassium clorazepate is a member of the benzodiazepine group (q.v.). Its principal use is in the treatment of anxiety.

Dosage
15 mg daily usually administered at night.

Nurse monitoring
See the section on benzodiazepines.

General note
Capsules containing potassium clorazepate may be stored at room temperature.

POTASSIUM PERCHLORATE (Peroidin)

Presentation
Tablets—200 mg

Actions and uses
Potassium perchlorate prevents the uptake of iodine by the thyroid gland and in this way inhibits the total amount of thyroxine produced by the gland. Its use in the treatment of thyrotoxicosis is limited by the occasional occurrence of severe side-effects.

Dosage
1. Adults: Initially 800 mg in divided doses daily with maintenance doses reduced to 200–400 mg daily.
2. Children: Up to 250 mg daily has been used in children over 5 years of age.
3. For specialized radioisotope brain scanning, a single dose of 200 mg is given.

Nurse monitoring
1. Hypersensitivity reactions, i.e. maculopapular rashes, fever and lymphadenopathy have been reported.

2. The drug can produce gastrointestinal upset and nausea may be severe.
3. Serious adverse effects include aplastic anaemia, pancytopenia, leucopenia and nephrotic syndrome.
4. Some thyrotoxic patients receive prior to operation a short course of potassium iodide. Potassium perchlorate should never be given at the same time as it negates the action of potassium iodide in this situation.

General notes
1. Potassium perchlorate tablets may be stored at room temperature.
2. The tablets should be protected from moisture.

PRAVASTATIN (Lipostat)

Presentation
Tablets—10 mg, 20 mg

Actions and uses
Pravastatin is one of a new range of lipid-lowering drugs which are frequently described as HMG-CoA reductase inhibitors (which refers to their inhibitory action on cholesterol synthesis). Drugs of this type produce a marked and sustained fall in cholesterol (particularly low density lipoprotein or LDL cholesterol) and triglyceride compared to that produced by other lipid-lowering agents and have consequently become very popular in recent years.

The drug may be used in patients with hypercholesterolaemia who are considered to be at risk of ischaemic heart disease and early cardiac death or hypertriglycerid-aemia in which case they are likely to develop peripheral vascular disease and pancreatitis. Usually such patients will have blood cholesterol levels well in excess of 7–8 mmol/litre or triglyceride levels above 3 mmol/litre. These may fall by up to 50% on treatment.

Dosage
Adults: A single evening dose of 10–40 mg is given.

Nurse monitoring
1. The use of lipid-lowering drugs is very controversial. In many cases, elevated blood cholesterol is the result of obesity, inappropriate diet or alcohol excess, and correction of these factors is more appropriate. It should be noted that treatment is lifelong and therefore very expensive.
2. A few patients present with a familial hypercholesterolaemia and history of early cardiac death in the family. In these patients, life may be markedly prolonged by treatment, Also, patients with extensive cardiac disease, especially after coronary artery bypass grafting, should have their cholesterol maintained in the normal range.
3. Pravastatin is effective within 2–4 weeks of commencing therapy.
4. Patients receiving warfarin should have their anticoagulant status carefully checked after starting pravastatin therapy. In the past, lipid-lowering drugs have been shown to increase the risk of bleeding in such patients.

General note
Pravastatin tablets are stored at room temperature, and protected from light and moisture

PRAZOSIN (Hypovase)

Presentation
Tablets—0.5 mg, 1 mg, 2 mg, 5 mg

Actions and uses
Prazosin lowers the blood pressure by a direct action on the smooth muscle of blood vessels described as selective alpha$_1$-blockade. It is used in the management of hypertension.

Also prazosin produces a secondary effect on the urethral sphincter causing relaxation and thus permitting urine flow. This is of use in the treatment of dysuria associated with benign prostatic hypertrophy.

P

Dosage

A significant number of patients suffer from sudden collapse within 30–90 minutes of receiving their first dose of prazosin. For this reason all patients are commenced on low doses (0.5 mg three times a day) and the dose is increased gradually until the required effect is obtained. The maximum dosage is 20 mg per day usually taken three times a day in divided doses.

Nurse monitoring

1. As noted above sudden collapse may follow the initial dose of prazosin and therefore the initial dose must be small and is usually given on retiring to bed on the first night of treatment.
2. Side-effects are numerous and include postural hypotension, drowsiness, headache, lethargy, weakness, palpitations/ tachycardia, dry mouth, blurred vision, urinary frequency, nasal congestion, fluid retention, nervousness, depression, vertigo, constipation and diarrhoea, nausea and vomiting, skin rashes, itching, sweating, abdominal pain, paraesthesia, impotence in males, nose bleeds, reddened eyes and tinnitus.
3. Prazosin may exacerbate depression and therefore is relatively contraindicated in patients with such problems.

General note

Prazosin tablets may be stored at room temperature.

PREDNISOLONE (Precortisyl, Prednesol, Predsol, Deltacortril)

Several other proprietary preparations containing prednisolone in many different formulations are also available.

Presentation

Tablets—1 mg, 5 mg, 25 mg
—2.5 mg and 5 mg (enteric coated)
Injection—32 mg in 2 ml (intravenous or intramuscular)
Eye/ear drops—0.5%
Suppositories—5 mg
Enema—20 mg in 100 ml

Actions and uses

Prednisolone is a corticosteroid drug and has actions and uses similar to other corticosteroids (q.v.).

Dosage

Dose ranges vary widely depending on the type of illness, the severity of the disease and the route of administration. It is therefore impossible to outline possible dosage regimes in this text.

Nurse monitoring

See the section on corticosteroids.

General notes

1. Preparations containing prednisolone may be stored at room temperature.
2. In common with other eye drops, containers should not be used for more than 7 days for in-patients in a hospital ward or 4 weeks in the domestic situation or the risk of bacterial contamination becomes too great.

PREDNISONE (Decortisyl, Deltacortone)

Presentation

Tablets—1 mg, 5 mg

Actions and uses

Prednisone is a corticosteroid drug and its actions and uses are described in the section on these drugs. It is worth noting that in the body prednisone is converted to the active substance prednisolone.

Dosage

Dose ranges vary widely depending on the type of illness, the severity of the disease and the route of administration. It is therefore impossible to outline possible dosage regimes in this text.

Nurse monitoring

See the section on corticosteroids.

General note
> Prednisone tablets may be stored at room temperature.

PRILOCAINE (Citanest)

Presentation
> Injection— 1. Plain: 0.5%, 1% and 4%
> 2. With adrenaline: 3%
> 3. With felypressin: 3%

Actions and uses
> This drug is a local anaesthetic. Adrenaline and felypressin are vasoconstrictor substances which prolong the duration of its effects.

Dosage
> There is considerable variation in the optimum dosage for individual use. It should be noted, however, that the maximum adult dose should not exceed 400 mg.

Nurse monitoring
> 1. The nurse monitoring aspects of lignocaine (local anaesthetic) (q.v.) apply to this drug.
> 2. At maximum dosage a chemical called methaemoglobin may be produced in the blood. This may lead to an appearance of cyanosis.

General note
> The drug may be stored at room temperature.

PRIMIDONE (Mysoline)

Presentation
> Tablets—250 mg
> Suspension—250 mg in 5 ml

Actions and uses
> Primidone is an anticonvulsant drug which is converted in the body to the active component phenobarbitone. It is used primarily for the treatment of grand mal epilepsy. In the past combinations of primidone and phenobarbitone were used to treat epilepsy but as they are in effect the same drug this practice is now discouraged.

Dosage
> As individual doses are extremely variable, the following are simply guidelines for treatment and dosages should always be adjusted to individual requirements. Initiation of treatment is the same for both adults and children. It is recommended that 125 mg be given once daily late in the evening and every 3 days thereafter the dose should be increased by 125 mg until the daily dosage is 1500 mg in adults and 500 mg in children. Thereafter the dosage should be adjusted until control is obtained or side-effects occur. Average daily maintenance doses are as follows:
> 1. Adults and children over 9 years: 750–1500 mg.
> 2. Children: Up to 2 years—250–500 mg; 2–5 years—500–750 mg; 6–9 years—750–1000 mg.
> It should be noted that although initial treatment is given once daily in the evening, by the time the dosage exceeds 250 mg in total it should be split into a twice daily regime.

Nurse monitoring
> 1. The nurse monitoring aspects of anticonvulsant drugs in general are discussed in the section on these drugs.
> 2. Primidone is converted in the body to phenobarbitone and therefore further nurse monitoring aspects of this drug may be found in the section dealing with this drug.

General note
> The drug may be stored at room temperature.

PROBENECID (Benemid)

Presentation
> Tablets—500 mg

Actions and uses
> Probenecid acts directly on the kidney tubules to produce two main effects:
> 1. It blocks the excretion of penicillin and some cephalosporin drugs from the renal tubules and may

therefore be used to maintain high blood levels of these drugs.

2. It promotes the excretion of uric acid and urate from the renal tubules and may therefore be used to reduce the blood urate concentration in hyperuricaemia and gout.

Dosage

1. Hyperuricaemia and gout: Adults usually receive 250 mg twice daily initially. The dose is increased after a week to 500 mg twice daily. Up to 2 g per day may be given in 2–4 divided doses where necessary.
2. Adjunct therapy with penicillin and cephalosporins:
   a. Adults: 2 g daily in divided doses.
   b. Children:
      i. Children under 50 kg: 25 mg/kg daily in divided doses.
      ii. Children over 50 kg should receive the adult dose.

Nurse monitoring

1. The nurse may play a major role in preventing the occurrence of renal stone formation or renal colic in patients on this drug by continually monitoring their fluid intake and encouraging them to take an adequate amount of fluid each day as this reduces the incidence of such side-effects.
2. Aspirin blocks the effect of probenecid and as patients may frequently be taking this drug in addition to prescribed medication the nurse may contribute to the management of such patients by ensuring that they know that they should never take aspirin when taking probenecid.
3. Common side-effects include anorexia, nausea, vomiting, headache and frequency of micturition.
4. More rarely allergic reactions may occur when patients are given this drug. They include anaphylactic shock, dermatitis, pruritus, fever, sore gums and occasionally haemolytic anaemia.
5. Rare serious side-effects include

nephrotic syndrome, liver damage and aplastic anaemia.
6. Probenecid must be used with caution in patients with a history of peptic ulcer disease.
7. Probenecid must never be given to patients receiving methotrexate as it may induce methotrexate toxicity.
8. Although probenecid reduces blood urate levels it may at the onset of treatment actually precipitate an acute attack of gout. It is common practice, therefore, to give concurrent therapy with an anti-inflammatory drug e.g. naproxen or colchicine at the beginning of treatment.

General note

Probenecid tablets may be stored at room temperature.

PROBUCOL (Lurselle)

Presentation

Tablets—250 mg

Actions and uses

Probucol is a lipid-lowering agent used in combination with dietary control in the management of hypercholesterolaemia (where significant coronary risk is associated with elevated cholesterol levels). It has a specific use in Type II hyperlipoproteinaemia.

Dosage

Adults: 500 mg taken twice daily with the morning and evening meals.

Nurse monitoring

1. Gastrointestinal upsets (diarrhoea, flatulence, abdominal pain, nausea) are the most common side-effects noted with this drug,
2. Some patients may develop hyper-sensitivity reactions including dizziness, palpitations, and syncope.
3. In common with other lipid-lowering drugs, probucol should not be used during pregnancy.
4. The drug should be taken with food when maximum absorption occurs.

General note
Probucol tablets may be stored at room temperature and should be protected from light.

PROCAINAMIDE (Pronestyl)

Presentation
Tablets—250 mg
Injection—1 g in 10 ml (multidose vials)

Actions and uses
Procainamide has a depressant action on the heart and reduces contractility and excitability of heart muscle and conductivity of the electrical conducting tissues. It is therefore useful in the treatment of ventricular and supraventricular dysrhythmias. It may be given in an emergency either intravenously or intramuscularly and for long-term treatment it may be given orally.

Dosage
Adults only:
1. Intravenously: 25–50 mg per minute up to a total of 1 g with continuous ECG and blood pressure monitoring.
2. Intramuscularly: 250 mg as a single intramuscular dose.
3. Oral dosage: Up to 50 mg/kg body weight daily is taken in divided doses at intervals ranging from 3-6-hourly. A serum concentration of between 4 and 8 microgram/ml has been found to be effective.

Nurse monitoring
1. The nurse will rarely see procainamide given intravenously outside the hospital setting. Rapid intravenous dosage of this drug can lead to hypotension, ventricular fibrillation and cardiac arrest. Constant monitoring of blood pressure and ECG monitoring is essential when the drug is given by the intravenous route.
2. Side-effects from procainamide occur most frequently after high dosage or in patients with heart failure or renal failure. The commonest side-effects are anorexia, diarrhoea, nausea and vomiting.
3. When patients have been on procainamide for a prolonged period of time, they may develop a syndrome similar to systemic lupus erythematosus with joint pains, skin lesions, pleuritic chest pain and the other features of this disease. The development of such symptoms in a patient on procainamide is an indication for blood tests to be carried out on the patient to detect LE cells and if these are present the drug should be stopped and if necessary an alternative anti-dysrhythmic drug should be substituted. This syndrome characteristically resolves after withdrawal of the drug.
4. Because procainamide depresses cardiac contractility it may lead to the development of heart failure. The nurse should therefore monitor the patient for symptoms of heart failure such as breathlessness on exertion or on lying flat in bed and ankle oedema.
5. Flushing, skin rash and pruritus, depression, psychotic reaction and hallucinations, bitter taste in the mouth, muscle weakness, leucopenia and agranulocytosis are other side-effects which have been encountered with this drug.

General note
Procainamide tablets and solution for injection may be stored at room temperature.

PROCARBAZINE (Natulan)

Presentation
Capsules—50 mg

Actions and uses
The mode of action of procarbazine remains unclear but it would appear to prevent cell division by interfering with one of the basic biochemical steps necessary for this process. Its main use is in the treatment of Hodgkin's disease, although very

rarely it may be indicated for the management of solid tumours.

Dosage
1. Adults: 50–200 mg orally divided in up to three doses daily.
2. Children: 100 mg per m^2 body surface area.

Nurse monitoring
1. Nearly all patients suffer from anorexia, nausea and vomiting. These symptoms may become less troublesome as treatment continues.
2. Bone marrow depression may produce thrombocytopenia and leucopenia. Regular blood counts are carried out during treatment to monitor this but should these effects arise the patient would be at an increased risk of severe infection or haemorrhage.
3. The drug should not be given to patients with severe liver or kidney disease.
4. Procarbazine is derived from the hydrazines which is one group of monoamine oxidase inhibitors used in the treatment of depression. This relationship leads to a number of important points:
   a. It has an action as a weak monoamine oxidase inhibitor and may produce hypertension if certain drugs and foodstuffs are taken concurrently (see the section on monoamine oxidase inhibitors). Patients should carry an appropriate monoamine oxidase inhibitor warning card while treated with procarbazine.
   b. Its mild monoamine oxidase inhibitor action may lead to side-effects of somnolence, confusion and ataxia.
5. It should not be given concurrently with other monoamine oxidase inhibitors.
6. The nurse should be constantly aware that cytotoxic drugs are highly dangerous and therefore must be handled with great care. Spillage and contamination of the skin of the patient or nurse may lead to a degree of absorption of the drug which, if chronically repeated, may cause damage and the skin may also be sensitized to the drug making it, in some cases, impossible for the nurse to continue working with the drug.

General note
Procarbazine capsules may be stored at room temperature.

PROCHLORPERAZINE (Buccastem, Stemetil)

Presentation
Tablets—5 mg, 25 mg
Buccal tablets—3 mg
Syrup—5 mg in 5 ml
Injection—12.5 mg in 1 ml; 25 mg in 2 ml
Suppositories—5 mg, 25 mg

Actions and uses
Prochlorperazine is a member of the phenothiazine group and its actions and uses are described in the section on these drugs. As this is a very widely used drug it is worth detailing its specific uses which are:
1. For the treatment of severe anxiety states.
2. For the treatment of behavioural disorders in schizophrenia and other psychotic states.
3. For the treatment of nausea and vomiting, particularly when this is due to other drug therapy.
4. For the symptomatic relief of vertigo and vomiting in neurological disorders such as Menière's disease.

Dosage
1. Psychosis: 75–100 mg in total daily is given in 2–3 divided doses by the oral, rectal or intramuscular route.
2. Nausea and vomiting:
   a. The oral dose is 10–20 mg
   b. The rectal dose is 25 mg
   c. The intramuscular dose is 12.5 mg
3. For the treatment of vertigo and nausea associated with neurological disorders such as Menière's disease: 5 mg three

times daily increased to 30 mg daily if required.
4. Children's doses are as follows:
   a. Less than 1 year:
      i. Orally 0.125 mg/kg three times per day.
   b. Children over 1 year:
      i. Orally 2.5–5 mg three times per day.
      ii. Rectally 2.5–5 mg once or twice per day.

Nurse monitoring
The nurse monitoring aspects of this drug are described under phenothiazines (q.v.).

General notes
1. Preparations containing prochlorperazine may be stored at room temperature but they should be protected from direct sunlight.
2. Prochlorperazine injection must not be mixed with other drugs.

PROCYCLIDINE (Kemadrin)

Presentation
Tablets—5 mg
Injection—10 mg in 2 ml

Actions and uses
The actions and uses of this drug are identical to those described for benzhexol (q.v.).

Dosage
Adults:
1. Orally: 20–30 mg in three or four divided doses daily.
2. Parenterally (by intravenous or intramuscular injection): 10–20 mg.

Nurse monitoring
The nurse monitoring aspects of benzhexol (q.v.) apply to this drug.

General note
The drug may be stored at room temperature.

PROGESTERONE (Cyclogest)

Presentation
Vaginal/rectal suppositories—200 mg and 400 mg

Actions and uses
The actions and uses of progestational hormones are discussed under hormones (2). In clinical practice progesterone is used most commonly for the treatment of premenstrual symptoms.

Dosage
200–400 mg rectally or vaginally once or twice daily from the 12th-14th day of the menstrual cycle or until menstruation recommences.

Nurse monitoring
See the section on progestational hormones.

General note
The drug may be stored at room temperature.

PROMAZINE (Sparine)

Presentation
Tablets—25 mg, 50 mg, 100 mg
Suspension—50 mg in 5 ml
Injection—50 mg in 1 ml

Actions and uses
Promazine is a member of the phenothiazine group of drugs and its actions and uses are described in the section dealing with these drugs.

Dosage
1. Adults:
   a. Orally: 25–100 mg three to four times per day.
   b. Intramuscularly: 25–50 mg repeated after 6–8 hours as required to a maximum of 100 mg per day.
2. Children's doses are usually calculated according to body weight.

Nurse monitoring
The nurse monitoring aspects of this drug are described under phenothiazines (q.v.).

General note
Preparations containing promazine may be stored at room temperature.

PROMETHAZINE (Phenergan, Avomine)

Presentation
Tablets—10 mg, 25 mg (as hydrochloride), 25 mg (as theoclate)
Elixir—5 mg in 5 ml
Injection—25 mg in 1 ml

Actions and uses
Promethazine is a member of the phenothiazine group of drugs but is unusual in that it has little if any appreciable tranquillizing activity. It is, however, found to be very useful for its anti-emetic, sedative and antihistaminic effects. It is particularly useful in the prevention and treatment of motion sickness and in the treatment of irradiation sickness, postoperative vomiting, the nausea and vomiting of pregnancy, drug-induced nausea and vomiting and for the symptomatic relief of nausea and vertigo in Menière's disease and other labyrinthine disturbances.

Dosage
1. For the treatment of nausea and vomiting:
   a. Adults: Adult doses are as follows:
      i. Orally: 25–75 mg at night with two or three additional daytime doses of 10–20 mg
      ii. Intramuscularly: Up to 100 mg may be given
      iii. Intravenously: Up to 100 mg may be given. The drug must be diluted to 10 times its volume with water for injection and administered very slowly.
   b. Children:
      i. Less than 1 year old: Doses of 1.5 mg/kg are given.
      ii. In older children 15–25 mg is administered in a single dose as necessary.
2. For the prevention of motion sickness, promethazine theoclate is administered in a dose of 25 mg on the night prior to undertaking a journey and a further 25 mg 1 to 2 hours prior to commencing the journey.

Nurse monitoring
1. Promethazine is a phenothiazine drug but in the dosages recommended and when used for the treatment of conditions described above, the problems encountered with phenothiazine drugs in general (q.v.) are rarely encountered.
2. It is important to remember that sedation may commonly occur and patients must be warned about the dangers of taking this drug while operating heavy machinery or driving.

General note
Preparations containing promethazine may be stored at room temperature.

PROPAFENONE (Arythmol)

Presentation
Tablets—150 mg, 300 mg

Actions and uses
In order to understand the anti-arrhythmic action of propafenone, a knowledge of cardiac conduction is required. However, since propafenone is likely to be prescribed, initially at least, in the acute coronary care setting, a description of its action is included for nurses working in this speciality. Propafenone is a class 1C agent, so-called because of the nature of its action on the conducting tissues of the myocardium. It acts primarily on the rapid depolarization phase of the cardiac action potential (i.e. it inhibits the fast inward sodium channel), and exerts a potent membrane stabilizing effect. Conduction is slowed in the atria, at the atrioventricular node and, in particular, the His-Purkinje system. Changes which may be seen on the ECG include prolongation of the PR interval and QRS complex duration. In addition, propafenone possesses beta-blocking activity but is much less potent than recognised beta-blockers in this respect, e.g. only about 1/40th the potency of propranolol.

Propafenone is indicated for the prevention and management of ventricular arrhythmias.

Dosage

Adults: Initially 150 mg three times daily, increasing gradually to 300 mg twice daily and up to three times daily.

Nurse monitoring

1. Patients may complain of a bitter taste.
2. Common side-effects of propafenone include dizziness, fatigue, nausea and vomiting, headache, constipation (and diarrhoea), allergic skin reactions, blurred vision and dry mouth.
3. Propafenone is extensively metabolized in the liver and readily accumulates in patients with liver impairment. A suitable dosage reduction is frequently necessary.
4. It should be avoided or administered with extreme caution in patients with marked hypotension, bradycardia, uncontrolled heart failure (unless related to the arrhythmia for which treatment is indicated) and cardiogenic shock, severe obstructive airways disease and uncontrolled electrolyte disturbances.
5. Patients with depression of the sinus node, atrial conduction, and 2nd or 3rd degree atrioventricular block should be adequately paced before treatment is administered.
6. Note that propafenone possesses beta-blocking activity, albeit weakly so, and may precipitate heart failure in patients with poor cardiac reserve.
7. Propafenone increases plasma levels of digoxin and warfarin, and patients receiving such combinations should be carefully monitored for signs of digoxin intoxication or excessive anticoagulation.

Raised levels of propranolol and metoprolol, but not of other beta-blockers, have also been noted and excessive beta-blockade may result.
8. Plasma levels of propafenone may be increased by co-administration of cimetidine due to its inhibitory action on the metabolizing enzymes of the liver.

General note

Propafenone tablets may be stored at room temperature. An injection is available, though only on a named patient basis at present.

PROPANTHELINE (Pro-Banthine)

Dosage

Tablets—15 mg
Injection—30 mg

Actions and uses

1. It has an anticholinergic effect similar to poldine (q.v.) and is therefore useful for the symptomatic relief and healing of peptic ulceration.
2. One of this drug's side-effects is to produce urinary retention and for this reason it is used occasionally in the treatment of enuresis.

Dosage

1. Peptic ulcer:
   a. Adults: The usual oral dose is 15 mg three times a day and at bedtime. By intravenous injection 30 mg in 10 ml sodium chloride injection 0.9% is given at a rate not exceeding 6 mg per minute. 30 mg in 1 ml of water may be given by the intramuscular route.
2. Enuresis: In children 15–45 mg may be taken at night as a single dose.

Nurse monitoring

The nurse monitoring notes on this drug are identical to those for hyoscine-N-butylbromide (Buscopan) (q.v.)

General note
Preparations containing propantheline may be stored at room temperature.

PROPRANOLOL (Inderal)

Presentation
Tablets—10 mg, 40 mg, 80 mg, 160 mg
Capsules—80 mg, 160 mg slow release
Injection—1 mg in 1 ml

Actions and uses
Propranolol is a non-selective beta-adrenoreceptor blocking drug. Its actions and uses are described under beta-adrenoreceptor blocking drugs (q.v.).

Dosage
1. By intravenous injection in an emergency situation, up to 1 mg may be given over 1 minute. Pulse, blood pressure and cardiac (ECG) monitoring must be continuous during the period of injection and injection must be stopped if profound bradycardia, hypotension or widening of the QRS complex occurs.
2. Adult oral maintenance dosage ranges from 80–480 mg per day. In the treatment of hypertension slow release capsules are available and total dosage is given once daily. In the treatment of dysrhythmias and angina the dosage is usually divided and given twice, three or four times a day.
3. The dosage for children is as follows: Up to 1 year—1 mg/kg; 1–6 years—10 mg; 7 years plus—20 mg.
   These oral doses may be doubled if necessary.
4. Dosage for intravenous injection in children is as follows: The intravenous dosage for the treatment of acute cardiac dysrhythmias is: Age 1–5—0.3 mg; Age 6–12—0.5 mg
   Note: The intravenous dose should be halved if a patient is anaesthetized.

Nurse monitoring
See the section on beta-adrenoreceptor blocking drugs.

General notes
1. Propranolol tablets, capsules and injection may be stored at room temperature.
2. Injection solution may be diluted for ease of administration with 5% dextrose, 0.9% sodium chloride or dextrose/saline mixtures immediately before use but no other drugs should be mixed in the same syringe.

PROSTAGLANDIN E$_2$ (Prostin E$_2$, Dinoprostone)

Presentation
Tablets—0.5 mg
Sterile solutions—1 mg in 1 ml alcohol (0.75 ml ampoule); 10 mg in 1 ml alcohol (0.5 ml ampoule)

Actions and uses
Prostaglandin E$_2$ has the capacity to induce contraction of the uterus. It, therefore, has the following uses:
1. The induction of labour.
2. Termination of pregnancy.
3. The induction of labour in missed abortion.
4. Treatment of hydatidiform mole.

Dosage
1. For the induction of labour:
   a. Orally: 0.5 mg initially and thereafter 1 mg at hourly intervals until an adequate uterine response has been achieved. Thereafter the dose may be reduced to 0.5 mg hourly.
   b. Intravenously: 1 mg/ml solution in alcohol is diluted with 0.9% sodium chloride or 5% dextrose to produce a solution containing 1.5 microgram/ml. This is infused intravenously at a rate of 0.25 microgram /minute for 30 minutes, the dose being subsequently maintained or increased according to patient response.
2. For the termination of pregnancy or treatment of missed abortion or

hydatidiform mole: A solution containing 5 microgram/ml is infused intravenously at a rate of 2.5 microgram/minute for 30 minutes and then maintained or increased to 5 microgram/minute. This higher concentration should be administered for at least 4 hours before further increases are made.

3. For the termination of pregnancy: 1 ml of a solution containing 100 microgram/ml may be instilled extra-amniotically through a suitable Foley catheter. Subsequent doses of 1 or 2 ml of the same concentration solution should be given at intervals usually of 2 hours according to uterine response.

Nurse monitoring

1. Nausea, vomiting and diarrhoea occur commonly at doses required to terminate pregnancy by the intravenous route but are less common after the extra-amniotic route for termination. Such symptoms are rare when the concentrations administered by the intravenous route for induction of labour are used.

2. Transient cardiovascular symptoms have been noticed including flushing, shivering, headache, dizziness.

3. Very rarely convulsions and changes in the electroencephalogram have occurred.

4. Local tissue irritation or erythema may follow intravenous infusion. This will disappear within 2–5 hours of stopping the infusion.

5. Infusion of this compound may occasionally lead to pyrexia.

6. Uterine rupture has occurred only rarely with this substance.

7. The drug should be used with caution in patients who have glaucoma or suffer from asthma.

General notes

1. Prostaglandin preparations should be refrigerated.

2. Once diluted the solutions should be used within 24 hours.

PROSTAGLANDIN F$_2$ ALPHA (Dinoprost)

Presentation

Sterile solutions—5 mg/ml: 1.5 ml, 4 ml and 5 ml ampoules

Actions and uses

The actions and uses of prostaglandin F$_2$ alpha are identical to those described for prostaglandin E$_2$ (q.v.)

Dosage

1. For the induction of labour: The drug is administered intravenously. It is diluted in normal saline or 5% dextrose to a concentration of 15 microgram/ml and administered initially in a dosage of 2.5 microgram/minute. This regime is maintained for at least 30 minutes and subsequent dose changes depend on patient response.

2. For the induction of labour after fetal death: An initial infusion concentration of 5 microgram/minute may be given and increases should be at intervals of not less than 1 hour.

3. For the termination of pregnancy, missed abortion or hydatidiform mole: A solution containing the equivalent of 50 microgram/ml is infused intravenously at a rate of 25 microgram/minute for at least 30 minutes, then maintained or increased to 50 microgram/minute according to response. This rate should be maintained for at least 4 hours before further increases are made.

4. For the termination of pregnancy by extra-amniotic administration: A solution containing 375 microgram may be injected via a catheter.

5. For intra-amniotic termination of pregnancy: 40 mg may be injected slowly into the amniotic sac.

Nurse monitoring

The nurse monitoring aspects of this drug are identical to those described for prostaglandin E$_2$ (q.v.)

General notes
1. The drug may be stored at room temperature.
2. Diluted solutions should be used within 24 hours if the intravenous or intra-amniotic route is contemplated. Solutions may be retained for up to 48 hours if they are to be given by the extra-aminiotic route.

PROTRIPTYLINE (Concordin)

Presentation
Tablets—5 mg, 10 mg
Actions and uses
Protriptyline is a tricyclic antidepressant drug. Its actions and uses are described in the section on these drugs.
Dosage
For the treatment of depression in adults the total daily dose is 15–60 mg given in three divided doses.

Nurse monitoring
See the section on tricyclic antidepressant drugs.

General note
Tablets containing protriptyline may be stored at room temperature.

PYRAZINAMIDE (Zinamide)

Presentation
Tablets—500 mg
Actions and uses
Pyrazinamide has been found to be effective against the organism *Mycobacterium tuberculosis* and is therefore used for the treatment of tuberculosis. It is rarely used as the first choice for treatment of this disease and is reserved for cases where resistance develops to the more commonly used drugs, or where severe side-effects are experienced with more commonly used drugs.
Dosage
The recommended dosage is 20–35 mg/kg body weight in total per day given in divided doses. The maximum daily dose should not exceed 3 g.

Nurse monitoring
1. Patients undergoing treatment for tuberculosis receive their drugs for considerable periods of time. The nurse may play an important role in reminding patients that their drug therapy must be taken regularly for as long as recommended by medical staff, whether or not they themselves feel that they have recovered.
2. Common side-effects experienced by patients on this drug include anorexia, nausea, vomiting, fever, tiredness, difficulty with micturition and arthralgia which may be due to gout (see below).
3. Photosensitivity and skin rash may occur.
4. The drug may effect concentration in the blood of uric acid and may precipitate attacks of joint pain due to gout.
5. The main drawback to the drug's use is that it may cause serious disturbance of liver function.
6. The drug should be used with caution in patients with diabetes as loss of control has occurred when the drug has been introduced.
7. The drug may occasionally cause some impairment of renal function.

General note
The drug may be stored at room temperature.

PYRIDOSTIGMINE (Mestinon)

Presentation
Tablets—60 mg
Injection—1 mg in 1 ml
Actions and uses
The actions of pyridostigmine are identical to those described for neostigmine (q.v.). In clinical practice its principal use is in the management of myasthenia gravis, where it has the advantage over neostigmine of having a longer duration of action. It may also be given intramuscularly in the treatment of paralytic ileus or postoperative urinary retention.

Dosage

1. For the treatment of myasthenia gravis:
   a. Adults. 60–240 mg 4 to 6-hourly according to individual response.
   b. Children: Up to 7 mg/kg body weight in total per day is given in six divided doses.
2. For the treatment of paralytic ileus or postoperative urinary retention: A dose of 1–2 mg may be given intramuscularly.

Nurse monitoring

1. The nurse monitoring aspects of pyridostigmine are identical to those described for neostigmine (q.v.).
2. It is worth noting that in practice there are fewer problems with gastrointestinal upset with pyridostigmine as compared with neostigmine.

General note

The drug may be stored at room temperature.

PYRIMETHAMINE (Daraprim)

Presentation

Tablets—25 mg

Actions and uses

Pyrimethamine is an antimalarial used, normally in combination with other drugs, in the prevention of malaria. It also possesses useful action against other parasitic organisms and is used in combination with a sulphonamide in the control of toxoplasmosis.

Dosage

1. For antimalarial prophylaxis (in combination with other drugs).
   a. Adults: 25 mg taken once per week.
   b. Children: Those over 5 years receive half the adult dosage.
2. For the treatment of toxoplasmosis:
   a. Adults: 50–75 mg daily (in combination with sulphonamide) reduced according to the patient's response after 1–3 weeks. Treatment is then continued for a further 4–5 weeks.

Nurse monitoring

1. Once weekly administration for the suppression of malaria is not usually associated with side-effects.
2. Patients undergoing malaria prophylaxis must ensure that regular weekly doses are taken. It should be stressed that treatment must be continued for a period of 4 weeks after return from an area where malaria is endemic.
3. With larger doses used in the treatment of toxoplasmosis, side-effects may arise. These include megaloblastic anaemia, leucopenia, thrombocytopenia and aplastic anaemia. Very high doses have produced vomiting, convulsions and respiratory failure.

General note

Tablets may be stored at room temperature.

P

Q

QUINALBARBITONE (Seconal)

Presentation
Capsules—50 mg, 100 mg
Actions and uses
Quinalbarbitone is a barbiturate drug
(q.v.) which is taken at night as a
hypnotic.
Dosage
50–100 mg on retiring.

> **Nurse monitoring**
> See the section on barbiturate
> drugs.

General note
Quinalbarbitone capsules may be
stored at room temperature.

QUINAPRIL (Accupro)

Presentation
Tablets—5 mg, 10 mg, 20 mg
Actions and uses
See section on ACE inhibitors.
Dosage
Range: 20–40 mg as a single daily
dose.

> **Nurse monitoring**
> See section on ACE inhibitors

General note
Quinapril tablets may be stored at
room temperature.

QUINIDINE (Kinidin)

Presentation
Tablets—200 mg as sulphate
(250 mg as bisulphate)

Sustained release tablets (Durules)
containing 250 mg quinidine
bisulphate
Actions and uses
Quinidine depresses heart function
by reducing the excitability of the
heart muscle and prolonging its
refractory period. It is therefore
useful in the treatment of cardiac
dysrhythmias. Conventional tablets
require to be taken in large and
frequent dosage to maintain an
effective blood level and it is
therefore advantageous to use the
sustained release tablet to guaran-
tee effectiveness of the drug.
Dosage
1. Adults: 200–400 mg 3–4 times
   daily as conventional tablets or
   500 mg to 1.25 g taken twice daily
   as sustained release tablets.
2. Children: The recommended
   dosage of quinidine sulphate is
   6 mg/kg body weight five times
   daily.
It should be noted that to avoid
hypersensitivity (as mentioned
below) all patients should be
given a small test dose prior to
commencement of the above
regimes.

> **Nurse monitoring**
> 1. As mentioned above, it is
>   essential to give a minute dose of
>   quinidine to all patients prior to
>   commencement of normal
>   therapy to detect those who may
>   be likely to suffer a hyper-
>   sensitivity reaction. Symptoms
>   which have been found to be
>   associated with such hyper-
>   sensitivity are as follows: tinnitus,
>   vertigo, visual disturbance,

headache, confusion, erythema-tous skin rashes, anorexia, nausea, vomiting, diarrhoea, chest pain, abdominal pain, fever, respiratory distress, cyanosis, hypotension and shock. Thrombocytopenic purpura has also occurred.
2. Side-effects which may occur in patients not hypersensitive to the drug include tinnitus, deafness, blurred vision, headache, dizziness and vomiting.
3. Excess dosage of the drug may lead to cardiac arrhythmias including heart block, paroxysmal ventricular tachycardia, ventricular fibrillation and cardiac arrest. As symptoms described in section (2) may precede these serious cardiac arrhythmias, the nurse may play a vital role in their prevention by detecting such symptoms in patients on the drug and advising medical staff accordingly.

General note
Quinidine tablets may be stored at room temperature.

QUININE (Sulphate and Bisulphate)

Presentation
Tablets—200 mg and 300 mg
Actions and uses
This drug was originally used for the treatment of malaria. It is now rarely used as an anti-malarial drug as more effective preparations have been developed. However, it was noted that when quinine was used it was effective in reducing painful night cramps suffered by a fair proportion of the older population. Its use nowadays is limited to the treatment of this condition.
Dosage
200–600 mg as a single dose on retiring.

Nurse monitoring
1. Perhaps the most important point to note about quinine sulphate is that it must not under any circumstances be confused with quinidine which is a drug that is used for the treatment of serious abnormalities in cardiac rhythm.
2. Certain individuals may prove hypersensitive to this drug and may suffer the following symptoms:
   a. Tinnitus, headache, visual disturbance and blindness.
   b. Nausea and abdominal pain.
   c. Skin rash.
   d. Blood disorders including haemolytic anaemia and thrombocytopenia.
3. It is recommended that the drug be avoided or used with extreme caution in patients with optic neuritis, heart disease or abnormalities of blood coagulation.
4. The drug may enhance the effect of oral anticoagulants (q.v.) producing an increased bleeding tendency.

General note
The tablets may be stored at room temperature.

R

RAMIPRIL (Tritace)

Presentation
Tablets—1.25 mg, 2.5 mg, 5 mg
Actions and uses
See section on ACE inhibitors.
Dosage
Range: 2.5–10 mg as a single daily dose.

Nurse monitoring
See section on ACE inhibitors

General note
Ramipril tablets may be stored at room temperature.

RANITIDINE (Zantac)

Presentation
Tablets—150 mg, 300 mg (both plain and effervescent)
Syrup—150 mg in 10 ml
Injection—50 mg in 2 ml
Actions and uses
See histamine H_2-receptor antagonists.
Dosage
Dosage for all indications is based on that used in the treatment of peptic ulceration, as follows:
1. Adults:
   a. Oral, treatment: 300 mg daily, in two divided doses or as a single evening dose.
   b. Oral, maintenance: usually a single bedtime dose of 150 mg or 300 mg since it appears that overnight acid output is important in determining ulcer relapse rates.
   c. Injection: Intramuscular therapy can be substituted for oral

treatment when necessary. Intravenous bolus doses of 50 mg, given over 1 minute, repeated at intervals of 6–8 hours, or intravenous infusion in a dose of 50 mg given over 2 hours, can be used in the acute stage.
2. Children 8 years and over: 2–4 mg/kg twice daily up to a maximum daily dose of 300 mg.

Nurse monitoring
The nurse monitoring aspects described for histamine H_2-receptor antagonists apply.

General notes
1. Ranitidine preparations may be stored at room temperature. The injection solution should be protected from light during storage.
2. Ranitidine intravenous infusions may be administered in sodium chloride or glucose solutions or mixtures thereof.

RAZOXANE (Razoxin)

Presentation
Tablets—125 mg
Actions and uses
Razoxane is a cytotoxic drug which prevents growth of malignant cells by interfering with the processes involved in cellular division. It is used in the treatment of acute myeloid leukaemia and sarcomata.
Dosage
1. In acute myeloid leukaemia: 3-day courses of 125 mg three times daily are used.

2. For the treatment of sarcomata: 125 mg once or twice daily is given in combination with radiotherapy.

Nurse monitoring
1. Common symptoms encountered with this drug include nausea, vomiting and diarrhoea.
2. Skin rashes and alopecia may occur with this drug.
3. When used in combination with radiotherapy, subcutaneous fibrosis, oesophagitis and pneumonitis may be produced.
4. The nurse should be constantly aware that most cytotoxic drugs are irritant to the skin and mucous surfaces, and are in general very toxic. Great care should therefore be exercised when handling these drugs, and in particular spillage or contamination of personnel or the environment must be avoided. If cytotoxic drugs are handled regularly it is theoretically possible that repeated skin contact or inhalation may produce systemic toxic effects and in nurses who have developed hypersensitivity, severe local and general hypersensitivity reactions.

General notes
1. Razoxane tablets may be stored at room temperature.
2. They should be protected from moisture and light.

REPROTEROL (Bronchodil)

Presentation
Inhaler—500 microgram per dose of metered aerosol

Actions and uses
This drug has a highly selective action on receptors in bronchial smooth muscle, causing relaxation of muscle tone. It is used, therefore, for the treatment of reversible airways obstruction (bronchospasm) in asthma and other conditions such as bronchitis and emphysema.

Dosage
Adults and children: One or two inhalations three times daily. More frequent, 3 to 6-hourly administration may be required to treat an acute attack.

Nurse monitoring
1. Rarely, this drug may cause palpitation, tachycardia, headache and fine muscle tremor.
2. The drug should be used with caution in patients with heart disease manifest by rhythm disturbances, angina, hyperthyroidism and hypertension.

General note
Reproterol aerosols should never be punctured or incinerated after use.

RIBAVARIN (Virazid)

Presentation
Nasal aerosol—6 g

Actions and uses
Ribavarin is an antiviral agent which is active against a range of viruses including influenza A and B viruses and para-influenza. It is used exclusively, however, in the treatment of infections due to respiratory syncytial virus (RSV), a common cause of chronic recurring lower respiratory infections in the first few years of life. In infants and children with established cardiorespiratory disease, RSV infections may present a special hazard: in otherwise healthy children it produces only mild symptoms. The precise mechanism whereby ribavarin prevents viral replication is unknown.

Dosage
The drug is delivered by aerosol or nebulization as a 20 mg/ml solution for 12 hours or longer daily over 3–7 days.

Nurse monitoring
1. Ribavarin solution may be delivered via an oxygen mask, or in a tent or hood. It is administered via a special small particle aerosol generator.

2. Patients must be monitored closely for signs of worsening respiratory function.

General note

Ribavarin vials may be stored at room temperature. The solution is prepared with water for injection and should be used within 24 hours of reconstitution.

RIFABUTIN (Mycobutin)

Presentation

Capsules—150 mg

Actions and uses

1. This drug is a member of the 'Rifamycin' group and has the same actions and potential uses as those of rifampicin.
2. In clinical practice rifabutin is most commonly indicated in the treatment of pulmonary tuberculosis and in other atypical mycobacterial infections.
3. It has a special role in preventing MAC (Mycobacterium Avium intracellular Comlex), a condition resembling Whipples disease which causes extensive problems in AIDS patients and is very difficult to treat. Rifabutin prophylaxis may be commenced as soon as the CD4 lymphocyte count falls to below 0.2 x 10^9/litre.

Dosage

Adults

1. Treatment of TB: 150–450 mg once daily administered in combination with other anti-tuberculous therapy for at least 6 months.
2. Other non-tuberculous mycobacterial disease: 450–600 mg once daily in combination therapy for up to 6 months after negative cultures are obtained.
3. MAC prophylaxis in immunodeficiency: 300 mg once daily as monotherapy.

Nurse monitoring

The nurse monitoring section on rifampicin also applies to this drug.

General note

Rifabutin capsules are stored at room temperature.

RIFAMPICIN (Rifadin, Rimactane)

Rifampicin is available in combination with isoniazid as Rifinah or Rimactazid.

Presentation

Capsules—150 mg, 300 mg
Syrup—100 mg in 5 ml
Injection—600 mg powder in vial plus special solvent

Actions and uses

1. Rifampicin is an anti-bacterial drug which is particularly effective against the tubercle bacillis (*Mycobacterium tuberculosis*). It has a bacteriostatic action inhibiting further growth and replication of the organism at low dose, and a bactericidal action (killing the organisms) at high dosage. The drug is usually used in combination with other anti-tuberculous agents (q.v.) for the prophylaxis and treatment of tuberculosis.
2. The drug is used in combination with other antibiotics in the treatment of other infections including brucellosis, legionnaires' disease and serious staphylococcal infections.
3. It is effective in the eradication of the organism *Neisseria meningitidis* (which causes bacterial meningitis) from the nasopharynx of carriers of the organism, and it is also used to prevent the occurrence of meningococcal meningitis in patients who have been in close contact with a case or carrier.
4. It is similarly used as in 3 above for prophylaxis of *Haemophilus influenzae*, type B infection.

Dosage

1. Tuberculosis (in multiple drug regimen):
   a. Adults: 600 mg (450 mg if body weight under 50 kg) taken daily in a single dose. To ensure rapid and complete absorption, the drug should preferably be taken before meals.

b. Children: 10 mg/kg as above.
Taken for 6 months, combined with isoniazid and pyrazinamide and, if resistance suspected, with ethambutol and streptomycin.

2. Brucellosis, legionnaires' disease, staphyloccocal infection:
   a. Adults: 600–1200 mg daily in two or four divided doses.

3. Prophylaxis of meningococcal meningitis:
   a. Adults: 600 mg twice daily for 2 days.
   b. Children: (over 3 months)—5 mg/kg (up to 1 year) or 10 mg/kg (1–12 years) twice daily for 2 days.

4. Haemophilus influenzae (Type B) prophylaxis:
   a. Adults: 20 mg/kg once daily for 4 days.
   b. Children: 20 mg/kg once daily for 4 days.
   c. Neonates: 10 mg/kg once daily for 4 days.

Nurse monitoring

1. Patients undergoing treatment for tuberculosis receive their drugs for considerable periods of time. The nurse plays an important role in reminding patients that their drug therapy must be taken regularly for as long as recommended by medical staff, whether or not they themselves feel that they have recovered.

2. As noted above, it is important that the drug should be administered prior to meals as it is rapidly and better absorbed if taken in this way.

3. The drug is usually well tolerated but occasionally patients experience gastrointestinal upset which may be manifest as anorexia, nausea, vomiting or diarrhoea.

4. Rarely abnormal liver or kidney function may be detected in patients on this drug and regular blood tests are usually performed to detect the occurrence of this side-effect.

5. This drug may cause a reddish discolouration of urine, sputum and tears, and to avoid potential worry and distress, patients should be warned to expect such an effect. In particular patients should avoid use of soft contact lenses which might become permanently discoloured.

6. Skin rashes and blood dyscrasias (leucopenia, thrombocytopenia or haemolytic anaemia) occasionally occur.

7. Other rare side-effects felt by the patient include dizziness, confusion, drowsiness, ataxia, peripheral neuropathy, blurred vision, hearing loss and menstrual disturbance.

8. Rifampicin is a potent inducer of the liver microsomal enzyme system the consequence of which is the more rapid metabolism of certain drugs normally inactivated by the liver. Thus the actions of warfarin, theophylline, phenytoin, oral anti-diabetic agents, anti-arrhythmics and other drugs may be reduced in the presence of rifampicin.

9. In particular, the action of the oral contraceptive pill can be impaired and breakthrough (mid-cycle) bleeding or even unexpected pregnancy result. Double the dose (i.e. 2 pills daily) may be tried for 30 microgram or less oestrogen containing pills and/or further contraception used.

10. There is no evidence that nursing meningitis patients increases the risk of infection to medical and nursing staff sufficient to warrant prophylaxis with rifampicin. This is reserved for family contacts.

General notes

1. The drug may be stored at room temperature.

2. Rifampicin injection (used in severe infections) is first reconstituted with the solvent provided then further diluted in 500 ml sodium chloride or glucose injection and administered over 2–3 hours.

RIMITEROL (Pulmadil)

Presentation
Inhaler—200 microgram/dose as a pressurized aerosol or 'breath activated' auto-inhaler.

Actions and uses
Rimiterol stimulates the beta$_2$ adrenergic sites in the smooth muscle of the airways. This causes relaxation of muscle tone and alleviation of bronchospasm. In clinical practice it is used for the prevention and treatment of asthma and other conditions producing bronchospasm.

Dosage
One to three inhalations three or four times a day for both adults and children (a maximum of eight treatments of three puffs in any 24-hour period is recommended).

Nurse monitoring
1. Occasionally palpitations, tachycardia, headache and muscle tremor may be produced as side-effects.
2. The drug should be administered with great caution in patients who also suffer from hypertension, coronary artery disease or thyrotoxicosis.

General notes
1. Preparations may be stored at room temperature.
2. Aerosols must never be punctured or incinerated after use.

RITODRINE (Yutopar)

Presentation
Tablets—10 mg
Injection—10 mg in 1 ml

Actions and uses
Ritodrine has a direct action on the uterine smooth muscle causing it to relax and therefore reducing contractions. It is used to prevent labour in the management of:
1. Uncomplicated premature labour.
2. Fetal asphyxia in labour when relaxation is required to improve the condition of the baby before planned, assisted delivery.

Dosage
1. For the treatment of uncomplicated premature labour: Ritodrine is administered as soon as possible at the onset of labour as follows:
   a. Initially, 50 microgram/minute by intravenous infusion in sodium chloride 0.9% injection, dextrose 5% injection or dextrose/saline mixtures. The infusion rate is increased gradually by 50 microgram/minute every 10 minutes until the required response is obtained or the heart rate reaches 140 beats/minute. This level of dosage is generally in the range, 150–350 microgram/minute. Intravenous infusions are continued for 12–48 hours after uterine contractions have ceased. If intravenous therapy is not possible, 10 mg ritodrine every 3–8 hours may be given by intramuscular injection and continued for 12–48 hours as above.
   b. Maintenance: Oral ritodrine is started about 30 minutes before intravenous therapy is completed. Up to 10 mg every 2 hours is given for the initial 24 hours and reduced thereafter to 10–20 mg or less, 4 to 6-hourly depending upon response or the presence of troublesome side-effects. The total oral dose must not exceed 120 mg/day. Oral therapy is continued for as long as it is required to prolong pregnancy.
2. The treatment of fetal asphyxia prior to planned assisted delivery: Initially, 50 microgram/minute by intravenous infusion increased rapidly until uterine activity is suppressed or the maternal heart rate reaches 140 beats/minute. The required dose level is usually of the order 350 microgram/minute or less. Delivery of the baby is carried out 15 minutes to 1 hour after infusions are started depending upon fetal scalp blood pH.

Nurse monitoring
1. The drug may affect maternal pulse rate leading to tachycardia and palpitations. The nurse may play an important role in titrating intravenous infusion dosage and preventing excess administration of the drug. It is important to note that a maternal tachycardia of up to 140 beats/minute is generally acceptable in a healthy patient.
2. Other side-effects seen with this drug are flushing, sweating, tremor, nausea and vomiting.
3. Extremely careful patient monitoring is essential in patients who have heart disease or for those who are receiving other drugs which may increase or reduce the response to ritodrine, e.g. monoamine oxidase inhibitors, tricyclic anti-depressants, and other drugs which stimulate the sympathetic nervous system and beta-adrenoreceptor blockers.
4. It should be noted that the drug should be used with great care in patients on co-incident treatment with corticosteroid drugs as pulmonary oedema may occur in the mother.

5. The drug should be avoided or used with great caution in the following situations:
   a. Antepartum haemorrhage requiring immediate delivery.
   b. Intra-uterine fetal death.
   c. Chorioamnionitis.
   d. Maternal cardiac disease.
   e. Cord compression.
   f. Diabetes mellitus.
   g. Hypertension.
   h. Hyperthyroidism.
6. It is important to note that the drug is much less effective if the membranes have been ruptured or if the cervix has dilated greater than 4 cm.

General notes
1. Ritodrine tablets and injection solution may be stored at room temperature though they should be protected from light.
2. Deterioration of the injection is evident if the solution is discoloured or else a precipitate may appear in the solution. Solutions with any evidence of deterioration should be immediately discarded.

R

S

SALBUTAMOL (Ventolin, Volmax)

Presentation
Tablets —2 mg, 4 mg
     —4 mg, 8 mg (slow release)
Syrup—2 mg in 5 ml
Injection—0.5 mg in 1 ml, 0.25 mg in 5 ml, 5 mg in 5 ml (for intravenous infusion)
Inhalation —100 microgram/dose of metered aerosol
    —200 microgram and 400 microgram as Rotacaps
    —0.5% as respirator solution
Nebules for inhalation—2.5 mg in 2.5 ml unit

Actions and uses
1. This drug stimulates receptors known as $beta_2$ adrenergic receptors. The effect of this stimulation is to relax bronchial muscle and relieve bronchospasm. Salbutamol is, therefore, used for the acute and chronic relief of bronchospasm in asthma and other conditions such as chronic bronchitis, where reversible airways obstruction has been shown to exist.
2. It has an additional use in that it may be given by intravenous infusion for the management of premature labour. In this case the $beta_2$ adrenergic stimulant action reduces contraction of uterine muscle.

Dosage
1. For the treatment of asthma:
   a. By inhalation:
      i. Using a metered aerosol: 2 inhalations 3 or 4 times a day.
      ii. Using Rotacaps: 200–400 microgram three or four times a day.
      iii. For acute severe conditions the respirator solution is administered by intermittent positive pressure using oxygen rich air or via a suitable nebulizer.
      iv. Alternatively, in acute severe conditions 1 or 2 'nebules' may be inhaled via a nebulizer 4 or 5 times daily.
   b. Orally:
      i. Adults: 2–8 mg three or four times a day.
      ii. Children: 2–6 years—1–2 mg three or four times daily; 6–12 years—2 mg three or four times daily; Over 12 years—2–4 mg three or four times daily.
   c. Parenteral:
      i. By subcutaneous or intramuscular injection for adults: 0.5 mg 4-hourly as required.
      ii. By slow intravenous injection for adults: 4 microgram/kg body weight.
      iii. By intravenous infusion: 3–20 microgram/minute.
2. For the treatment of premature labour: An intravenous infusion is administered at a rate of 10–45 microgram/minute and adjusted to control uterine contractions. It is usual to commence with a rate of 10 microgram/minute and increase accordingly. Once uterine contractions have ceased the infusion rate should be maintained for 1 hour and then reduced by 50% decrements at 6-hourly intervals. Treatment may be continued orally with Ventolin tablets, 4 mg given three or four times daily.

Nurse monitoring

1. Common side-effects include fine muscle tremor, palpitations, tachycardia, flushing and headache.
2. The drug should be used with caution in patients who have heart disease manifest by rhythm disturbance or angina, hyperthyroidism and hypertension.
3. When intravenously administered elevation of blood glucose may be caused and care, therefore, should be exercised when diabetic patients are being treated.
4. Intramuscular use of the undiluted injection produces slight pain and stinging.
5. In the management of premature labour intravenous infusion of salbutamol has occasionally caused nausea, vomiting and headache.

General notes

1. Preparations of salbutamol may be stored at room temperature.
2. Preparations should be protected from light.
3. Solutions for injection can be diluted using water for injection.
4. Intravenous infusions are prepared in 0.9% sodium chloride or dextrose 5% or dextrose/saline injections.
5. Aerosols should never be punctured or incinerated after use.

SALCATONIN (Calsynar, Miacalcic)

Presentation

Injection—50 units, 100 units in 1ml, 400 units in 2 ml (multidose)

Actions and uses

Salcatonin is a synthetic form of calcitonin based on a polypeptide derived from the salmon. In this form it is much less immunogenic than porcine calcitonin over which it is generally preferred.

Calcitonin is a hormone secreted by the thyroid and parathyroid glands which regulates bone turnover. It does so by lowering plasma calcium and phosphate levels, and antagonizing the actions of parathyroid hormone on bone. In particular, calcitonin:

1. Inhibits the activity of bone cells called osteoclasts which continuously digest bone tissue releasing free calcium and phosphate.
2. Promotes the renal excretion of calcium and phosphate.
3. Inhibits the activation of vitamin D and hence calcium absorption from the gut.

It is used in conditions associated with rapid bone turnover including Paget's disease (to relieve pain and neurological complications), postmenopausal osteoporosis, hypercalcaemia of malignancy, and for pain relief in metastatic disease of the bone.

Dosage

Administration is usually by subcutaneous (occasionally i.m.) injection.

1. Adults:
    a. Paget's disease: dose ranges from 50 units two or three times daily to single daily doses of 50–100 units.
    b. Osteoporosis: 100 units once daily.
    c. Malignant hypercalcaemia: A short course of injections of 400 units 6-hourly or 8-hourly.
    d. Bone metastases: Two day course of injections, either 200 units 6-hourly or 400 units 12-hourly.

Nurse monitoring

1. As described above, calcitonin is to some extent immunogenic and injections may be poorly tolerated by some patients in whom it causes nausea, vomiting, flushing, diarrhoea, tingling sensation and skin rashes. Anaphylaxis has occurred.
2. As a result of the above, patients may be assessed for likely allergy by prior skin prick or scratch testing.
3. If used to arrest the rate of bone turnover in osteoporotic women it is important that supplementary calcium and vitamin D be given also.

S

General note
Ampoules and multidose vials retain their potency for 2 years when stored in a refrigerator. Solutions must not be frozen.

SALSALATE (Disalcid)

Presentation
Capsules—500 mg
Actions and uses
1. See the section on aspirin.
2. Salsalate is converted to aspirin in the blood following absorption. It may therefore be used as an alternative to aspirin in patients who have experienced intolerable gastrointestinal upsets caused by that drug.
Dosage
1. Adults: The dose range is 2–4 g daily in three or four divided doses which are usually taken with meals and at bedtime.
2. Children: It is not recommended that children receive this form of aspirin.

Nurse monitoring
See the section on aspirin.

General note
Salsalate capsules may be stored at room temperature.

SELEGILINE (Eldepryl)

Presentation
Tablets—5 mg
Actions and uses
Selegiline, by complex actions in the brain, potentiates the action of levodopa (in Madopar and Sinemet) in the treatment of Parkinson's disease and it is used in conjunction with these drugs.
Dosage
Adults: Initially 5 mg once daily, increased to 10 mg if necessary.

Nurse monitoring
Selegiline is used in conjunction with Madopar or Sinemet (or levodopa alone) and it should be noted that a reduction in dosage of these drugs

is often possible. The nurse must therefore be vigilant for the occurrence of levodopa side-effects which indicate the need to reduce levodopa dosage.

General note
Selegiline tablets may be stored at room temperature.

SENNOSIDE (Senokot, X-Prep)

Presentation
Tablets—7.5 mg
Granules—5.5 mg in 1 g
Syrup—15 mg in 10 ml
Actions and uses
See the section on laxatives for general discussion. Sennoside acts by action 1, i.e. it has an irritant effect on the gut wall. It is used for the treatment of constipation.
Dosage
1. Adults: 15–30 mg or 1–25 ml spoonfuls of granules taken as a single dose at bedtime.
2. Children: Under 2 years—Up to 5 mg; 2–6 years—One-quarter of the adult dose; Over 6 years—One half of the adult dose.
3. X-Prep is a single dose of sennoside (142 mg in 71 ml of fluid) which is taken between 2 and 4 p.m. on the day prior to radiographic procedures involving the bowel.

Nurse monitoring
1. The granular form of this drug may be stirred into hot milk, sprinkled on food or eaten plain and as it is more acceptable to the patient, better compliance may be achieved.
2. Because of its irritant effect on the bowel it may produce cramping abdominal pain.

General notes
1. Preparations containing sennoside may be stored at room temperature.
2. Liquid preparations are sensitive to light and should be kept in amber bottles.

---

3. Granules should be kept in a closed, air-tight container since they may absorb moisture from the air.

SIMVASTATIN (Zocor)

Presentation

Tablets—10 mg, 20 mg

Actions and uses

Simvastatin is one of a new range of lipid-lowering drugs which are frequently described as HMG-CoA reductase inhibitors (which refers to their inhibitory action on cholesterol synthesis). Drugs of this type produce a marked and sustained fall in cholesterol (particularly low density lipoprotein or LDL cholesterol) and triglyceride compared to that produced by other lipid-lowering agents and have consequently become very popular in recent years.

The drug may be used in patients with hypercholesterolaemia, who are considered to be at risk of ischaemic heart disease and early cardiac death, or hypertriglyceridaemia in which case they are likely to develop peripheral vascular disease and pancreatitis. Usually such patients will have blood cholesterol levels well in excess of 7–8 mmol/l or triglyceride levels above 3 mmol/l. These may fall by up to 50% on treatment.

Dosage

Adults: A single evening dose of 10–40 mg is given.

Nurse monitoring

1. The use of lipid-lowering drugs is very controversial. In many cases, elevated blood cholesterol is the result of obesity, inappropriate diet or alcohol excess, and correction of these factors is more appropriate. It should be noted that treatment is lifelong and therefore very expensive.
2. A few patients present with a familial hypercholesterolaemia and history of early cardiac death in the family. In these patients life may be markedly prolonged by

treatment. Also, patients with extensive cardiac disease, especially after coronary artery bypass grafting, should have their cholesterol maintained in the normal range.
3. Simvastatin is effective within 2–4 weeks of commencing therapy.
4. Patients receiving warfarin should have their anticoagulant status carefully checked after starting simvastatin therapy. In the past, lipid-lowering drugs have been shown to increase the risk of bleeding in such patients.

General note

Simvastatin tablets are stored at room temperature, and protected from light and moisture.

SINEMET

Note: This combination now officially named Co-careldopa

Presentation

Sinemet L.S. containing 12.5 mg of carbidopa and 50 mg of levodopa (Co-careldopa 62.5)
Sinemet 110 containing 10 mg of carbidopa and 100 mg of levodopa (Co-careldopa 110)
Sinemet 275 containing 25 mg of carbidopa and 250 mg of levodopa (Co-careldopa 275)
Sinemet Plus containing 25 mg of carbidopa and 100 mg of levodopa (Co-careldopa 125)

Actions and uses

Sinemet contains levodopa: See the description of the actions and uses of this drug. It is used in clinical practice principally for the treatment of Parkinsonism. The advantages of combining carbidopa with levodopa are thought to be improved control throughout the day and a reduced overall dose of levodopa.

Dosage

N.B. Dosages for individual patients are carefully titrated using low initial dosages with gradual increments. The following is only one example of such a scheme using Sinemet 275:

S

1. Patients not receiving levodopa: Initially a half tablet of Sinemet 275 is given once or twice a day. This is subsequently increased by half a tablet every day or every other day until optimum response is achieved.
2. Patients receiving levodopa: At least 12 hours before sinemet is started (or 24 hours if slow release preparations of levodopa are used), all levodopa-containing medication should be discontinued. The starting dose of sinemet should be equivalent to 20% of the previous levodopa dose. The dosage should be gradually increased and most patients can be maintained on a dosage of 3–6 tablets of Sinemet 275 per day. It is recommended that no patient should receive more than eight tablets of Sinemet 275 per day.

Nurse monitoring
The nurse monitoring aspects of levodopa (q.v.) apply to this drug.

General note
The drugs may be stored at room temperature.

SODIUM AUROTHIOMALATE (Myocrisin)

Presentation
Injection—0.5 ml ampoules containing 10 mg, 20 mg and 50 mg

Actions and uses
This drug is a gold salt and is used in the treatment of chronic rheumatoid disease which has not responded adequately to conventional anti-inflammatory analgesic therapy. It is not in itself an analgesic but by modifying the autoimmune inflammatory process involved in the disease, it may lead to a reduction in pain.

Dosage
1. Adults: A course of injections each of 50 mg is usually given at weekly intervals to a total dose of 1 g. For the first few weeks less than 50 mg may be given so that patients who suffer severe side-effects may be detected before they have received large doses.
2. Children: This drug is only used for the treatment of Still's disease. Graded doses at weekly intervals are used up to a maximum which is based on body weight, i.e. less than 25 kg—10 mg; 25–50 kg—20 mg; 50 kg or over—50 mg.

Nurse monitoring
1. Early side-effects from this drug may precede the more serious life-threatening side-effects and the nurse may play an important part in managing these patients by helping to detect the early side-effects which include skin rashes, pruritus, a metallic taste in the mouth, a painful throat or tongue, mouth ulcers, bruising, bleeding gums, menorrhagia, nose bleeds, dry cough or progressive breathlessness.
2. Serious side-effects include skin eruptions, pulmonary fibrosis, renal toxicity, blood dyscrasia such as agranulocytosis, thrombocytopenia and aplastic anaemia.
3. The drug should never be given to patients with liver or kidney disease, diabetes, history of toxaemia during pregnancy, blood dyscrasias or exfoliative dermatitis.
4. Laboratory tests such as blood counts, urine tests for protein and chest X-rays are carried out regularly during a course of treatment. It is essential that these tests are performed regularly and the nurse may again contribute by emphasizing the importance of having these tests done to the patient.
5. During treatment the details of the course of treatment and laboratory results are usually recorded together on a pre-designed 'gold card'. The nurse may contribute by ensuring such cards are fully and accurately filled out.

General notes

1. Sodium Aurothiomalate injection may be stored at room temperature.
2. As the solution is light-sensitive any darkening in the usual straw colour indicates degradation and such solutions must be discarded.

SODIUM CROMOGLYCATE (Intal, Nalcrom, Opticrom, Rynacrom)

Presentation

Spincaps for Inhalation—20 mg plain: 20 mg compound (with isoprenaline 0.1 mg)
Capsules—100 mg
Nasal Spray and Drops—2%
Nasal Insufflation—capsules containing 10 mg
Nebulizer Solution—20 mg in 2 ml
Eye Drops—2%

Actions and uses

1. This drug binds to cells present in the airways which under certain conditions would normally release chemicals which would cause an increase in muscle tone in the airways causing bronchospasm manifest as dyspnoea and wheezing. It is, therefore, useful for the prophylactic treatment of conditions associated with bronchospasm.
2. The drug has been postulated to be effective orally in the management of ulcerative colitis, proctitis, proctocolitis and food allergy.
3. When rhinitis and conjunctivitis is caused by an allergic reaction, the cells which release the chemicals causing the symptoms may be prevented from releasing these chemicals by the application of this drug directly to the nasal or conjunctival surfaces.

Dosage

1. For the treatment of bronchospasm: For adults and children the normal dose is 1 spincap (contents of each capsule are inhaled through a spinhaler) at intervals ranging from 3–6 hours.
2. For the treatment of ulcerative colitis, proctitis, proctocolitis and food allergy:

a. Adults: 200 mg orally four times a day before meals.
b. Children (over 2 years): Up to 100 mg orally four times daily before meals.
3. For the treatment of allergic rhinitis instil into the nostrils 6 times daily.
4. For conjunctivitis, 1 or 2 drops into the eye 4 times daily using 2% eye drops.

Nurse monitoring

1. It is essential to note that this drug is only useful for the prophylaxis, i.e. prevention of attacks of bronchospasm, and it is no use in the acute attack.
2. A special whistle-type spinhaler is available to encourage proper use of spincaps in young children.
3. Administration of the drug as noted above does not produce any immediate effect, patients may therefore come to the conclusion that the drug is doing them no good and may stop taking it. The nurse may play an important role in educating the patient on the benefits of continuing with treatment.
4. When the drug is taken orally for the management of ulcerative colitis, proctitis, proctocolitis or food allergy it may be either swallowed whole or taken in a solution. It is worth noting that when food allergy is being treated, administration in a solution is preferred.
5. As with other eye drops, the drug itself may produce slight irritation to the eyes.
6. Eye drops should be discarded 4 weeks after opening.

General notes

1. Preparations containing sodium cromoglycate may be stored at room temperature.
2. Capsules and solutions should be stored in moisture-proof containers and protected from light.
3. It should be clearly understood that the spincaps are for inhalation and should not be swallowed.

SODIUM IRONEDETATE (Sytron)

Presentation
Liquid—55 mg of elemental iron in 10 ml

Actions and uses
See the section on iron (oral).

Dosage
1. For the treatment of iron deficiency anaemia:
   a. Adults: 10–20 ml per day.
   b. Children: Less than 1 year—5–10 ml per day; 1–7 years—10–15 ml per day; 7–12 years—15–20 ml per day; Over 12 years—adult doses apply.
2. For the prevention of iron deficiency anaemia in pregnancy: 10 ml twice a day.

Nurse monitoring
See the section on iron (oral).

General note
The drug may be stored at room temperature.

SODIUM NITROPRUSSIDE (Nipride)

Presentation
Injection—50 mg ampoules

Actions and uses
Sodium nitroprusside has a direct action on blood vessels causing peripheral vasodilation and a reduction in peripheral resistance. It is therefore useful in the management of hypertension. It is available for intravenous infusion only and has been found to be of use in the treatment of hypertensive crises.

Dosage
The drug is usually given by continuous infusion of a 0.01 or 0.05% solution in dextrose. The initial rate is between 0.5 and 8 microgram/kg body weight per minute. Maintenance dosage depends on the control obtained but 3 microgram/kg per minute has been found to be the average infusion required to maintain the blood pressure at 30–40% below the pre-treatment blood pressure. The maximum recommended rate of infusion is 11 microgram/kg per minute.

Nurse monitoring
1. Once sodium nitroprusside has been diluted in dextrose for infusion it will deteriorate, if exposed to sunlight. Some of the products of deterioration are harmful and therefore it is essential that the nurse ensures that the infusion bottle and as much of the infusion apparatus as possible is completely shielded from exposure to light.
2. During the initial period of treatment the blood pressure must be monitored on an almost continuous basis.
3. Sodium nitroprusside has a very short duration of action and therefore infusions must be constantly monitored to ensure that accidental reduction or increase in infusion rate does not occur as drastic effects may ensue.
4. Prolonged therapy may be associated with cyanide intoxication. This is characterized by tachycardia, sweating, hyperventilation, cardiac dysrhythmia and metabolic acidosis.
5. Common side-effects with this drug include nausea, vomiting, anorexia, abdominal pain, apprehension, restlessness, muscle twitching, retrosternal chest pain, palpitations and dizziness.

General notes
1. Sodium nitroprusside ampoules may be stored at room temperature.
2. The injection solution is prepared by first mixing with dextrose 5% in ampoules which are usually provided, then the required amount is added to dextrose 5% for infusion. Any unused solution should be immediately discarded. The drug is sensitive to sunlight and during infusion the bottle should be covered by a protective opaque bag.

SODIUM PICOSULPHATE (Laxoberal)

Presentation
Syrup—5 mg in 5 ml

Actions and uses
The actions and uses of laxative drugs are described in the section on these drugs. Sodium picosulphate falls into group 1. It is converted by bacterial action into an active substance in the gut and tends to produce bowel evacuation 10–14 hours after administration.

Dosage
1. Adults: 5–15 ml
2. Children: 0–5 years—2.5 ml; 5–10 years—2.5–5 ml

In all cases a single night-time dose is taken.

Nurse monitoring
1. In common with most laxatives, excessive doses may produce abdominal discomfort.
2. As the drug requires the presence of gut bacteria to convert it to its active component its effectiveness may be lost in patients who are taking broad-spectrum antibiotics.

General notes
1. Sodium picosulphate may be stored at room temperature.
2. It should be protected from light.
3. For ease of administration the syrup should be diluted with water.

SODIUM VALPROATE (Epilim)

Presentation
Tablets—200 mg and 500 mg (enteric-coated)
—100 mg (crushable tablets)
—200 mg, 300 mg, 500 mg (slow release tablets)
Syrup—200 mg in 5 ml
Injection—400 mg vial

Actions and uses
The actions and uses of anti-convulsant drugs are discussed in the section on these drugs.

Dosage
N.B. Individual dosage requirements vary greatly. The following doses are given as a guideline only.
1. Oral:
   a. Adults: An initial dose of 600 mg is given increasing each day until an optimum response is achieved. The usual dose range is 1000–2000 mg per day.
   b. Children:
      i. Over 20 kg body weight: 400 mg daily initially increasing to maintenance doses usually in the range 20–30 mg/kg body weight per day in total.
      ii. Under 20 kg body weight: 20–50 mg/kg body weight per day in total.
2. Injection:
   a. Adults: 400–800 mg by slow intravenous injection or intravenous infusion, up to a maximum of 2.5 g total dose daily.
   b. Children: 20–30 mg/kg body weight daily by slow intravenous injection or intravenous infusion.

Nurse monitoring
1. The nurse monitoring aspects of anticonvulsant drugs in general are discussed in the section on these drugs.
2. This drug should preferably be taken with or immediately after food in order to minimize the common side-effect of gastrointestinal irritation. Enteric-coated tablets may have to be used if gastric upset still occurs.
3. Metabolites of sodium valproate are excreted in the urine and may give false positive results for ketones. It is especially important that this effect be recognized in diabetic patients where the presence of ketonuria usually leads to hospital referral.
4. As this drug may reduce the number of platelets circulating in the blood, unexplained bruising or haemorrhage should always

S

be taken as an indication to check the patient's blood and if thrombocytopenia (reduced platelets) has been produced, the drug should be stopped.
5. Liver damage may occasionally occur.
6. A few patients suffer from hair loss.
7. When the drug is used in high dosage tremor may be a problem.

General notes
1. The drug should be stored at room temperature.
2. If for ease of administration dilution of sodium valproate syrup is necessary, syrup BP should be used and the diluted preparation discarded after 14 days if not used.

SOTALOL (Beta-Cardone, Sotacor)

Presentation
Tablets—40 mg, 80 mg, 160 mg, 200 mg
Injection—10 mg in 5 ml

Actions and uses
Sotalol is a non-selective beta-adrenoreceptor blocking drug. Its actions are described in the section on these drugs.

Dosage
1. It may be given intravenously in emergency situations for cardiac dysrhythmias in a dosage of 10–20 mg. This is usually given over 5 minutes and is repeated as necessary. Careful monitoring of pulse, blood pressure and electrocardiogram is necessary during administration (see equivalent section for propranolol, q.v.).
2. The oral daily adult maintenance dose range is 120–640 mg and it may be given as a single dose or in three or four divided doses.

Nurse monitoring
See the section on beta-adrenoreceptor blocking drugs.

General note
Sotalol tablets and injection may be stored at room temperature.

SPIRONOLACTONE (Aldactone, Spiroctan)

Presentation
Tablets—25 mg, 100 mg
Injection—200 mg in 20 ml (as Canrenoate potassium).

Actions and uses
Spironolactone inhibits the adrenal hormone aldosterone and thus is a 'potassium-sparing' diuretic which prevents excessive potassium loss. It is usually given together with other diuretics to prevent the development of hypokalaemia (excessive blood potassium loss) which often occurs in patients treated with diuretic drugs. It is usually unnecessary for patients treated with spironolactone to be given potassium supplement tablets such as Slow K or Sando K.

Dosage
1. Oral:
   The usual adult dose range of spironolactone is 50–500 mg daily; it is occasionally given in divided doses though a single dose is usually adequate. It takes about three days of treatment before the maximum effect of spironolactone is achieved and this effect may persist for 2–3 days after therapy is discontinued. Children's doses are:
   a. Up to 1 year: 0.6 mg/kg four times daily.
   b. 1–6 years: 6.25 mg four times daily.
   c. 7 years plus: 12.5 mg four times daily.
2. Injection:
   Adults may receive up to 800 mg daily by slow intravenous injection either as a single dose or in divided dosage. The injection period should be at least 2–3 minutes per 200 mg dose.

Nurse monitoring
Patients receiving spironolactone should be observed for the occasional occurrence of excessive

S

potassium retention (hyperkalae-mia). This is particularly important in patients with renal failure. This may be manifest by confusion, drowsiness, anorexia, nausea, vomiting and other features of uraemia. Less common side-effects include breast enlargement in the male (gynaecomastia), milk secretion in the female (galactorrhoea) and skin rashes.

General note
Spironolactone tablets may be stored at room temperature.

STANOZOLOL (Stromba)

Presentation
Tablets—5 mg

Actions and uses
1. See the section discussing the actions and uses of anabolic steroids.
2. This drug is occasionally used to aid recovery from prolonged and debilitating illness or following major surgery.
3. Stanozolol has a particular use in treating vascular symptoms of Bechet's disease and in angio-oedema.

Dosage
1. To aid metabolic recovery: 5 mg daily with food.
2. Bechet's disease: 10 mg daily
3. Angio-oedema: 2.5–10 mg daily (low dose in children).

Nurse monitoring
See the hormones (4) section on androgenic hormones and anabolic steroids.

General note
The drug may be stored at room temperature.

STILBOESTROL (Tampovagan)

Presentation
Tablets—0.5 mg, 1 mg and 5 mg
Pessaries—0.5 mg

Actions and uses
Stilboestrol is an oestrogenic substance which has the following uses in clinical practice.
1. For the treatment of menopausal symptoms.
2. For the treatment of secondary amenorrhoea due to ovarian insufficiency.
3. For the inhibition of lactation.
4. For palliative treatment of malignant neoplasm.
5. For post-coital contraception.

Dosage
1. For the treatment of menopausal symptoms: 0.1–1 mg by mouth daily.
2. For the treatment of secondary amenorrhoea: 0.25–1 mg daily during the proliferative phase of the menstrual cycle.
3. For the inhibition of lactation: 5 mg is given twice or thrice daily initially with subsequent reduction in dosage.
4. For the palliative treatment of malignant neoplasm of the breast: 10–20 mg is usually given daily. For carcinoma of the prostate between 1 and 3 mg is given daily.
5. For post-coital contraception: 25 mg is given twice daily for 5 days starting within 72 hours of intercourse.

Nurse monitoring
See the hormones (1) section on oestrogenic hormones.

General note
The drug may be stored at room temperature.

STREPTOKINASE (Kabikinase)

Presentation
Vials for intravascular administration contain either 250 000, 750 000 and 1500 000 (1.5 million) international units (i.u.).

Actions and uses
This enzyme stimulates the action of the fibrinolytic system in man and, therefore, promotes the dissolution of clots. In clinical practice it has been used as a thrombolytic agent:

S

1. Following acute myocardial infarction (see thrombolytic drugs, q.v.) and following monograph.
2. Venous thrombosis.
3. Pulmonary embolism.
4. Acute arterial thromboembolism.
5. Clotted haemodialysis shunts.
6. Occlusion of the retinal vessels.

Dosage
1. Adults: An initial dose of 600 000 i.u. over a period of 30–60 minutes is given followed by maintenance doses of 100 000 i.u. hourly for 3 or more days. The initial and maintenance doses may be titrated by measuring the anti-streptokinase antibody level of the individual.
2. Children: There are no absolute recommendations on dosage for children other than that the adult scheme should be used and reduced according to the size of the patient.

Nurse monitoring
1. Allergic reactions ranging from fever to anaphylactic shock may occur.
2. The drug should not be used in patients with severe hypertension, defects of blood coagulation, peptic ulceration and during menstruation.
3. The nurse should note that the preparation normally has a faint straw colour and such discolouration does not indicate degeneration of the preparation.

General notes
1. Vials of streptokinase should be stored below 25°C before reconstitution.
2. The vial containing a prepared concentrated solution may be stored for 24 hours in a refrigerator.
3. Diluted solution should be used within 12 hours of preparation.

4. The diluents of choice are physiological saline and 5% dextrose but other diluents should not be used.

STREPTOKINASE (Streptase)

Presentation
Freeze-dried powder in vials containing 250 000, 750 000 and 1500 000 (1.5 million) international units (i.u.).

Actions and uses
See thrombolytic drugs.

Dosage
The drug should be given by intravenous infusion in 50–200 ml physiological saline, 5% glucose or Haemaccel.
1. Acute myocardial infarction:
   a. Adults: A single dose with 1.5 million i.u. may be given intravenously over 1 hour.
   b. Children: There are no recommendations for the use of streptase in acute myocardial infarction in children.
2. Intravenous dissolution of thrombi and emboli:
   a. Adults:
      i. Loading dose: a dose of 250 000 units infused into a peripheral vein over 30 minutes.
      ii. Maintenance dose: a maintenance infusion of 100 000 units per hour for 72 hours following DVT; 24–72 hours following arterial thrombosis; and 24 hours following pulmonary embolism.
   b. Children: The loading dose should be calculated by means of a streptokinase resistance test, and the recommended maintenance dose should be 20 units/ml of blood volume per hour.

Nurse monitoring
1. Nurse monitoring notes on thrombolytic drugs (q.v.) apply to this medicine.

2. There is an increased risk of haemorrhage in patients who are receiving, or who have recently received, other anticoagulant drugs.
3. The drug is contraindicated in pregnancy.
4. Early reactions to the drug include headache, backpain and allergic anaphylactic reactions with flushing and dyspnoea. Allergic reactions can be largely avoided by giving the intravenous dose slowly. Corticosteroids can also be given prophylactically.

General notes

1. Streptokinase is stable for at least three years when stored at 2–25°C. After being dissolved in 5 ml of sterile physiological saline, it can be stored in a refrigerator at 2–8°C for 24 hours without loss of activity.
2. To ensure that the contents of the vial are rapidly and completely dissolved, 5 ml of physiological saline should be injected into the vial and the residual vacuum abolished by loosening the needle from the syringe.
3. For administration with an infusion pump, physiological saline, Ringer-lactate solution, 5% glucose or fructose solution can be used as diluent. For higher dilutions Haemaccel may be used as diluent.

STREPTOKINASE/STREPTODOR-NASE (Varidase)

Presentation

Vials containing streptokinase 100 000 units, streptodornase 25 000 units
Oral tablets each containing 10 000 units of streptokinase and 2500 units of streptodornase

Actions and uses

1. The combination of these two enzymes in solution is suitable for use by local application to help in the dissolution of clotted blood and fibrinous or purulent accumulations.
2. Application as a desloughing agent, mixed with hydrocolloid dressing e.g. Intrasite Gel to chronic wounds.

Dosage

1. For local administration: The dosage depends on the condition under treatment. Some examples are as follows:
   a. For treatment of a pneumothorax or thoracic empyema: An initial dose of 200 000 units of streptokinase and 50 000 units of streptodornase is suggested.
   This amount should be applied to single or multiple sites as the case warrants.
   b. For treatment of maxillary sinus empyema: Recommended doses would be from 10 000 to 15 000 units of streptokinase and 2500 to 3750 units of streptodornase in a volume of 2–3 ml.
2. As a desloughing agent applied to wound: 1 vial mixed with hydrocolloid dressing.

Nurse monitoring

1. It is essential to note that vials of Varidase powder are for local application only and should never be administered parenterally.
2. Occasional allergic skin reactions may occur.

General notes

1. Varidase topical:
   a. Must be kept in its original pack in a refrigerator.
   b. Once reconstituted, solutions are stable for 1 week.
   c. For reconstitution sterile water or sterile physiological saline should be used.

STREPTOMYCIN

(See Note 3, p. 362)

Presentation

Injection—1 g

Actions and uses

This aminoglycoside antibiotic is primarily reserved for the treatment of tuberculosis and more rarely for the treatment and prevention of chronic respiratory infections and bacterial endocarditis.

Dosage

1. For the treatment of tuberculosis:
   a. Adults receive 0.75–1 g per day by a single intramuscular injection.
   b. Children receive 30 mg/kg daily by a single intramuscular injection.
   c. In the treatment of tuberculous meningitis intrathecal doses of 50 mg for adults or 1 mg/kg for children may be given daily.
2. Non-tuberculous infections:
   a. Adults: Intramuscular doses of 0.75–1 g per day are administered.
   b. Children receive 25 mg/kg daily.

Nurse monitoring

1. The most important toxic effect of this drug is damage to the auditory nerve with resultant deafness and loss of balance. The risk of this increases with high dosage, prolonged duration of treatment, or when the patient is over 40 years of age. Recovery may occur over weeks or months but is often incomplete. The development of any symptoms suggestive of damage to the auditory nerve is an indication immediately to stop treatment.
2. Allergic reactions may occur, including rash and fever.
3. Vague feelings of paraesthesia of the lips, headache, lassitude, and dizziness may occur after each injection. They are less common if the patient is kept at rest after an injection. This is because with muscular activity absorption from the intramuscular injection site is increased and high plasma concentrations may occur.
4. These injections are particularly painful and the patient may

usefully receive support and encouragement from the attending nurse.
5. It is essential that the nurse notes that streptomycin is a potent skin sensitizer and severe skin reactions may occur in nurses who handle the drug if they are sensitive to it. The wearing of protective gloves during handling of the drug is therefore advised.

General notes

1. Streptomycin powder and vials may be stored at room temperature.
2. After reconstitution the solutions may be kept for several days in a refrigerator.
3. Streptomycin is for deep intra-muscular injection and occasionally intrathecal injection only.

SUCRALFATE (Antepsin)

Presentation

Tablets—1 g
Suspension—1 g in 5 ml

Actions and uses

Sucralfate is used in the treatment of gastric and duodenal ulcer and chronic gastritis, and for prophylaxis of gastrointestinal haemorrhage from stress ulceration in very ill patients. It exerts an action which is similar to that of Tri-potassium Di-citrato Bismuthate (De-Nol). Briefly, the drug binds to protein in the ulcer crater, thereby forming a protective layer of a chemically complex substance which resists further digestion of the ulcer by gastric acid and pepsin and therefore aids healing.

Dosage

1. Adults:
   a. 1–2 g four times a day for up to 6 weeks.
   b. 1 g 6–8 times daily to prevent GI haemorrhage from stress ulceration.

Nurse monitoring

1. Patients should be instructed to take dosages 1 hour before meals with a single dose at bedtime.
2. The absorption of tetracycline drugs may be impaired by the presence of sucralfate and such combination should be avoided or, if necessary, doses of tetracycline drugs should not be given within 2 hours of sucralfate administration.
3. The drug should be used with caution in patients with kidney impairment due to the possibility of aluminium retention. However, it is interesting to note that sucralfate has been administered to a patient with renal failure in an attempt to bind phosphate in the gut and so reduce hyperphosphataemia.
4. The only side-effect of note is constipation.

General note

Tablets may be stored at room temperature.

SULINDAC (Clinoril)

Presentation

Tablets—100 mg, 200 mg

Actions and uses

See the section on non-steroidal anti-inflammatory analgesic drugs.

Dosage

The usual adult dose is 100–200 mg twice daily usually taken with fluids at meal-times.

Nurse monitoring

See the section on non-steroidal anti-inflammatory analgesic drugs.

General note

Sulindac tablets may be stored at room temperature,

SULPHASALAZINE (Salazopyrin)

Presentation

Tablets—500 mg plain and enteric-coated
Suspension—250 mg in 5 ml
Suppositories—500 mg
Enema—3 g in 100 ml

Actions and uses

Sulphasalazine is a combination of two drugs:
1. An anti-inflammatory salicylic acid derivative.
2. An anti-infective sulphonamide derivative, sulphapyridine.

It is used for the induction and maintenance of remission in ulcerative colitis, distal proctocolitis, stump proctitis and Crohn's disease. It is further used as a disease modifying drug in the treatment of rheumatoid arthritis.

Dosage

1. Adults: 1–2 g four times per day initially orally. Once remission of the disease has been obtained lower daily dosages, i.e. 1.5–2 g in total per day may be sufficient. In rheumatoid arthritis: the required dose is gradually adjusted to the individual starting with 500 mg daily, then twice daily, three times daily, etc up to a total daily dose, if necessary, of 3 g. Enteric-coated tablets are used for this indication.
2. Children: 40–60 mg/kg body weight daily initially, reducing to a maintenance dose of 20–30 mg/kg body weight. Not recommended in juvenile arthritis.
3. The drug may also be given for a local effect via suppositories. These should be given morning and night after defaecation. An alternative local treatment is one enema given daily usually at bedtime.

Nurse monitoring

1. It is important to note that sulphasalazine is a combination of a salicylate and sulphonamide and therefore is contraindicated in patients with a history of allergy to sulphonamide drugs or salicylates.

2. The salicylate component may give any of the side-effects described in the section on non-steroidal anti-inflammatory analgesic drugs (q.v.).
3. The sulphonamide component of sulphasalazine can produce any of the side-effects associated with sulphonamides (q.v.).

General note
Preparations containing sulphasalazine may be stored at room temperature. It is important that suppositories are not stored in a warm place, e.g. near or above a radiator since they will readily melt.

SULPHINPYRAZONE (Anturan)

Presentation
Tablets—100 mg, 200 mg
Actions and uses
Sulphinpyrazone has two important actions:
1. It increases the urinary excretion of uric acid and urate and is therefore useful for the treatment of hyperuricaemia and gout. It has no analgesic properties and is therefore only useful for reducing blood urate in the long-term.
2. It has an additional quite separate action in that it inhibits platelet breakdown, adhesion and aggregation and thus reduces the tendency for blood to clot. In clinical practice this action has led to it being given to patients after myocardial infarction to reduce the incidence of reinfarction or sudden death.
Dosage
1. Hyperuricaemia and gout: The initial dose of sulphinpyrazone is 100–200 mg daily taken with meals or milk. The dosage is gradually increased over a week until the daily dosage of 600 mg is reached. After the blood urate concentration has been controlled the maintenance dose may be reduced to as low as 200 mg.
2. Following myocardial infarction: 200 mg four times daily is the prescribed dose. It is usual to commence this about one month after the initial myocardial infarction.
The above doses are for adults only.

Nurse monitoring
1. The nurse may play an important role in helping to prevent the serious side-effect of urate stone formation by monitoring carefully patients' fluid intake and encouraging them to drink large quantities of fluid daily.
2. As aspirin antagonizes the uricosuric action of this drug the nurse may play an important role in detecting patients who are taking this drug in addition to prescribed medicines and advising them to stop, and also by educating all patients as to the necessity to avoid taking aspirin at the same time as sulphinpyrazone.
3. The drug may occasionally produce gastrointestinal upset and gastric bleeding and therefore must be used with caution in patients with a history of peptic ulcer disease.
4. Rare side-effects for which withdrawal of treatment is necessary include skin rashes and blood dyscrasias (aplastic anaemia, leucopenia and thrombocytopenia).

General note
Sulphinpyrazone tablets may be stored at room temperature.

SULPHONAMIDES

Presentation
See individual compounds.
Actions and uses
The sulphonamide group of drugs, although chemically unrelated to antibiotics, were once widely used for the prevention and treatment of a wide variety of diseases due to bacterial infection. They are in fact the forerunner to the modern antibiotics which have now largely replaced them in clinical use. The

following sulphonamides are however still used:
1. Sulphamethoxazole (in Co-trimoxazole),
2. Sulphasalazine (which contains sulphapyridine).

All bacteria require folic acid in order to be able to grow and multiply. This folic acid is usually synthesized by bacteria themselves within cells. Sulphonamides act by preventing the production of folic acid in bacterial cells. The sulphonamides have a bacteriostatic rather than bactericidal action. The former term means that they prevent further growth and reduplication of cells whereas the latter term implies that the drug actually kills cells already present in the body. In practice many organisms are found to be resistant to sulphonamides. This is because these organisms have developed alternative means of synthesizing folic acid to the pathway of synthesis that is blocked by the drug. Sulphonamides have a wide range of action against both Gram-positive and Gram-negative organisms (see the section on antibiotics). They are used to treat a wide range of infections including bacterial diarrhoea, urinary infection, chest infection, bacterial meningitis, venereal disease and various dermatological infections.

Dosage
See individual drugs.

Nurse monitoring
1. Unless a high fluid intake and urine output is achieved there is a danger that patients receiving these drugs may suffer kidney damage due to crystallization of the drug in the renal tract. However this is now rarely a real concern given the disappearance of many drugs from the group. Nevertheless, the nurse may play an important role in both encouraging a high fluid intake and in monitoring urine output so that early warning of inadequate fluid intake may be obtained.

2. There are two important instances in which sulphonamides may affect the action of other drugs concurrently being administered to patients:
   a. In diabetic patients on oral anti-diabetic drugs the sulphonamides may precipitate hypoglycaemia with dizziness, sweating, tachycardia, fainting and eventually coma. Such patients should be carefully observed and warned of the dangers of this potential complication.
   b. In patients receiving the drug warfarin for the purpose of anticoagulation the coincident administration of sulphonamides may lead to an increase in warfarin's action with the resultant danger of severe haemorrhage. Regular checks on clotting function should therefore be made when sulphonamides are instituted in such cases.
3. Hypersensitivity reactions to sulphonamides may occur and these include skin rash, fever, joint pains and the more severe erythema multiforme and Stevens-Johnson syndrome.
4. As well as the danger of the drug precipitating into the kidney substance when fluid intake is poor, sulphonamides may have a direct damaging action on the kidney.
5. Sulphonamides may exert a wide range of toxic effects on the blood and bone marrow leading to megaloblastic anaemia, haemolytic anaemia, thrombocytopenia and aplastic anaemia. More rarely agranulocytosis (complete absence of white cells) with resultant risk of overwhelming infection may occur. As a result they are now rarely used in the elderly.
6. Liver damage and jaundice may occasionally occur. Jaundice is specially likely to occur in very young children, and may be dangerous. Such patients should not, therefore, receive sulphonamides.

SULPIRIDE (Dolmatil, Suliptil)

Presentation
Tablets—200 mg

Actions and uses
Sulpiride has actions and uses similar to those described for the phenothiazines although it has major chemical differences to drugs such as chlorpromazine. It is a neuroleptic (major tranquillizer) therefore and is used in the management of psychosis, e.g. acute and chronic schizophrenia, mania, etc. Sulpiride also possesses anti-emetic properties and has a relaxant effect on gut smooth muscle which has led to its occasional use in functional intestinal spasm.

Dosage
Adult dose in acute and chronic schizophrenia: 50–900 mg twice daily according to response.

Nurse monitoring
The nurse monitoring aspects described for the phenothiazines also apply to this drug.

General note
Sulpiride tablets may be stored at room temperature.

SUMATRIPTAN (Imigran)

Presentation
Tablets—100 mg
Injection—6 mg in 0.6 ml prefilled syringe

Actions and uses
This drug stimulates 5-HT$_1$ receptors which are specific target sites for the naturally occurring neurotransmitter 5-hydroxytryptamine (serotonin). Stimulation of these receptors which are found in abundance in the cranial blood vessels results in constriction of the carotid arterial circulation and a consequent reduction in blood flow through the intracranial and extracranial vessels which are dilated during a migraine attack. Thus sumatriptan rapidly aborts migraine attacks and cluster headaches; within 10–15 minutes by subcutaneous injection or 30–40 minutes after oral administration. It is ineffective for migraine prophylaxis.

Dosage
Adults only: A single oral dose of 100 mg or 6 mg by subcutaneous injection.

Nurse monitoring
1. Note that a second dose is not advised in the event that no response to the first dose is obtained. However patients may take one further dose to abort a subsequent attack within any 24 hour period.
2. Subcutaneous injections are administered by the patients themselves using a special 'Auto-Injector' device which is also available on prescription. Tablets should be swallowed whole with water.
3. As a result of the possible widespread vasocontrictor action of sumatriptan at other receptor sites patients with angina or a history of ischaemic heart disease or uncontrolled hypertension should not receive this drug.
4. Ergotamine, another widely used drug in migraine attacks, must not be taken concurrently. The combined vasoconstrictor action of the two drugs may produce severe vasospasm. Also patients with depression who are treated with monoamine oxidase inhibitors or newer selective serotonin re-uptake inhibitors (fluoxetine, fluvoxamine, paroxetine and sertreline) should not take sumatriptan since a potentially serious 'serotonin syndrome' may result.
5. Reported side-effects include ischaemic pain and tingling sensations which indicate developing ischaemia often affecting the chest and throat; flushing, dizziness, paraesthesia and weakness. Nausea and vomiting and altered liver function has also been reported.

General note

Sumatriptan tablets and injection should be stored at room temperature and protected from light.

SYNTOMETRINE (A combination of ergometrine and oxytocin)

Presentation

Syntometrine is available as a parenteral solution containing 500 microgram of ergometrine maleate and 5 units of oxytocin in 1 ml.

Actions and uses

The combination of these two drugs is effective by intramuscular injection in the stimulation of uterine contraction. In clinical practice it is used mainly to stimulate uterine contraction and it may also be given to prevent or treat postpartum haemorrhage and to stimulate uterine contraction in labour.

Dosage

1. To stimulate uterine contraction and cessation of bleeding after birth of the placenta: An intramuscular injection of 1 ml is usually administered.
2. When used for the other reasons described above dosage varies according to the clinical practice of the centre concerned and the nurse is advised to seek advice from her local obstetric unit.

Nurse monitoring

1. High doses may cause excessive uterine contraction and dosage should therefore be carefully monitored to prevent the potentially disastrous occurrence of a ruptured uterus.
2. When high doses of syntometrine are given with large volumes of electrolyte-free fluid, water intoxication may occur. Initially headache, anorexia, nausea, vomiting and abdominal pain may be the presenting features and this progresses to lethargy, drowsiness, unconsciousness and grand mal type seizures. The concentration of blood electrolytes may be markedly disturbed.

General notes

1. The drug should be protected from light.
2. The drug should be stored at room temperature.

S

T

TALAMPICILLIN (Talpen)

(See Note 3, p. 362)

Presentation
Tablets—250 mg

Actions and uses
After absorption from the gastrointestinal tract, talampicillin is converted to ampicillin. Its actions and uses are therefore identical to ampicillin (q.v)

Dosage
Adults: 250 mg three times per day.

Nurse monitoring
See the section on ampicillin.

General note
Talampicillin tablets may be stored at room temperature.

TAMOXIFEN (Nolvadex, Tamofen)

Presentation
Tablets—10 mg, 20 mg, 40 mg

Actions and uses
Tamoxifen is an oestrogen antagonist which has two major uses:
1. It is used in the treatment of breast cancer.
2. It is used to stimulate ovulation in patients suffering from infertility.

Dosage
1. For the treatment of breast cancer: 20–40 mg is given once daily or divided into twice daily dosage.
2. For the treatment of infertility: 10 mg is given twice daily on the second, third, fourth and fifth days of the menstrual cycles if patients are menstruating regularly. In women who are not menstruating the initial course may begin on any day.

Nurse monitoring
1. Because of its oestrogen antagonist action it frequently produces hot flushing, vaginal bleeding and pruritus vulvae.
2. Gastrointestinal upset, light headedness and fluid retention may occur.
3. Thrombocytopenia has been rarely reported.
4. When used for the treatment of breast cancer it may produce pain at the site of the tumour.

General notes
1. Tamoxifen tablets may be stored at room temperature.
2. The drug should be protected from light.

TEMAZEPAM (Normison)

Presentation
Tablets—10 mg, 20 mg
Capsules—10 mg, 15 mg, 20 mg
Liquid—10 mg in 5 ml

Actions and uses
Temazepam is a benzodiazepine drug (q.v.). It has a marked sedative effect and is therefore taken at night as an hypnotic. It is particularly interesting to note that this drug has a very short action. It therefore tends to produce less hang-over effect the following day and is particularly useful in treating insomnia in elderly patients where daytime confusion can be avoided.
Temazepam is also used for pre-anaesthetic medication because of its sedative and anxiolytic properties.

Dosage

1. As a hypnotic: 10–60 mg taken on retiring. It is recommended that as low a dose as possible be used for elderly patients.
2. For pre-medication: 20–40 mg single dose 30 minutes to 1 hour before the surgical procedure.

Nurse monitoring

See the section on benzodiazepines.

General note

Preparations containing temazepam may be stored at room temperature.

TERAZOSIN (Hytrin)

Presentation

Tablets—1 mg, 2 mg, 5 mg, 10 mg

Actions and uses

Terazosin is a selective alpha₁-blocking drug which is chemically related to prazosin and has the actions and uses described for that drug.

Dosage

1. Hypertension: 2–10 mg taken as a single daily dose.
2. Benign prostatic hypertrophy: 1 mg initially increasing until symptoms are controlled. Up to 10 mg daily may be required.

Nurse monitoring

1. As with prazosin, patients may experience an early rapid fall in blood pressure and care is required when introducing therapy in those with a history of syncope.
2. Dizziness and postural hypotension are therefore possible common side-effects.
3. Some patients may experience lethargy and the vasodilator action may result in development of peripheral oedema.
4. Patients with impaired liver function are less able to inactivate terazosin and may be particularly sensitive to the action.

General note

Terazosin tablets may be stored at room temperature.

TERBINAFINE (Lamisil)

Presentation

Tablets—250 mg
Cream—1%

Actions and uses

Terbinafine is a new class of antifungal drug used specifically in the treatment of dermatophytic skin and nail infections including ring-worm: Tinea pedis, T. cruris, and T. corporis.

Dosage

1. Adults only
   a. Oral: When topical therapy is ineffective, 250 mg once daily for up to 4 weeks (*T. cruris*); up to 6 weeks (*T. pedis*); and for 4 weeks (*T. corporis*). Nail infections require treatment for up to 3 months.
   b. Topical: For more easily treated dermatophyte and yeast infections cream is rubbed well into the skin once or twice daily for periods of 1–2 weeks.

Nurse monitoring

1. Patients may complain of gastrointestinal upsets and, in particular, disturbances of taste.
2. Other side-effects include allergic skin reactions, headaches, arthralgia and myalgia. In the event of altered liver function the drug must be immediately discontinued.
3. Avoid use in established liver disease and the concurrent use with drugs which may also cause changes in liver enzyme levels.

General note

Terbinafine preparations are stored at room temperature.

TERBUTALINE (Bricanyl)

Presentation

Tablets—5 mg, 7.5 mg sustained release

Syrup—0.3 mg (300 microgram) in 1 ml

Inhalation—250 microgram/dose of metered aerosol or 'spacer' inhaler.

Respirator solution—10 mg in 1 ml (10 ml bottle)

'Respules' unit dose—5 mg in 2 ml

Injection—0.5 mg (500 microgram) in 1 ml

Actions and uses

1. This drug stimulates receptors known as beta$_2$ adrenergic receptors in the smooth muscle of the airways with the result that the airways dilate. It is used in clinical practice for the prevention and treatment of conditions such as asthma and chronic bronchitis which produce bronchospasm.
2. The drug may be administered to reduce uterine contraction in the management of premature labour.

Dosage

1. For the treatment of bronchospasm:
   a. By inhalation:
      i. Via metered aerosol: 1 or 2 inhalations three or four times a day.
      ii. For acute severe conditions respirator solution is administered via a suitable nebulizer.
   b. Orally: 5 mg two or three times daily for adults. Infants and children: 0.75–2.5 mg three times per day.
   c. Parenteral:
      i. By subcutaneous intramuscular and slow intravenous injection: 0.2–0.5 mg four times daily for adults. 0.01 mg/kg to a maximum dose of 0.3 mg in children.
      ii. By intravenous infusion: For adults 1.5–2.5 mg should be dissolved in 500 ml and administered at a rate of 10 to 20 drops per minute for 8–10 hours.
2. For the management of premature labour: 10–25 microgram/minute by intravenous infusion is recommended.

Nurse monitoring

1. Common side-effects produced are muscle tremor, palpitation, tachycardia, flushing and headache.
2. The drug should be used with great caution in patients who have heart disease manifest by rhythm disturbance or angina thyrotoxicosis and hypertension.

General notes

1. Preparations may be stored at room temperature.
2. Syrup may be diluted with water.
3. Injections may be diluted with water for injection, sodium chloride or dextrose.
4. Aerosols must not be punctured or incinerated after use.

TERFENADINE (Triludan)

Presentation

Tablets—60 mg, 120 mg
Suspension—30 mg in 5 ml

Actions and uses

Terfenadine is an antihistamine. The actions and uses of antihistamines in general are described in the antihistamine section. Terfenadine is used specifically:

1. To suppress generalized minor allergic responses to allergens such as foodstuffs and drugs.
2. To suppress local allergic reactions, i.e. inflammatory skin responses to insect stings and bites, contact allergens, urticaria, etc.
3. Orally for other allergic conditions. e.g. hay fever and allergic rhinitis.

Dosage

1. Adults: 60 mg twice daily or 120 mg once daily.
2. Children: 6–12 years should receive only half the adult dose.

Nurse monitoring

1. See the section on antihistamines.
2. Studies with this drug indicate that sedation is less of a problem than with other antihistamines.

General notes

1. The drug may be stored at room temperature.
2. During 1992 the Committee on Safety of Medicines drew attention to the possibility that serious cardiac dysrhythmias may arise in patients who receive excessive doses or in whom plasma concentrations are otherwise likely to be raised. The latter may arise if erythromycin is co-prescribed with terfenadine. The drug is best avoided in patients with heart disease who may be pre-disposed to ventricular rhythm disturbances.

TERLIPRESSIN (Glypressin)

Presentation

Injection—1 mg vial with 5 ml diluent

Actions and uses

Terlipressin is chemically related to vasopressin and is used for its ability to constrict blood vessels in the hepatic portal circulation thereby reducing blood flow. It is administered in the treatment of bleeding associated with portal hypertension and oesophageal varices. Unlike vasopressin, terlipressin can be administered as bolus intravenous injections and the risk of reduction in coronary blood flow (producing angina and even infarction) is minimized.

Dosage

Adults: 2 mg by i.v. bolus injection followed by 1–2 mg repeat doses every 4–6 hours until bleeding is controlled.

Nurse monitoring

1. Although terlipressin is less likely than vasopressin to produce coronary artery constriction and hypertension, patients with cardiovascular disease must nevertheless be carefully monitored during treatment.
2. Terlipressin may produce abdominal cramping, blanching and headache due to its action

on gut smooth muscle and surface and cerebral blood vessels.
3. Failure to achieve rapid control of variceal haemorrhage is an indication for surgical intervention.

General note

Terlipressin injection may be stored at room temperature.

TESTOSTERONE (Sustanon, Testoral, Primoteston)

Presentation

Capsules—Restandol contains 40 mg testosterone undecanoate
Injection—Sustanon 100 contains testosterone proprionate 20 mg, testosterone phenyl-proprionate 40 mg and testosterone isocaproate 40 mg in 1 ml ampoule
Injection—Primoteston contains 250 mg of testosterone enanthate in 1 ml
Injection—Virormone contains 100 mg testosterone propirionate in 2 ml
Subcutaneous implants—100 mg, 200 mg

Actions and uses

The actions of this and other androgenic hormones are discussed in the section dealing with these drugs. In practice the above preparations are used in the following:

1. Male hypogonadism, cryptor-chism and delayed puberty.
2. Osteoporosis in males due to androgen deficiency.
3. Prostatic cancer and breast cancer in men.
4. Post-menopausal breast cancer.

Dosage

1. For the treatment of hypogonadism in males:
   a. Restandol capsules 120–160 mg daily for 2–3 weeks reducing therafter to a daily maintenance dose from 40 mg to 120 mg.
   b. Promoteston depot injection: 250 mg initially every 2–3 weeks then a maintenance dose of 250 mg every 3–6 weeks.

T

c. Sustanon depot injection: 1 ml is injected every 2 weeks.
d. Virormone injection 50 mg 2 or 3 times weekly or every week in cryptorchism or delayed puberty.

2. For the treatment of mammary carcinoma schedules vary: For example Virormone injection 100 mg 2–3 times weekly.

3. Osteoporosis in males: Oral Restandol as above.

4. Implants are only occasionally used: 600 mg every 6 months in male hypogonadism or very rarely 100 mg every 6 months in post-menopausal breast cancer.

Nurse monitoring

See the hormones (4) section on androgenic hormones.

General notes

1. Preparations may be stored at room temperature.
2. Preparations should be protected from light.

TETRACYCLINE (Achromycin)

(See Note 3, p. 362)

Presentation

Tablets—250 mg
Capsules—250 mg
Injection—250 mg and 500 mg (intravenous); 100 mg (intramuscular)
Ointment—3%
Eye/ear ointments—1%

Actions and uses

1. For general notes on actions and uses see tetracyclines (q.v.).
2. Topical applications are available for use in skin, eye and ear infections. The drug is effective against local infections caused by both Gram-positive and Gram-negative organisms including streptococci, staphylococci and coliform organisms.

Dosage

1. Adults:
   a. Orally: 1–2 g daily in total taken in four divided doses half an hour before meals.
   b. By intramuscular injection: 200–300 mg in total daily administered in divided doses either 8 or 12-hourly.
   c. By intravenous injection: 1–2 g daily in total administered in divided doses either 8 or 12-hourly. When administered intravenously the drug should be dissolved in sodium chloride 0.9% or dextrose 5% injections, and infused over 6–12 hours. See nurse monitoring notes below.

2. Children:
N.B. Tetracyclines must be avoided by systemic routes if at all possible in children under 8 years, see tetracyclines.

3. Application to eye in treatment of trachoma and chlamydia infection: apply to both eyes twice daily for 5 days. Repeat every month for up to 6 months.

4. Skin application: 1–3 times daily in susceptible infections.

Nurse monitoring

1. See the section on tetracyclines.
2. It should be noted that intramuscular tetracycline injections contain procaine (a local anaesthetic) to reduce pain at the injection site.
3. When given intravenously, the injections should be reconstituted by adding 5 ml of water for injection to the 250 mg vial or 10 ml to the 500 mg vial. The solution should then be diluted to a concentration not exceeding 500 mg in 500 ml with normal saline or 5% dextrose or sodium lactate compound injection B.P. The infusion should then be given over 6–12 hours to provide the dosage required.

General notes

1. The drug may be stored at room temperature.
2. Reconstituted injections for intravenous administration are stable at room temperature for 12 hours only.

TETRACYCLINES

(See Note 3, p. 362)

This group of antibiotics includes:

Chlortetracycline
Demeclocycline
Doxycycline
Minocycline
Oxytetracycline
Tetracycline

Actions and uses

The tetracycline group of antibiotics are bacteriostatic, i.e. they prevent further growth and multiplication of bacteria but do not kill them. The mechanism of action is by interfering with the synthesis of proteins necessary for growth and division of bacterial cells. Tetracyclines have a broad spectrum of activity against both Gram-positive and Gram-negative organisms. It is important to note that infections due to Proteus and *Pseudomonas aeruginosa* are usually not sensitive to Tetracyclines. They are used for the following conditions:

1. They are frequently used to treat acute exacerbations of chronic bronchitis and upper and lower respiratory tract infections.

2. They are effective in the treatment of the following specific infections:
   a. Brucellosis
   b. Q-fever
   c. Infections due to rickettsia (typhus)
   d. Non-specific urethritis
   e. Sinusitis
   f. Pustular acne vulgaris
   g. Pneumonia due to mycoplasma and psittacosis
   h. Trachoma.

3. Topical applications for skin, eye and ear infections due to staphylococcal, streptococcal and coliform organisms are available.

Dosage

See specific drugs.

Nurse monitoring

1. Gastrointestinal upsets including heartburn, anorexia, nausea and vomiting may commonly occur with this drug. It is important to note that if the drug is given with milk or food to try to reduce these symptoms, the actual concentration absorbed may be reduced and therefore the treatment may be rendered ineffective. The nurse may play an important role in discouraging the patient from taking the tablets with milk or especially antacids.

2. Diarrhoea may sometimes occur. This may be due to a change in the flora of the gut caused by tetracyclines but it may also be due to superinfection with Proteus, Pseudomonas or Staphylococcus or *Clostridium difficile* (the latter organism causing pseudomembranous enterocolitis). It is therefore recommended that the drug be discontinued if patients develop severe and persistent diarrhoea.

3. If the drug is taken during late pregnancy or administered to young children (less than 12 years of age), permanent staining of the teeth and bones may occur. This is because tetracyclines have been found to be taken up by growing bones and teeth. This group of drugs is therefore, for this reason, contraindicated in pregnant women and young children.

4. The drug is not recommended for administration to pregnant women for the following reasons:
   a. Their children's teeth may be permanently stained
   b. There is a risk of liver and pancreatic damage. Liver damage is especially likely if tetracyclines are given during pregnancy by the intravenous route.

5. Patients with impaired renal function should not be given tetracyclines as they may worsen the degree of renal failure by inhibiting body protein synthesis.

6. Other adverse effects include photosensitivity reactions and hypersensitivity producing urticaria, asthma, dyspnoea, itching, oedema and hypotension.
7. Tetracyclines affect blood clotting function and therefore if they are given to patients already on anticoagulants, the anticoagulant dose may have to be altered.
8. The coincident administration of antacids, iron tablets and milk will all reduce the amount of tetracycline absorbed from the gut and may render its administration ineffective.
9. Superinfection with fungi, i.e. oral candidiasis, or Proteus, Pseudomonas and Staphylococcus may occur.

General note
See specific drugs.

THEOPHYLLINE (Lasma, Nuelin, Slo-Phyllin, Theo-Dur, Uniphyllin)

Presentation
Tablets—125 mg
Tablets (slow release)—175 mg, 200 mg, 250 mg, 300 mg, and 400 mg.
Capsules, slow release—60 mg, 125 mg, and 250 mg.
Syrup—60 mg in 5 ml
Suppositories—300 mg

Actions and uses
Theophylline has the actions and uses described for aminophylline though it is not itself water soluble and cannot therefore be produced in an injectable form.

Dosage
1. Adults:
   a. Oral: 125–250 mg (conventional tablets) taken 3 or 4 times daily. In most cases, slow release tablets or capsules are taken twice daily (once daily in the case of Uniphylline); the usual dose is one or two slow release tablets or capsules.
   b. Rectal: One or two suppositories, usually inserted at night for nocturnal wheeze.

2. Children:
Oral: Initially a dose of up to 5 mg/kg body weight is given followed by maintenance doses of 2.5 mg/kg or more every 6 hours. Children aged 3–5 years or more should if possible take slow release preparations, e.g. one or two tablets or capsules twice daily. For this purpose Slo-phyllin capsules may be preferred since they can be opened and taken as small pellets to facilitate administration.
3. Premature infants:
Oral: For the management of apnoea, 3 mg/kg body weight is taken every 8 hours.

Nurse monitoring
1. See the section on aminophylline.
2. Note that different slow release preparations may produce different plasma concentration profiles (i.e. are not necessarilly bio-equivalent). Patients should ideally continue to receive a given brand whether in hospital or the community.
3. The individual dosage is determined by the plasma theophylline concentration. The target range is 55–110 micromol/litre (10–20 mg/litre).

General note
See the section on aminophylline.

THIABENDAZOLE (Mintezol)

Presentation
Tablets—500 mg
Actions and uses
Thiabendazole is an antihelminthic drug which is used both in the United Kingdom and in tropical countries for the treatment of:
1. Threadworm disease (enterobiasis)
2. Roundworm disease (Ascariasis)
3. Hookworm disease (due to Necator americanis or *Ankylostoma duodenale*)
4. Whipworm disease (Trichiniasis).

Dosage

Each dose given is dependent on body weight. The number of doses given is dependent on the disease under treatment.

Dosage with respect to weight is as follows:

10 kg: 250 mg
20 kg: 500 mg
30 kg: 750 mg
40 kg: 1 g
50 kg: 1.25 g
60 kg or over: 1.5 g

1. For the treatment of threadworm: Two doses are given on one day and again one week later.
2. For the treatment of strongyloid-iasis, roundworm and hookworm disease and whipworm disease: Two doses are given each day for two successive days. Alterna-tively a single dose of 50 mg/kg may be given but this produces a higher incidence of side-effects.
3. For the treatment of cutaneous larva migrans: Two doses per day for two successive days.
4. For the treatment of trichinosis: Two doses a day for 2–4 successive days.

Nurse monitoring

1. Patients should be reminded that tablets should be chewed prior to swallowing.
2. There is no need for dietary restriction, complementary medication or cleansing enemata.
3. Side-effects are common especially with high single dosage treatment regimes and include anorexia, nausea, vomiting, dizziness, diarrhoea, epigastric pain, pruritus, weariness, giddiness, headache and drowsiness.
4. Hypersensitivity to the drug may result in fever, facial flushing, chills, angioneurotic oedema and more rarely anaphylactic shock.

General note

The drug may be stored at room temperature.

THIAZIDE AND RELATED DIURETICS

Bendrofluazide
Chlorothiazide
Chlorthalidone
Cyclopethiazide
Hydrochlorothiazide
Hydroflumethiazide
Mefruside
Metolazone
Polythiazide
Xipamide

Actions and uses

Most of the plasma passing through the kidney is reabsorbed at various sites along the tubules of the kidney. Thiazide diuretics decrease the ability of the kidney to reabsorb sodium and water in the distal part of the tubules, thus increasing urine output. They are therefore useful in diseases where fluid accumulates in the form of oedema, i.e. heart failure, nephrotic syndrome, and liver cell failure. In addition they have a direct action on blood vessel walls which leads to a reduction in blood pressure, and they may therefore be used in the treatment of hypertension.

Onset of action is within 1 to 2 hours and duration of action tends to be for some hours. They therefore produce a more gentle, and long lasting diuresis than 'loop' diuretics, such as frusemide (q.v.).

Dosage

See individual drugs.

Nurse monitoring

This group of drugs can cause important side-effects which must be detected as early as possible to prevent their potentially serious consequences.

1. Hypokalaemia: The patient may become apathetic and confused and may develop muscle weakness or abdominal disten-sion. If these signs are noticed more serious effects of hypok-alaemia such as potentially fatal cardiac arrhythmias in patients on digoxin and coma in patients with liver cell failure, may be

prevented. (In patients on digoxin or with liver cell failure coincident administration of potassium supplements or a potassium-sparing diuretic such as spironolactone is recommended.)
2. Dehydration may occur causing postural hypotension and collapse.
3. An increase in blood urate may occur causing gout. Joint pains in patients on these drugs should always make the nurse suspect this complication.
4. The drugs may alter glucose metabolism leading to hyperglycaemia and glycosuria. Thus any diabetic patient receiving these drugs should be followed up closely in case change in treatment is required.
5. Thrombocytopenia may occur very rarely. This may be detected initially by observing small haemorrhages or bruises in the skin and if confirmed by checking the platelet count the drug should be stopped.

THIOGUANINE (Lanvis)

Presentation
Tablets—40 mg
Actions and uses
Thioguanine is a cytotoxic drug which is used for the treatment of acute leukaemia and chronic myeloid leukaemia.
Dosage
Adults and children: A single oral daily dose of 2–2.5 mg/kg body weight is usually given. Treatment courses may last from 5–20 days.

Nurse monitoring
1. Bone marrow suppression with resultant increased risk of haemorrhage, anaemia and infection is the most serious adverse effect from this drug. Frequent blood counts are usually performed during treatment courses.

2. Symptoms commonly produced include nausea, vomiting, anorexia.
3. Stomatitis and jaundice due to altered liver function may occur with this drug.
4. Hyperuricaemia occasionally resulting in gout and impairment of renal function may be produced.

General note
Thioguanine tablets may be stored at room temperature.

THIOPENTONE (Intraval)

Presentation
Injection—500 mg, 1 g, 2.5 g, 5 g vials for preparation of 2.5 or 5% solutions
Rectal—Thiopentone sodium solution has been administered rectally to produce sleep within 10–12 minutes.
Actions and uses
Thiopentone sodium is a barbiturate drug (q.v.) with a rapid onset and short duration of action. It has the following uses:
1. It may be administered intravenously to induce anaesthesia. The anaesthesia produced is of short duration when the drug is given alone.
2. It may be administered rectally to produce sleep, its onset of action being approximately 10–12 minutes.
Dosage
1. For induction of anaesthesia: 2.5% or more occasionally a 5% solution is used and injected very slowly into a superficial vein. The total dosage administered is that required to induce anaesthesia and in general is not likely to be more than 500 mg. Doses in excess of 500 mg may be associated with an unnecessarily prolonged recovery time and other complications (see the section on barbiturates).
2. The dosage required for rectal administration to induce sleep is

calculated on the basis of 1 g per 23 kg body weight. The required quantity is dissolved in 25 ml of water and instilled through a rectal catheter.

Nurse monitoring
See the section on barbiturates.

General notes
1. Vials containing thiopentone sodium as dry powder may be stored at room temperature. When reconstituted however solutions readily break down producing cloudiness and precipitation or crystallization. Solutions are therefore not suitable for prolonged storage and should be discarded immediately after use.
2. Solutions are strongly alkaline and therefore should not be mixed with other drugs in the same syringe.

THIORIDAZINE (Melleril)

Presentation
Tablets—10 mg, 25 mg, 50 mg, 100 mg
Syrup/suspension—25 mg in 5 ml, 100 mg in 5 ml

Actions and uses
Thioridazine is a member of the phenothiazine group of drugs and its actions and uses are described in the section dealing with these drugs.

Dosage
1. Adults: According to individual requirements and the reason for treatment. The adult oral dose ranges from 30–600 mg daily in total. It is administered in three or four divided doses.
2. Children: Under 5 years—1 mg/kg body weight; Over 5 years—one-quarter to one-half of the adult dose is administered.

Nurse monitoring
See the section on phenothiazines.

General notes
1. The drug should be stored at room temperature.
2. The drug should be protected from direct sunlight.

THROMBOLYTIC DRUGS

Presentation
See the individual sections for:
1. Streptokinase (Kabikinase, Streptase)
2. Alteplase (Actilyse; TpA; Recombinant Human Tissue-Type Plasminogen Activator)
3. Anistreplase (Eminase; APSAC; Anisoylated Plasminogen-Streptokinase Activator Complex).

Actions and uses
1. All three of the above drugs are indicated for the acute treatment of myocardial infarction. They act by dissolving clots in coronary arteries, thus allowing reperfusion of cardiac muscle and reduction in infarct size and a diminution in mortality.
2. Streptokinase (Streptase, Kabikinase) is additionally indicated for the intravascular dissolution of thrombi and emboli in extensive deep venous thrombosis, pulmonary embolism, acute or sub-acute occlusion of peripheral arteries, and central retinal venous or arterial thrombosis.

Dosage
See individual drugs.

Nurse monitoring
1. In the treatment of myocardial infarction it has been demonstrated that the earlier the drug is given, the better the effect. This holds for all three treatments.
2. The nurse may play an important role in identifying contraindications to treatment; these are as follows:
   a. History of cerebrovascular disease.
   b. Uncontrolled hypertension.
   c. Known bleeding diathesis.

d. Recent severe internal bleeding, major surgery or trauma or puncture of major non-compressible blood vessels.

e. Active peptic ulceration.

f. Other known contraindications to fibrinolytic therapy, e.g. acute pancreatitis, bacterial endocarditis.

g. Severe liver disease including hepatic failure, sclerosis, portal hypertension and active hepatitis.

h. Recent prolonged or traumatic resuscitation.

3. The commonest and most serious complication after administration of these drugs is bleeding. Careful control by pressure of the site where the drug or other intravenous therapy may be administered is essential.

4. Side-effects specific to each of the three therapies are listed under the individual drugs.

General note

See specific drugs.

THYMOXAMINE (Opilon)

Presentation

Tablets—40 mg

Actions and uses

Thymoxamine acts on the sympathetic nervous system and produces peripheral vasodilation. It is used in the treatment of peripheral vascular disease including Raynaud's disease, intermittent claudication, chilblains and frostbite.

Dosage

Adults: Orally: 40 mg four times a day.

Nurse monitoring

1. Nurse monitoring aspects of vasodilator drugs discussed under nicofuranose apply to this drug.

2. The drug should be used with great caution in patients who have had a recent myocardial infarction, those who are at present on anti-hypertensive therapy and in diabetics (when insulin requirements may be altered).

General note

Tablets should be stored at room temperature.

THYROXINE (Eltroxin)

Presentation

Tablets—25 microgram (0.025 mg), 50 microgram (0.05 mg), 100 microgram (0.1 mg)

Actions and uses

Thyroxine is the hormone released by the thyroid gland which is essential for maintaining a normal metabolic rate. Deficiency leads to obesity, coarse skin and hair, hoarseness, constipation, impairment of intellect, an inability to tolerate cold temperatures and in severe cases it may lead to psychosis or coma. Thyroxine's primary use is in the treatment of disorders associated with under-production of thyroid hormone.

Dosage

1. Replacement therapy may be taken orally once daily in the morning. It is not essential to take the drug any more than once a day as it takes a particularly long time for it to be metabolized and multiple daily dosages are of no benefit.

2. The actual dose necessary for patients is variable and is usually adjusted by observing clinical improvement and measuring thyroid hormone in the blood. Normal adult replacement doses vary between 0.05 and 0.2 mg per day.

3. It is essential that replacement therapy should be commenced at very low dosages and very cautiously in elderly patients and patients with ischaemic heart disease (see below).

Nurse monitoring

1. Any patient receiving thyroxine is likely to be on this drug for life. As the effects of stopping taking the drug take some time to manifest themselves, patients may come to believe that the drug is unnecessary. As hypothyroidism has many effects on physical and mental function and in the long-term may lead to death due to ischaemic heart disease, it is essential that all patients be encouraged to take replacement dosage regularly and the nurse may play a major role in encouraging patients to do this.

2. Thyroxine has no adverse effects when given in appropriate dosage. However, if too much is given too quickly, especially to elderly patients or patients with angina, severe angina or myocardial infarction may be precipitated. Such patients should receive initially as low doses as 0.025 mg on alternate days for the first 1–2 months followed by cautious increases in dose over the next 6 months or so to a full replacement regime.

3. Excessive dosage may produce anginal pain, cardiac dysrhythmias, palpitations, cramps, tachycardia, diarrhoea, restlessness, excitability, headache, flushing, sweating, weight loss and muscle weakness.

4. Any patients who have hypothyroidism due to inadequate pituitary function (hypopituitarism) should always have steroid replacement treatment commenced before thyroxine is commenced. Failure to do this may lead to death.

General notes

1. Tablets containing thyroxine may be stored at room temperature.
2. The tablets should be protected from light.

TIAPROFENIC ACID (Surgam)

Presentation
Tablets—200 mg, 300 mg
Capsules—300 mg (sustained release)
Sachets—300 mg

Actions and uses
Tiaprofenic acid is a member of the propionic acid group of non-steroidal anti-inflammatory drugs. It therefore has the actions and uses of drugs described under non-steroidal anti-inflammatory analgesics.

Dosage
Adults: 600 mg daily in divided doses.

Nurse monitoring
The nurse monitoring notes for non-steroidal anti-inflammatory analgesics apply to this drug.

General note
Tiaprofenic acid tablets may be stored at room temperature.

TICARCILLIN (Ticar)

(See Note 3, p. 362)

Presentation
Injection—1 g and 5 g vials
Injection—5 g intravenous infusion pack

Actions and uses
Ticarcillin is a derivative of the penicillin group of antibiotics. It has a wider spectrum of activity than the parent drug benzylpenicillin and is effective against many Gram-positive and Gram-negative organisms. Its mode of action is identical to that described for benzylpenicillin (q.v.). The indications for its use are for the treatment of infection at any site in the body where it is caused by an organism sensitive to ticarcillin. It is of particular interest to note that ticarcillin is often effective in the treatment of serious infections due to Pseudomonas species which are commonly resistant to other antibiotics.

Dosage
1. Adults:
   a. For severe infection: 15–20 g daily at intervals of 6–8 hours

b. For urinary tract infection: 4 g
6-hourly.
2. Children:
a. For serious infection: 200–300
mg/kg body weight in total per
day given in divided doses
either 6 or 8-hourly
b. For the treatment of urinary
tract infection: 50–100 mg/kg
body weight in total daily given
in divided doses.

Nurse monitoring
See the section on benzylpenicillin.

General notes
1. Ticarcillin injection may be stored
at room temperature.
2. For intramuscular injection: 1 g
vials are reconstituted with 2 ml of
water for injection.
3. For intravenous bolus injection:
Vials are prepared initially with
2 ml water for injection and diluted
to 20 ml solution. They should be
given over 3–4 minutes.
4. For intravenous infusion: The vials
are diluted in the diluent provided.
It is interesting to note that the
solution warms as ticarcillin
dissolves. Rapid intravenous
infusion should be given over
30–40 minutes.

TIMENTIN

(See Note 3, p. 362)
Timentin is a combination of
ticarcillin and clavulanic acid.
Presentation
Injection—

Ticarcillin	750 mg,	1.6 g,	3.2g
+	+	+
Clavulanic	50 mg,	100 mg,	200 mg
Acid			

Actions and uses
The actions and uses of ticarcillin are
described elsewhere: by adding
clavulanic acid, the spectrum of
activity of ticarcillin may be
broadened as clavulanic acid
prevents the breakdown and
therefore the inactivation of ticarcillin
by penicillinase (beta-lactamase).
This substance is produced by a

number of bacteria and effectively
renders them penicillin-resistant.
Some bacteria, therefore, resistant to
ticarcillin alone, may be effectively
treated by timentin. In practice this
may prove particularly important in
the treatment of urinary tract
infections due to *E. coli* and
Pseudomonas sp., skin and soft
tissue infections due to *Staphylococcus aureus* and general systemic
and respiratory infections due to
Gram-negative microorganisms.
Dosage
1. Adults: Usually 3.2 g (as ticarcillin)
by intravenous injection at
intervals of 4, 6 or 8 hours
depending upon severity of
infection and susceptibility of the
pathogen involved.
2. Children: Usually based on a dose
of 80 mg timentin (i.e. 75 mg
timentin + 5 mg clavulanic acid)
by intravenous injection at
8-hourly intervals.

Nurse monitoring
1. Timentin is administered by rapid
intravenous infusion in 50–100
ml minibags containing glucose
5% over 30–40 minutes.
2. Lower doses, e.g. adult doses of
1.6 mg 8 to 12-hourly are used
for patients with moderate to
severe renal impairment.
3. Timentin should not be administered by direct intravenous bolus
or intramuscular injection.
4. Note that heat is produced when
powder is dissolved and also that
the resulting solution has a
straw-coloured appearance.
5. Timentin is often prescribed
together with gentamicin or a
related aminoglycoside antibiotic
and while such combinations are
useful, these drugs must not be
mixed in solution.
6. Other nurse monitoring aspects
are as those described for
ticarcillin.

General notes
1. Timentin injection may be stored
at room temperature.
2. Solutions should normally be
prepared immediately before use

but if necessary can be refrigerated for up to 72 hours without significant loss of activity.

TIMOLOL (Betim, Blocadren, Timoptol)

Presentation
Tablets—10 mg
Eye drops—0.25%, 0.5%

Actions and uses
Timolol is a non-selective beta-adrenoreceptor blocking drug and its actions are described in the section on these drugs.

In addition, it is applied to the eye in the treatment of glaucoma (ocular hypertension). In this condition it lowers intra-ocular pressure by reducing aqueous humor production.

Dosage
1. The adult oral range is 15–60 mg daily in 2 or 3 divided doses.
2. Glaucoma: One drop instilled in the eye twice daily, starting with the lower strength and increasing to 0.5% if required.

Nurse monitoring
See the section on beta-adrenoreceptor blocking drugs.

General notes
1. Timolol tablets may be stored at room temperature.
2. Note that eye drops, after opening, should be used within 7 days for hospitalized patients and 4 weeks for others. This is due to the risk of bacterial contamination which exists.

TINIDAZOLE (Fasigyn)

Presentation
Tablets—500 mg

Actions and uses
This drug is a member of the nitromidazole group of which metronidazole is the forerunner. It therefore has the actions and uses of metronidazole but its action is more prolonged so that once or twice daily dosing is possible. In practice it is used for prophylaxis and treatment of anaerobic infections, and treatment of bacterial vaginosis and acute ulcerative gingivitis.

Dosage
Adults:
1. Anaerobic infections: Initially 2 g followed by doses of 1 g daily or 500 mg twice daily for 5–6 days.
2. Vaginosis/gingivitis: A single 2 g dose is used.
3. Prophylaxis prior to abdominal surgery: A single 2 g dose 12 hours before surgery.

Nurse monitoring
The nurse monitoring section under metronidazole applies to this drug.

General note
Tinidazole tablets are stored at room temperature.

TOBRAMYCIN (Nebcin)

(See Note 3, p. 362)

Presentation
Injection—40 mg in 1 ml, 20 mg in 2 ml, 80 mg in 2 ml

Actions and uses
Tobramycin is an aminoglycoside antibiotic. Its actions and uses are described in the section on these drugs. It may occasionally be effective for the treatment of micro-organisms resistant to gentamicin.

Dosage
The dosage for adults and children is calculated on the basis of 2–5 mg/kg in total per day usually given in three or four divided doses by the intramuscular or intravenous route. For the treatment of severe infection in neonates 4 mg/kg per day in total given in two divided doses may be used.

Nurse monitoring
1. The nurse monitoring notes on aminoglycoside antibiotics (q.v.) apply to this drug, other than that tobramycin may be administered by intravenous infusion.

2. When given by intravenous infusion the drug is diluted with 50–100 ml of normal saline or 5% dextrose in adults, and appropriately lower volumes in children. The infusion is administered over a period of 20–60 minutes.

General note
The drug may be stored at room temperature.

TOCAINIDE (Tonocard)

Presentation
Tablets—400 mg
Actions and uses
Tocainide has an antidysryhythmic action which resembles lignocaine. It is used in the treatment of serious ventricular dysrhythmias complicating severe left ventricular function, but only as a second line measure.
Dosage
Adults: 1.2–2.4 g daily taken in three divided doses.

Nurse monitoring
See the section on lignocaine.

General note
Preparations containing tocainide are stored at room temperature.

TOLAZAMIDE (Tolanase)

Presentation
Tablets—100 mg, 250 mg
Actions and uses
See the section on hypoglycaemic drugs, oral (1).
Dosage
100 mg–1 g daily in 2–3 divided doses.

Nurse monitoring
See the section on hypoglycaemic drugs, oral (1).

General note
Tablets may be stored at room temperature.

TOLBUTAMIDE (Rastinon)

Presentation
Tablets—500 mg
Actions and uses
See the section on hypoglycaemic drugs, oral (1).
Dosage
500 mg to 1.5 g daily in 2–3 divided doses is recommended.

Nurse monitoring
See the section on hypoglycaemic drugs, oral (1).

General note
Tablets may be stored at room temperature.

TRANDOLAPRIL (Gopten, Odrik)

Presentation
Capsules—0.5 mg, 1 mg, 2 mg
Actions and uses
See section on ACE inhibitors.
Dosage
Range: 1–4 mg as a single daily dose.

Nurse monitoring
See section on ACE inhibitors.

General note
Trandolapril capsules may be stored at room temperature.

TRANEXAMIC ACID (Cyklokapron)

Presentation
Tablets—500 mg
Injection—500 mg in 5 ml
Syrup—500 mg in 5 ml
Actions and uses
The actions and uses of tranexamic acid are identical to those described for aminocaproic acid (q.v.).
Dosage
1. Adults:
   a. Orally: 1–1.5 g two or three times per day
   b. Intravenously: 500 mg–1 g by slow intravenous injection (at a rate of 1 ml per minute)

c. As a bladder washout: 1 g in 1 litre of 0.9% sodium chloride irrigated at a rate of 1 ml per minute.
2. Children: Orally, 25 mg/kg two or three times per day.

Nurse monitoring
1. Common symptoms include gastrointestinal upset (nausea, vomiting and diarrhoea), postural hypotension and dizziness.
2. There is an increased incidence of thrombosis with this drug.
3. The risk of thrombosis is markedly increased if patients have reduced renal function or are concurrently receiving oral contraceptive medication.

General note
The drug may be stored at room temperature.

TRANYLCYPROMINE (Parnate)

Presentation
Tablets—10 mg
Actions and uses
Tranylcypromine is a monoamine oxidase inhibiting drug. Its actions and uses are described in the section on these drugs.
Dosage
10 mg two or three times daily.

Nurse monitoring
See the section on monoamine oxidase inhibiting drugs.

General note
Tranylcypromine tablets may be stored at room temperature.

TRAZODONE (Molipaxin)

Presentation
Tablets—150 mg
Capsules—50 mg and 100 mg
Liquid—50 mg in 5 ml
Actions and uses
Trazodone is an antidepressant drug which is derived from and is closely related chemically to tricyclic antidepressants. Its actions and uses are similar to those described for tricyclic antidepressants.
Dosage
Adults: 200–600 mg in total per day administered in two or three divided doses.

Nurse monitoring
1. See the section on tricyclic antidepressant drugs.
2. This drug in particular is associated with priapism in males.

General note
Tablets, capsules and liquid containing trazodone may be stored at room temperature.

TRIAMCINOLONE (Adcortyl, Kenalog, Ledercort, Lederspan)

Presentation
Tablets—4 mg
Deep intramuscular injection—40 mg in 1 ml, 80 mg in 2 ml
Intra-articular injection—10 mg in 1 ml, 50 mg in 5 ml
Cream, ointment, lotion and dental paste— 0.1%
Topical spray—0.006%
Actions and uses
Triamcinolone is a corticosteroid drug and has actions and uses as described in the section on these drugs. It is used by a number of routes for conditions as follows:
1. It is administered topically for the management of inflammatory skin conditions.
2. It may be given orally as a dental paste.
3. It may be taken orally or administered by deep intramuscular injection for hay fever or asthma.
4. Direct intra-articular injection may be given where appropriate for such conditions as arthritis, bursitis and tendonitis.
Dosage
1. Topical applications are applied two to four times daily sparingly.
2. Dental paste is applied two to four times daily.

3. Oral doses depend on the type of disease under treatment and the severity of the symptoms and it is impossible to give relevant instances.
4. For intra-articular injection, 2–20 mg is given according to joint size.

Nurse monitoring
See the section on corticosteroid drugs.

General notes
1. Preparations containing triamcinolone may be stored at room temperature.
2. Tablets must be protected from moisture.

TRIAMTERENE (Dytac)

Presentation
Capsules—50 mg
Also combined with thiazide diuretics in Dyazide and Dytide.

Actions and uses
Triamterene has a very mild diuretic action. It achieves this by inhibition of sodium excretion in the distal tubules with resultant sodium and water loss in the urine. As a diuretic alone it is of little use. However, it has an action on the renal tubule which reduces potassium excretion and it may therefore be used usefully in combination with thiazide diuretics to prevent the common dangerous side-effect of hypokalaemia encountered when thiazide diuretics are given alone. Hypokalaemia is particularly serious in patients who are on digoxin treatment or in those with serious hepatic dysfunction such as cirrhosis.

Dosage
The usual daily dose is 50 mg once or twice daily. Triamterene produces maximum effect after 8 hours and its actions may continue for 2–3 days after therapy is withdrawn.

Nurse monitoring
1. By far the most important problem which may arise in patients on triamterene is the development of hyperkalaemia which is especially likely to occur if patients have impaired renal function. Hyperkalaemia is difficult to detect clinically and is extremely dangerous because of the possibility of precipitation of cardiac arrest.
2. Side-effects are infrequent but nausea, vomiting, leg cramps and dizziness may occur.
3. In common with other diuretics triamterene may alter blood glucose levels and therefore treatment requirement in patients with diabetes mellitus may be altered.

General note
Triamterene capsules may be stored at room temperature.

TRICLOFOS

Presentation
Elixir—500 mg in 5 ml
Actions and uses
Triclofos is a general central nervous system sedative which is used to induce sleep and which is particularly favoured for young and elderly patients. It owes its activity to its conversion in the body to trichloroethanol and in this respect it is similar to chloral hydrate. Triclofos is, however, usually preferred to chloral hydrate since it is more palatable and produces a lower incidence of gastrointestinal upset.
Dosage
1. Adults: Usually 1 g on retiring though 2 g may occasionally be necessary.
2. Children: Up to 1 year—25–30 mg/kg body weight; 1–5 years—250–500 mg; Up to 12 years—500 mg–1 g

Nurse monitoring
1. Triclofos mixture is generally palatable and non-irritant to the gastrointestinal tract. There are therefore few patients who are unable to tolerate this drug.
2. Triclofos and chloral hydrate are converted in the body to the same active substance and, for this reason, patients unable to tolerate chloral hydrate may receive triclofos as an alternative. In such cases it should be noted that 1 g triclofos is equivalent to 600 mg chloral hydrate.
3. Where the standard mixture is diluted for ease of administration, e.g. young children, diluted elixir cannot be used more than 2 weeks after dilution and any unused quantity should therefore be discarded.

General note
Triclofos elixir should be stored at room temperature.

TRICYCLIC ANTIDEPRESSANTS

Amitriptyline
Butriptyline
Clomipramine
Desipramine
Dothiepin
Doxepin
Imipramine
Iprindole
Lofepramine
Maprotiline
Nortriptyline
Protriptyline
Trimipramine

Actions and uses
1. These drugs are used for the treatment of depression caused by either psychotic disturbance (endogenous depression) or as a reaction to a precipitating factor such as the death of a close relative (reactive depression). The precise mechanism of action of tricyclic antidepressants is not clearly understood.
2. Some tricyclic antidepressants have marked sedative properties and are therefore very effective in treating depressed patients who also have features of agitation or anxiety. Conversely other drugs in the group tend to be stimulant and are particularly useful when depression is accompanied by marked retardation.
3. This group of drugs has been used in other situations which are as follows:
   a. They have been used successfully in the treatment of enuresis in childhood
   b. Trimipramine has been used in the treatment of peptic ulcer disease.

Dosage
See individual drugs.

Nurse monitoring
1. Perhaps the most important point to make about tricyclic drugs is that they take a number of weeks to exert their antidepressant effect. As the effect is delayed and as depressed patients may be particularly prone to fail to comply with treatment, the nurse may play an important role in ensuring that the patient knows that the drug is not meant to take effect for a number of weeks and in encouraging the patient to continue with treatment during this period.
2. Tricyclic drugs lower the seizure threshold and therefore increase the frequency of fitting in epileptic patients. They should therefore be avoided in epileptic patients if at all possible.
3. The total daily dose may be taken once in the evening if a sedative effect during the day is not required. This has the added benefit of helping patients get to sleep.
4. Tricyclic drugs have anti-cholinergic or 'atropine-like' effects, which are particularly likely to occur during the early period of treatment and may be particularly troublesome in elderly patients. These effects

T

include dry mouth, blurred vision, constipation, urinary retention and tachycardia.
   a. Constipation may lead to paralytic ileus.
   b. Blurred vision is due to pupillary dilatation and these drugs should be used with caution in patients with glaucoma.
   c. Urinary retention may be particularly troublesome in patients with symptoms of prostatism.
5. Other side-effects include gastrointestinal upset such as gastric pain, anorexia, nausea and vomiting, fatigue, malaise, dizziness, confusion, cardiac conduction defects and hypotension. The latter two effects indicate that the drug should be used with caution in patients with a history of heart disease.
6. It is recommended that patients receiving tricyclic antidepressants should not concurrently receive a monoamine oxidase inhibitor antidepressant.
7. Large doses of tricyclic antidepressants have caused hyperpyrexia, convulsions, circulatory failure, cardiac arrest, respiratory failure, cyanosis, coma and death.
8. Deaths have also occurred from agranulocytosis and jaundice.

TRIFLUOPERAZINE (Stelazine)

Presentation
   Tablets—1 mg, 5 mg
   Capsules—2 mg, 10 mg, 15 mg (all slow release)
   Syrup—1 mg in 5 ml
   Concentrated syrup—10 mg in 1 ml
   Injection—1 mg in 1 ml
Actions and uses
   Trifluoperazine is a member of the phenothiazine group of drugs and its actions and uses are described in the section on these drugs.
Dosage
   1. Adults:
      a. Orally: 2–15 mg per day in total is given either in two divided doses or as a single dose of the slow release capsule.

b. 1–6 mg daily has been given by deep intramuscular injection.
2. Children:
   a. Less than 5 years: Up to 1 mg in total per day can be administered.
   b. 5–12 years: Up to 4 mg per day in divided doses is administered.
   c. Intramuscularly a dose of 1 mg/20 kg body weight daily should be administered and the dosage thereafter should be adjusted according to individual response.

Nurse monitoring
   See the section on phenothiazines.

General notes
   1. The drug should be stored at room temperature.
   2. Liquid preparations should be protected from direct sunlight.

TRILOSTANE (Modrenal)

Presentation
   Capsules—60 mg, 120 mg
Actions and uses
   Trilostane inhibits steroid synthesis by an action on the adrenal cortex reducing levels of both hydrocortisone (cortisol) and aldosterone. It is of use in conditions associated with overproduction of these steroids, i.e. Cushing's syndrome and primary hyperaldosteronism.
Dosage
   The dose must be carefully adjusted in the individual but usually lies in the range 120–480 mg daily or more, taken in up to four divided doses.

Nurse monitoring
   1. Trilostane must not be used for the treatment of pregnant patients.
   2. Some patients may experience flushing, some nausea and nasal stuffiness.
   3. It is important to avoid co-administration of trilostane and potassium-conserving diuretics

(amiloride, spironolactone and triamterene) which may produce a marked retention of potassium. Patients who receive such combinations must be carefully monitored for developing hyperkalaemia.

General note

Trilostane capsules may be stored at room temperature.

TRIMEPRAZINE (Vallergan)

Presentation

Tablets—10 mg
Syrup—7.5 mg in 5 ml; 30 mg in 5 ml

Actions and uses

Trimeprazine is a member of the phenothiazine group of drugs which is particularly valuable in the following situations:

1. It is widely used for its anti-emetic and sedative effect in the treatment of children with vomiting.
2. It is widely used as an antipruritic drug for the treatment of itch associated with dermatological conditions such as urticaria and jaundice.
3. It is also used for the pre-operative medication of children.

Dosage

1. When used as a sedative in children:
   a. Less than 1 year old: 0.25 mg/ kg is administered three times daily.
   b. Between 1 and 7 years of age: 2.5–5 mg is administered three times daily.
2. For the treatment of pruritus: 10– 40 mg per day for adults and 7.5– 25 mg daily for children in three or four divided doses is given. In severe cases adults may receive up to 100 mg per day.
3. For pre-operative medication of children either 2–5 mg/kg body weight by mouth or 600–900 microgram/kg by deep intramuscular injection is administered.

Nurse monitoring

Apart from unwanted drowsiness or sedation trimeprazine does not cause any of the many problems caused by other phenothiazines (q.v.).

General notes

1. The drug should be stored at room temperature.
2. Liquid preparations should be protected from direct sunlight.

TRIMETHOPRIM (Ipral, Trimopan)

See also Co-trimoxazole and Note 3, p.362.

Presentation

Tablets—100 mg
Suspension—10 mg in 1 ml

Actions and uses

Trimethoprim is an antibacterial agent which prevents the growth of bacteria by inhibiting the synthesis of the cellular constituent folinic acid within the cell. This substance is essential for growth and division of bacteria. The drug has two main uses:

1. It is used in combination with a sulphonamide under the name co-trimoxazole (q.v.).
2. It can be used alone for the prevention and treatment of urinary tract infections.

Dosage

1. For the treatment of urinary tract infection:
   a. The adult dose is 200 mg twice daily orally
   b. Children's dosages should be calculated on the basis of 3 mg/kg twice daily.
2. For prophylaxis of urinary tract infections:
   a. The adult dose should be 100 mg at night.
   b. Children's doses should be calculated on the basis of 2.5 mg/kg given in a single dose at night.

Nurse monitoring

1. If taken in short courses, very few problems are encountered with this drug. Occasionally nausea and vomiting occur and more rarely megaloblastic anaemia. This latter effect may be prevented by concurrent administration of folinic acid.
2. Because of its potential to interfere with the metabolism of folic acid in cells, the drug is not recommended for use during pregnancy nor for administration to very young children.

General note

The drug may be stored at room temperature.

TRIMIPRAMINE (Surmontil)

Presentation

Tablets—10 mg, 25 mg
Capsules—50 mg

Actions and uses

Trimipramine is a tricyclic antidepressant drug. Its actions and uses in general are described in the section on these drugs. It should be noted that trimipramine has a marked sedative action and is particularly useful where depression is associated with sleep disturbance, anxiety or agitation.

Dosage

For the treatment of depression in adults 50–100 mg is given at night two hours before retiring.
Alternatively the dose may be given twice a day, i.e. 25 mg at mid-day and 50 mg late in the evening.

Nurse monitoring

1. See the general nurse monitoring notes in the section on tricyclic antidepressant drugs.
2. As this drug has a marked sedative action it should only be given during the day if it is felt that the sedative action would be advantageous, i.e. if patients are particularly anxious or agitated.

General note

Trimipramine tablets may be stored at room temperature.

TRIPROLIDINE (Pro-Actidil)

Presentation

Tablets—10 mg (slow release)

Actions and uses

Triprolidine is an antihistamine. The actions and uses of antihistamines in general are described in the section on these drugs. In clinical practice it is used as a nasal decongestant, i.e. in the treatment of allergic rhinitis and hay fever. It is occasionally added to proprietary cough preparations, again because of its decongestant action.

Dosage

Adults: 10 mg slow release tablet once per day.

Nurse monitoring

See the section on antihistamines.

General note

The drug may be stored at room temperature.

TRI-POTASSIUM DI-CITRATO BISMUTHATE (De-Nol)

Presentation

Tablets—120 mg
Liquid—120 mg in 5 ml

Actions and uses

When this drug is exposed to the acid in the stomach it forms a complex which is thought to coat the surface of the ulcer bed preventing further acid from reaching it and therefore reducing further damage to that area. It is effective in the treatment of both gastric and duodenal ulcers.
An interesting development is the use of short course De-Nol (e.g. 14 days) in combination with metronidazole and amoxycillin (or tetracycline)—so-called 'Triple Therapy'—or other combinations with antibiotics to eradicate the micro-organism *Helicobacter pylori*

from the gastric mucosa. This pathogen is found in the mucosa of a large proportion of patients with peptic ulcer disease which does not readily respond to conventional therapy. Bismuth chaelate (i.e. De-Nol) appears to have a major bactericidal action agains this bacterium.

Dosage

1. Adults: 120 mg (5 ml) is diluted to 15 ml with water and taken four times a day on an empty stomach half an hour before each of the three main meals and two hours after the last meal of the day. A higher dosage, i.e. 240 mg six times daily taken half an hour before and two hours after each of the main meals is sometimes necessary, especially in the treatment of duodenal ulcers. The recommended length of treatment is 28 days.
2. Adults: One tablet is chewed and swallowed with water four times a day 30 minutes before meals and 2 hours after the last meal of the day.
3. Children: Adult dosages have been used.
4. See individual policies on eradication of *Helicobacter* as a treatment for resistant peptic ulcer disease.

Nurse monitoring

1. It is important to note that the drug causes a dark staining of the tongue and tends to blacken the colour of the stool. Patients may find this distressing especially if they have not been warned of the possibility of these effects occurring prior to starting the drug.
2. Difficulties with compliance are often experienced because the drug has a foul taste and ammoniacal odour.
3. Apart from the inconvenient effects mentioned above, the drug is not associated with any major side-effects.

General note

Tri-potassium di-citrato bismuthate tablets and liquid may be stored at room temperature.

TROPISETRON (Navoban)

Presentation

Capsules—5 mg
Injection—5 mg in 5 ml

Actions and uses

Trapisetron is a member of the group of drugs including ondansetron and granisetron which selectively inhibit the effects of 5-hydroxytryptamine (5-HT, serotonin) at specific binding sites called $5-Ht_1$ receptors. Stimulation of these receptors in the gastrointestinal tract and chemoreceptor trigger zone induces nausea and triggers the vomiting reflex. Drugs of this type are therefore used to prevent and treat nausea and vomiting in patients who are exposed to various emetogenic stimuli including anti-cancer drugs and radiotherapy. More recently they have been shown to be similarly effective in the control of post-operative nausea and vomiting.

Dosage

Adults: Acutely, 5 mg by slow i.v. injection or infusion followed by 5 mg orally once daily for a further 5 days.

Nurse monitoring

The nurse monitoring aspects for ondansetron also apply to this drug.

General notes

1. Tropisetron capsules and injection are stored at room temperature but must be protected from light during storage.
2. The drug may be injected slowly via the drip tubing of a running infusion fluid or added to 100 ml sodium chloride 0.9% or glucose 5% injection and administered over 30 minutes.

U

UROKINASE (Ukidan)

Presentation
Injection—5000, 25 000 international unit vials

Actions and uses
This enzyme stimulates the process by which blood clots are dissolved. In clinical practice it is administered locally for the treatment of secondary hyphema, vitreous haemorrhage and clotted arterio-venous shunts. It is given by injection to promote dissolution of blood clots in DVT, pulmonary embolism and peripheral vascular occlusion. Further assessment of a role in acute myocardial infarction is possible in the future (see the section on thrombolytic drugs).

Dosage
1. Hyphema: 5000 units are dissolved in 2 ml of sterile saline and instilled locally.
2. Vitreous haemorrhage: 5000–25 000 units of urokinase dissolved in 0.5–1.5 ml of sterile water are introduced into the eye.
3. Clotted arterio-venous shunt: 5000–25 000 units of urokinase in 2–3 ml of saline are instilled into the effective limb of the shunt which is then clamped off for 2–4 hours.
4. Intravenous injection: 4400 units/kg administered over 10 minutes followed by the same dose over 12 hours in pulmonary embolism or 24 hours in DVT.

Nurse monitoring
1. Any evidence of active bleeding or a bleeding disorder is an absolute contraindication to the administration of this drug.
2. High-dosage urokinase therapy carries the risk of inducing haemorrhage, particularly cerebral haemorrhage in patients with severe hypertension.

General notes
1. Lyophilized urokinase is extremely stable and may be stored at 4°C for at least 5 years.
2. Aqueous solutions at 4°C retain their activity for 3–4 days.

URSODEOXYCHOLIC ACID (Destolit)

Presentation
Tablets—150 mg

Actions and uses
This drug is chemically related to chenodeoxycholic acid and has the actions and uses described in the section on chenodeoxycholic acid.

Dosage
Adults: The effective range is 4–10 mg/kg body weight which approximates to 3 or 4 tablets daily in two divided doses (after meals) for most cases. Treatment should not extend beyond 2 years and should continue for 3–4 months after radiological disappearance of the gallstones.

Nurse monitoring
1. The nurse monitoring aspects of chenodeoxycholic acid apply to this drug.
2. It should be noted that diarrhoea occurs to a lesser extent than with chenodeoxycholic acid.

General note
Tablets should be stored at room temperature when they have a shelf life of 3 years.

V

VALPROIC ACID (Convulex)

Presentation

Capsules—150 mg, 300 mg, 500 mg

Actions and uses

This drug is an anticonvulsant with the actions and uses described under sodium valproate, of which this is its acidic form. Both sodium valproate and valproic acid are interchangeable on a dose for dose basis but there may be differences in bioavailability and close serum level monitoring is recommended if transferring from one drug to the other.

Dosage

Adults and children: Initially a dose of 15 mg/kg daily is administered and carefully adjusted upwards by increments of 5–10 mg/kg daily until seizure control is obtained or a maximum of 30 mg/kg reached. This drug is administered twice, three times or four times daily.

Nurse monitoring

The nurse monitoring section under sodium valproate also applies to this drug.

General note

Valproic acid capsules are stored at room temperature.

VANCOMYCIN (Vancocin)

(See Note 3, p. 362)

Presentation

Capsules—125 mg, 250 mg
Injection—500 mg vial

Actions and uses

This antibiotic has a bactericidal action and is effective against a wide range of Gram-positive bacteria. At present its use is limited to situations where other less toxic antibiotics such as penicillins or cephalosporins have been shown to be ineffective or where patients with severe infection are known to be allergic to penicillin or cephalosporins.

Vancomycin is not sufficiently well absorbed after oral administration and this route is used exclusively for the treatment of gastrointestinal infections, notably pseudomembranous colitis due to the anaerobic organism, *Clostridium difficile*. This may develop in patients who receive broad spectrum antibiotics when it manifests as intense bloody diarrhoea.

Dosage

1. Oral: The adult oral dosage for *Clostridium difficile* infection is 125 mg four times daily for 7–10 days. Children should receive half the adult dose.
2. Intravenous infusion:
   a. Adults: 500 mg 6-hourly or 1 g 12-hourly.
   b. Babies less than 1 week: 15 mg/kg as a single loading dose, then 10 mg/kg 12-hourly.
   c. Older children should receive a 15 mg/kg loading dose, then 10 mg/kg 8-hourly.

Nurse monitoring

1. As noted above, vancomycin is a highly toxic drug and its use should be restricted to the situations described above.

2. The intravenous administration of vancomycin leads to frequent toxic effects including nausea, chill, fever, urticaria, other skin rashes and occasionally anaphylaxis with resultant shock.
3. The intravenous injections are very irritant and frequently produce severe pain and thrombophlebitis at injection sites.
4. Intravenous injections should be diluted to a volume of at least 200 ml with normal saline or 5% dextrose and given over 60 minutes at appropriate intervals.
5. In high doses the drug is toxic to the auditory nerve (producing deafness) and the kidney. It is therefore contraindicated in patients with renal failure.
6. The oral drug is less well absorbed and produces less severe toxic effects.

General note

The drug may be stored at room temperature.

VERAPAMIL (Cordilox, Securon, Univer)

Presentation

Tablets—40 mg, 80 mg, 120 mg
Capsules (sustained release)—120 mg, 180 mg, 240 mg
Injection—5 mg in 2 ml

Actions and uses

The actions and uses of verapamil may be divided into two major groups:
1. It decreases the oxygen requirement of the heart muscle and also reduces peripheral resistance. These two actions make it useful in the treatment of angina pectoris.
2. It has also been found to be useful for the abolition of supra-ventricular dysrhythmias. It is thought that the drug acts by influencing the movement of calcium ions across cell membranes.

3. Peripheral vasodilatation is associated with a fall in blood pressure and it is also used in the treatment of hypertension.

Dosage

1. Adults:
   a. Intravenously for cardiac dysrhythmias: 5 mg repeated after intervals of 5–10 minutes until the dysrhythmia is controlled. It may also be given by infusion in a dose of 5–10 mg per hour up to a total daily dose of 25–100 mg.
   b. The oral maintenance dose for the prophylaxis of angina is 40–120 mg three times a day.
   c. The oral antihypertensive dose is in the range 120–160 mg twice daily.
   d. Single daily doses may be taken as slow release capsules.
2. Children: The intravenous dose for cardiac dysrhythmias is as follows: Neonates—0.75–1 mg; Infants—0.75–2 mg; 1–5 years—2–3 mg; 6–15 years—2.5–5 mg.

Nurse monitoring

1. The most important point to remember with this drug is that it should never be given to patients who are already receiving or have in the immediate past received beta-adrenergic blocking drugs as the combination of these two can lead to complete cessation of heart function.
2. As verapamil can produce hypotension when given intravenously, patients should be placed in the supine position prior to receiving such therapy.
3. The oral preparation of the drug is associated with few side-effects of which nausea and vomiting are the commonest.
4. If the drug is given to patients who have heart failure their symptoms are likely to be worsened.

General notes

Verapamil tablets, capsules and injection may be stored at room temperature. When given by intravenous infusion the solution may be added to sodium chloride, dextrose or laevulose injections.

VIDARABINE (Vira-A)

Presentation
Injection—200 mg/ml (5 ml vial)
Eye ointment—3%

Actions and uses
1. This anti-viral agent may be given by intravenous injection for the treatment of herpes zoster (shingles) and chickenpox. In normal individuals these diseases are not likely to be life-threatening and therefore the drug should only be given to patients whose body defence systems are compromised by drug treatment or other disease such as patients with immunosuppression disorders, cancer or leukaemia.
2. The eye ointment may be used successfully for the treatment of herpetic keratoconjunctivitis.

Dosage
1. By intravenous injection the drug should be diluted in 500 ml of 5% dextrose or 0.9% sodium chloride or dextrose/saline mixtures. Each 500 ml of infusion fluid should contain, at a maximum, 225 mg. A total daily dose of 10 mg/kg body weight should be administered, slowly over 12–24 hours.
2. Eye ointment should be instilled five times daily initially, reducing subsequently to twice daily.

Nurse monitoring
1. The ophthalmic preparation may lead to lacrimation (excess tear formation), a sense of irritation and a feeling as if there is a foreign body in the eye, a burning sensation, pain and photophobia (pain on exposure to light).
2. Intravenous administration is associated with the following problems:
   a. Anorexia, nausea, vomiting and diarrhoea may commonly occur.
   b. Tremors, dizziness, hallucinations, confusion, psychotic reaction and ataxia may also occur.
   c. The total number of white cells and platelets in the blood may be reduced leading to an increased susceptibility to infection and bleeding disorders.
   d. Less commonly, weight loss, malaise, pruritus, rash and haematemesis may occur.
   e. Pain at injection sites is common.
   f. The drug should be administered with great caution to patients with impaired renal function.

General notes
1. The injection may be stored at room temperature.
2. The ophthalmic preparation should be stored in a refrigerator.

VIGABATRIN (Sabril)

Presentation
Tablets—500 mg

Actions and uses
Vigabatrin is an anticonvulsant drug. It is chemically related to gamma-aminobutyric acid (GABA), a substance which is produced naturally in the brain and a deficiency of which is associated with epilepsy. After conversion to its active form, vigabatrin produces an irreversible inhibition of the enzyme responsible for inactivation of GABA thereby enhancing brain GABA levels. It has been used in the treatment of epilepsy associated with partial and generalized seizures, when resistant to established anticonvulsant drugs.

Dosage
1. Adults: Initially, a dose of 2 g is given in addition to existing anticonvulsant therapy and increased by increments of 500 mg until control of epilepsy is achieved. The usual upper dose limit is 4 g daily. Tablets may be taken as a single daily dose or in two divided daily doses.

V

2. Children: As above but lower starting doses, e.g. 1 g, are used in children less than 9 years old.

Nurse monitoring
1. Vigabatrin is a new drug unrelated chemically to other agents. The nurse can contribute greatly to the close monitoring of patients which is therefore necessary; not least for the early detection of adverse effects.
2. At present, the drug is known to cause drowsiness and dizziness and patients should be warned of this in the event of driving, operating machinery, etc.
3. Changes in mood, confusion, and other behavioural disturbances may arise. Children in particular may appear excited or agitated.
4. Vigabatrin is excreted unchanged by the kidney, and patients with renal impairment require lower doses.
5. When given in combination with phenytoin, a reduction of up to 20% in blood phenytoin levels has been reported. The mechanism for this interaction is unclear and adjustment of phenytoin dosage may be necessary.
6. In common with other anticonvulsant therapy, patients must be warned against sudden discontinuation of therapy which might precipitate serious convulsions.

General note
Vigabatrin tablets may be stored at room temperature.

VINBLASTINE (Velbe)

Presentation
Injection—10 mg vials with 10 ml special solvent.
Actions and uses
Vinblastine's actions are similar to those described for vincristine (q.v.). Its uses are as follows:
1. It has been found to be of most value in the management of Hodgkin's disease and other lymphomas.

2. It has also been used in combination with other drugs in the treatment of a variety of solid tumours including neuroblastoma, breast cancer, testicular cancer and resistant choriocarcinoma.
Dosage
The drug is given by intravenous injection at weekly intervals. The dose range is 1–10 mg and varies with the type of condition treated and the state of the patient.

Nurse monitoring
1. Vinblastine more commonly affects the bone marrow than vincristine and therefore patients receiving this drug are at increased risk of severe infection and haemorrhage.
2. Vinblastine may cause slight neurotoxicity but this effect is not as severe as that seen with vincristine.
3. Gastrointestinal effects include blistering in the mouth, anorexia, nausea, vomiting, constipation, paralytic ileus, abdominal pain, pharyngitis, and bleeding from the healed peptic ulcer sites.
4. Other adverse effects include hair loss, malaise, weakness, dizziness and pain at the tumour site.
5. Leakage from intravenous injection sites produces severe irritation, cellulitis and phlebitis.
6. The drug is contraindicated in pregnancy.
7. The nurse should be constantly aware that most cytotoxic drugs are irritant to the skin and mucous surfaces, and are in general very toxic. Great care should therefore be exercised when handling these drugs, and in particular spillage or contamination of personnel or the environment must be avoided. If cytotoxic drugs are handled regularly it is theoretically possible that repeated skin contact or inhalation may produce systemic toxic effects and in nurses who have developed hypersensitivity, severe local and general hypersensitivity reactions.

General notes
1. Vinblastine ampoules should be stored in a refrigerator.
2. It is given by intravenous injection either directly or via the drip tubing of a running 0.9% sodium chloride infusion.
3. Reconstituted solutions may be stored in a refrigerator for up to 30 days if the special diluent (containing a bactericide) is used. Alternatively reconstituted solution should not be used after 48 hours.

VINCRISTINE (Oncovin)

Presentation
Injection—1 mg, 2 mg and 5 mg vials with 10 ml special solvent. Also available as ready mixed solutions.

Actions and uses
Vincristine is a cytotoxic drug, the action of which is incompletely understood. It has, however, been shown to interfere with the synthesis of both DNA and RNA and to affect chromosome multiplication all of which are necessary for cell division. Its uses are as follows:
1. It has been found to be particularly of value in inducing remission in acute lymphatic leukaemia.
2. It has also been found particularly useful in the management of advanced Hodgkin's disease and other lymphomas.
3. Other malignancies which have been shown to respond to treatment with this drug include neuroblastoma, Wilms' tumour (kidney tumour occurring mainly in children) and rhabdomyosarcoma (a tumour affecting skeletal muscles).

Dosage
Vincristine is given by intravenous injection:
1. For the treatment of acute leukaemias in children:
   a. Initial dosage is 0.05 mg/kg body weight. This is gradually increased to a maximum of 0.15 mg/kg body weight by sequential injection.
   b. Weekly maintenance doses of 0.05–0.075 mg/kg body weight may be given following remission.
2. In the treatment of adult leukaemia: A weekly dose of 0.025–0.075 mg/kg body weight is used.
3. In the treatment of other malignancies: Weekly injections of 0.025 mg/kg are given until an effect is obtained and this effect may be maintained with lower weekly doses of about 0.005–0.01 mg/kg.

N.B. Because the difference between therapeutic and toxic doses is very small it is important to establish carefully dosage requirements for individual patients.

Nurse monitoring
1. Bone marrow suppression is less common with this drug than with many other cytotoxics but if it occurs the patient will be at risk of serious infection and haemorrhage.
2. The most important side-effect of vincristine is neurotoxicity which most frequently presents as peripheral neuropathy either sensory, motor or mixed. Initial symptoms may be slight and patients may complain of tingling or numbness in the fingers and toes. Subsequently tendon reflexes may disappear. If the early signs of neurotoxicity are ignored damage may progress and be irreversible. Thus patients must be closely questioned about the development of these symptoms and if present the drug should be immediately stopped.
3. Gastrointestinal effects may occur and include anorexia, nausea, vomiting, constipation or diarrhoea. Oral ulceration and abdominal cramps are also known to occur. Constipation may be particularly severe in the elderly and may give rise to intestinal obstruction.
4. The most common side-effects include diplopia, malaise,

V

depression, headache and psychotic reactions. Alopecia, weight loss and fluid retention, or low serum sodium due to inappropriate secretion of antidiuretic hormone have been known to occur.

5. Leakage into surrounding tissues after intravenous injection causes severe irritation. If administered via the drip tubing of a running 0.9% sodium chloride infusion it is important to check first whether the infusion is working correctly and to look for signs of local leakage before administering the drug.

6. The drug is contraindicated in pregnancy.

7. The nurse should be constantly aware that most cytotoxic drugs are irritant to the skin and mucous surfaces, and are in general very toxic. Great care should therefore be exercised when handling these drugs, and in particular spillage or contamination of personnel or the environment must be avoided. If cytotoxic drugs are handled regularly it is theoretically possible that repeated skin contact or inhalation may produce systemic toxic effects and in nurses who have developed hypersensitivity, severe local and general hypersensitivity reactions.

General notes

1. Vincristine vials should be stored in a refrigerator.

2. When given intravenously a suitable injection time is about 1 minute.

3. Reconstituted solution may be stored in a refrigerator for up to 14 days without significant loss of potency, providing the special solvent (containing a bactericide) is used in its preparation. If this is inconvenient, ready mixed solutions may be used.

VINDESINE (Eldisine)

Presentation

Injection—5 mg vials with 5 ml special solvent

Actions and uses

Vindesine's actions are similar to those described for vincristine. Its uses are as follows:

1. In the treatment of acute lympho-blastic leukaemia in childhood resistant to standard treatments.

2. In blast crisis phases of chronic myeloid leukaemia.

3. In malignant melanoma resistant to standard treatments.

Dosage

Usually 3–5 mg/m^2 body surface area, given by bolus intravenous injection at weekly intervals.

Nurse monitoring

See the section on vincristine.

General notes

1. Vindesine ampoules should be stored in a refrigerator.

2. It is given by intravenous injection either directly or via the drip tubing of a running 0.9% sodium chloride infusion.

3. Reconstituted solutions may be stored in a refrigerator for up to 30 days if the special diluent (containing a bactericide) is used. Alternatively reconstituted solution should not be used after 48 hours.

VITAMIN A (Retinol)

Presentation

Vitamin A is available in a preparation of fish liver oil in doses expressed in terms of international units.

Actions and uses

In the normal body vitamin A is produced from precursors in the diet and is essential for maintenance of healthy mucus secreting epithelial surfaces and for the maintenance of normal vision via the production of a retinal pigment known as rhodopsin. In clinical practice, vitamin A is indicated only for the treatment of deficiency states which are very rare in this country. Symptoms of deficiency states include night blindness, drying and change in the microscopic make-up of skin and other body surfaces, and drying and degeneration of the superficial layers of the eye.

Dosage

For the treatment of xerophthalmia: 50–70 000 international units should be given.

Nurse monitoring

Excessive doses of vitamin A may be toxic:

1. If large doses are taken acutely, nausea, vomiting, abdominal pain, drowsiness and headache may occur.
2. In chronic overdosage, fatigue, insomnia, bone pain, loss of hair and abnormal pigmentation of the skin may occur.

VITAMIN B COMPLEX

Presentation

Vitamin B complex is available either as preparations of its components (see below) or in multivitamin preparations. Vitamin B complex comprises B$_1$ (aneurine or thiamine), B$_2$ (riboflavin), B$_6$ (pyridoxine), B$_5$ (pantothenic acid), and nicotinamide.

Actions and uses

Vitamin B complex is indicated for the treatment of deficiency disorders of components of the complex. Symptoms of deficiency disorders are as follows:

1. Thiamine deficiency may present as:
   a. Beri-beri characterized by anorexia, emaciation, cardiac arrhythmias and in the 'wet' form of the disease oedema.
   b. Neurological symptoms due to thiamine deficiency are known as Wernicke's encephalopathy and these include: agitation, behavioural disturbance, loss of memory and confusion.
2. Riboflavine deficiency: Causes a rough scaly skin on the face, red swollen cracked lips, stomatitis

and a swollen red tongue. Congestion of conjunctival blood vessels may also be seen.

3. Nicotinamide deficiency produces diarrhoea, dermatitis and dementia.
4. Pyridoxine: Pyridoxine deficiency may produce roughening of the skin or anaemia.

Dosage

1. For the treatment of beri-beri: 5–10 mg of thiamine daily produces good clinical response.
2. For the treatment of nicotinamide deficiency: Between 40 and 200 mg per day produces good clinical response.

Nurse monitoring

No problems have been identified with the administration of these compounds.

VITAMIN C (Ascorbic Acid)

Presentation

Vitamin C is available in many preparations either singly or in combinations of multivitamins.

Actions and uses

Vitamin C is essential for the maintenance of normal body function. Its sole real indication in clinical practice is for the treatment of vitamin C deficiency known commonly as scurvy. The clinical features of this are weakness, tiredness, lassitude, bleeding and diseased gums, haemorrhage around the hairs of the legs, peripheral oedema and sudden cardiac failure. In addition wounds heal very poorly and bones may be affected by osteoporosis. Anaemia may also occur.

Dosage

For the treatment of scurvy: 500 mg–1 g three times daily in adults. Children over 12 years should receive three-quarters of the adult dose. Children of 4–12 years should receive half the adult dose. Children under 4 years should receive one-quarter of the adult dose.

Nurse monitoring

There are no problems associated with the administration of this drug.

VITAMIN D

Alfacalcidol (One-Alpha)
Calciferol (Ergocalciferol, Cholecalciferol, Sterogyl)
Calcitriol (Rocaltrol)
Dihydrotachysterol (Tachyrol, AT 10)

Presentation

See individual drugs.

Actions and uses

The drugs listed above are all preparations of various forms of vitamin D.

1. Vitamin D is essential for the normal growth of bones and teeth. It should only be used in clinical practice if vitamin D deficiency has been clearly demonstrated. Vitamin D deficiency causes rickets in children and osteo-malacia in adults. The commonest cause in European communities is steatorrhoea. In immigrants inadequate intake in the diet and poor exposure to sun (which stimulates the production of vitamin D in the body) may be contributory features.
2. Vitamin D may also be used to treat the rare condition of hypoparathyroidism.
3. In chronic renal disease the body is incapable of producing the active derivatives of vitamin D necessary to maintain normal healthy bones and it is for the treatment of the resultant condition, renal osteodystrophy, that One-Alpha Hydroxycalciferol is particularly indicated.

Dosage

See individual drugs.

Nurse monitoring

1. An excess of vitamin D causes high blood calcium. This may cause anorexia, nausea, vomiting, constipation, abdominal pain and increased urine output and subsequently renal stones and renal failure.
2. One-Alpha Hydroxycalciferol is the most active of the group of drugs which may be used in vitamin D deficiency states and, therefore, patients should be carefully monitored by regular estimations of blood calcium.
3. In clinical practice children appear to be at the greatest risk of receiving an excessive dose of vitamin D.

General note

All preparations of vitamin D may be stored at room temperature.

VITAMIN E (Ephynal)

Presentation

Tablets—3 mg, 10 mg, 50 mg, 200 mg
N.B. Vitamin E is also available in a number of proprietary multivitamin preparations.

Actions and uses

The actual function of vitamin E is yet to be identified. It has been used prophylactically to prevent habitual abortion but its efficacy in this context is in doubt.

Dosage

There are no dosage recommendations for this drug.

Nurse monitoring

There are no problems as yet identified in association with the administration of this drug.

VITAMIN K (Konakion, Synkovit)

Presentation

10 mg phytomenadione tablets (Konakion)
Ampoules—1 mg phytomenadione in 0.5 ml; 10 mg phytomenadione in 1 ml

Note

Synkavit is a synthetic water soluble form of vitamin K called menadiol sodium phosphate.

Actions and uses

1. Vitamin K is indicated for the treatment of vitamin K deficiency which is usually manifest as an increased bleeding tendency. The commonest cause of vitamin K deficiency is malabsorption.
2. Vitamin K may also be used to reverse the effect of warfarin.
3. Premature infants may have a relative deficiency of vitamin K and are often given therapeutic vitamin K to avoid the development of bleeding complications.
4. Synkavit is a water-soluble analogue of vitamin K which is better absorbed from the gut in fat malabsorption syndrome.

Dosage

1. To treat vitamin K deficiency due to malabsorption: 10 mg is given by intramuscular injection until clotting studies have been shown to be normalized.
2. As an antidote to anticoagulant drugs: 10–20 mg is given as a slow intravenous injection. The clotting function of the blood should be estimated 3 hours later and if still abnormal a second dose of 10–20 mg may be given but not more than 40 mg should be given intravenously in 24 hours.
3. For the prophylactic treatment of newborn infants: 1 mg should be administered by intramuscular injection.

Nurse monitoring

The too rapid intravenous administration of vitamin K has caused reactions including facial flushing, sweating, a sense of chest construction, cyanosis and peripheral vascular collapse.

General notes

1. Konakion and Synkavit ampoule solutions should be protected from light and should not be allowed to freeze.
2. Konakion and Synkavit tablets should be stored in a well closed container, protected from light and in a cool place.

W

WARFARIN (Marevan)

Presentation
Tablets—1 mg, 3 mg, 5 mg, 10 mg

Actions and uses
A number of the substances present in blood which play an important part in preventing bleeding by forming clots are produced by the liver from vitamin K. Warfarin inhibits the synthesis of these substances (known as clotting factors) and therefore reduces the ability of the blood to clot. Its principal uses are for the prevention and treatment of thromboembolic states such as deep venous thrombosis and pulmonary embolus. It is also used to prevent the formation of clot in cardio-vascular disease either on artificial heart valves or in the atria of patients who have atrial dysrhythmias.

Dosage
The general principle is to give a loading dose over 48 hours and subsequently adjust the dosage to the patient's individual requirements as gauged on the results of clotting tests such as the thrombotest or prothrombin time.

1. Adults:
   a. Loading dose: 10–20 mg on the first day followed by 10 mg on the second day. The dosage on the third day should depend on the result of the clotting test used.
   b. Maintenance: This depends on results of clotting tests.
2. Children:
   a. Loading dose: 2 weeks to 1 year—0.75 mg/kg; 1–7 years: 7.5–15 mg on the first day. On the second day half of the above dose. On the third day the dose should be adjusted according to the result of the clotting test.
   b. Maintenance dosage: depends on the results of clotting tests.

Nurse monitoring
1. The daily maintenance dose of warfarin is, as noted above, determined by the results of clotting studies. As the effects of bleeding due to overcoagulation or thrombosis due to undercoagulation can be so rapidly catastrophic strict adherence to the recommended dose is mandatory and the nurse may play an important role in ensuring that patients are aware of this.
2. The effects of warfarin may be influenced by a number of factors listed below and the nurse may play an important role by identifying their occurrence and alerting both the patient and medical staff. The following circumstances may lead to a requirement for alteration in dosage:
   a. Acute illness such as chest infection or viral infection.
   b. Sudden weight loss.
   c. The concurrent administration of other drugs: A number of drugs may affect the patient's dosage requirements. Where drugs are known to interfere with anticoagulant control this has been noted in the nurse monitoring sections of the drugs in this book.
3. The occurrence of haemorrhage in a patient on warfarin is an

indication for immediate withdrawal of the drug and if the haemorrhage is at all serious or repetitive the patient should be immediately referred to hospital for further assessment and, if necessary, they may be given vitamin K which accelerates a return to normal clotting function.

4. Warfarin is relatively contraindicated in patients with severe liver or kidney disease, haemorrhagic conditions or uncontrolled hypertension. It should also be used with great caution immediately after surgery or labour.

5. Hair loss, skin rash and diarrhoea may rarely occur.

General note

The drug may be stored at room temperature.

W

X

XAMOTEROL (Corwin)

Presentation
Tablets—200 mg

Actions and uses
Xamoterol is a beta-blocker and the section under beta-adrenoreceptor blocking drugs should be consulted for a general account of these compounds. However xamoterol is notably different from other beta-blockers, so far, in that it also possesses marked beta-stimulant properties and can actually stimulate resting heart rate and contractility. Thus the beta-blocking properties on the heart are only manifest when there is excessive sympathetic drive (i.e. when the heart is stressed) while the problem of resting bradycardia and hypotension commonly seen with other beta-blockers is much less likely to occur. Xamoterol is used for the treatment of mild heart failure in which its beta-stimulant properties support resting cardiac function while its beta-blocking properties protect the heart from sympathetic overactivity.

Dosage
Adults: Initially 200 mg daily (under hospitalization) for one week increasing to 200 mg twice daily therafter.

Nurse monitoring
1. The Committee on Safety of Medicines have stressed that xamoterol is only indicated in the treatment of mild heart failure. Early experience in more severe heart failure was associated with an increase in mortality!

For the above reason, xamoterol therapy is only initiated in hospitals where the facility for close monitoring exists.
2. Other side-effects include gastrointestinal disturbances, headaches, dizziness and bronchospasm. Palpitations, hypotension and chest pain have also been reported.

General note
Xamoterol tablets are stored at room temperature.

XIPAMIDE (Diurexan)

Presentation
Tablets—20 mg

Actions and uses
Xipamide is a drug which has both a useful diuretic and hypotensive action. It may therefore be used in the treatment of hypertension and also in the management of heart failure (see thiazide diuretics section, actions and uses).

Dosage
The usual daily adult dose is 20–40 mg taken once daily in the morning.

Nurse monitoring
1. The major points on nurse monitoring are identical to those for thiazide diuretics (q.v.).
2. This drug may also produce gastrointestinal upset and dizziness.

General note
Xipamide tablets may be stored at room temperature.

Z

ZIDOVUDINE (Retrovir)

Presentation
Capsules—100 mg, 250 mg
Syrup—50 mg in 5 ml

Actions and uses
Zidovudine is an anti-retroviral agent i.e. it is active against retroviruses of which the human immunodeficiency virus (HIV or AIDS virus) is perhaps the best known. Its mode of action is complex and the following is a simplified version only.

Zidovudine is a chemical analogue of thymidine which on entering human (normal and viral infected) cells is converted by intracellular enzymes to zidovudine triphosphate via a series of phosphorylation reactions. Zidovudine triphosphate in turn inhibits the formation of pro-viral DNA (which is essential for viral proliferation) by competitive inhibition of the enzyme viral reverse transcriptase.

Zidovudine is the first and (at the time of writing) only effective anti-retroviral agent for the treatment of HIV infection. However newer reverse transcriptase inhibitors (didanosine and zalcitabine) are under development and have been used in controlled studies in combinations with zidovudine.

Zidovudine is indicated for the following:

1. Asymptomatic HIV infection with a CD4 lymphocyte count of less than 0.5×10^9 and falling. Some specialists however prefer to delay treatment until disease progression occurs.
2. CD4 lymphocyte count of less than 0.5×10^9 accompanied by HIV-related symptoms.
3. HIV-related thrombocytopenia.
4. HIV dementia.

Dosage
Oral: The dose of zidovudine has been reduced over the past few years in order to limit toxicity and reduce the vast cost of treatment without seriously impairing its effectiveness. The usual dose is currently 250 mg twice daily but this is reduced to 200 mg twice daily for women weighing less than 50 kg. Higher doses e.g. 250 mg four times daily are required in the treatment of HIV dementia in which high CNS levels are necessary. Treatment is continued indefinitely.

Nurse monitoring
1. The very high cost of zidovudine (thousands of pounds per patient per year) must be stressed. Since it is the only drug active against the HIV virus to be marketed so far (although didanosine and/or zalcitabine are expected soon), there is overwhelming pressure on health authorities from those known to carry the virus or those exposed regularly to AIDS patients as well as patients in whom the syndrome is established to make the drug freely available. This must be seen against a background of unproven efficacy in certain situations and the urgent need for proper evaluation of the treatment. Special

Z

arrangements currently exist in the United Kingdom whereby the drug is obtained only after careful consideration of the individual case and is not freely prescribable.

2. Anaemia, leucopenia and neutropenia are the most common severe adverse reactions to zidovudine. Occasionally transfusions are required for severely anaemic patients.

3. The dose requires modification in patients who develop haematological toxicity, e.g. anaemia or neutropenia, and treatment should be suspended if haemoglobin and neutrophil counts fall below 7.5 g/decilitre and 0.75 x 10⁹ respectively.

4. Other commonly reported side-effects are anorexia, nausea, vomiting and abdominal pain: fever, myalgia, headache, and paraesthesia. A variety of other effects have been attributed to zidovudine including taste disturbance, diarrhoea, chest pain, lack of concentration, breathlessness, urinary frequency, pruritus, and flu-like symptoms. Severe neurological toxicity has resulted in convulsions. As well as the need for proper evaluation of the effectiveness of this drug it is equally important to establish a true picture of its toxic potential; a role for which the nurse is well placed.

5. Due to the possibility of serious haematological toxicity the administration of other drugs which are potentially toxic to the bone marrow should be avoided.

6. Accumulation of zidovudine is likely to occur in patients with kidney impairment and dosage adjustment may become necessary.

General notes

1. Zidovudine preparations may be stored at room temperature.
2. They must be protected from light.

ZINC SULPHATE (Zincomed, Solvazinc)

Presentation

Eye drops—0.25% (also in combinations with phenylephrine as 'Zincfrin' and adrenaline)
Capsules—220 mg
Tablets—200 mg effervescent
Lotion—1%
Mouthwash—2%

Actions and uses

1. Topical: Zinc sulphate possesses a soothing (astringent) action and aids granulation which renders it useful when applied locally in inflammatory conditions, e.g. applied to indolent ulcers and to the cornea in conjunctivitis.
2. Oral: Oral tablets or capsules are used to correct zinc deficiency (zinc is an essential trace element in the diet), to aid wound healing and in the treatment of acrodermatitis enteropathica.

Dosage

1. Topical:
   a. Lotion: Apply to inflammatory lesions twice daily.
   b. Eye drops: Apply up to 4 times daily.
2. Oral:
   a. Adults: One capsule or effervescent tablet is taken three times daily after meals.
   b. Children: Under 10 kg body weight—100 mg as dissolved tablet once daily; 10–30 kg— Take half adult dose.

Nurse monitoring

1. The only side-effect of note is the production of gastrointestinal upsets. It is for this reason that the drug was formerly used as an emetic, though at somewhat higher doses than described above.
2. Gastrointestinal upsets are reduced if dosages are taken immediately after meals.
3. Melaena and anaemia following haemorrhagic gastric erosion have been reported.
4. It is important to note that zinc sulphate was formerly used as an emetic but this indication is no longer valid.

General note
Preparations containing zinc sulphate may be stored at room temperature.

ZOPICLONE (Zimovane)

Presentation
Tablets—7.5 mg

Actions and uses
Zopiclone is chemically a new type of hypnotic which induces and maintains sleep of about six hours' duration without producing sedation or 'hangover' into the next day. Zopiclone is not itself a benzodiazepine. It is hoped that zopiclone will be free from the addictive effects associated with the benzodiazepines, and in some cases it has been used to assist withdrawal from these drugs.

Dosage
Adults: A single dose of 7.5–15 mg is taken on retiring.

Nurse monitoring

1. In view of problems of dependency with benzodiazepines in the past it must be stressed that all hypnotics should be prescribed for short-term use only. Although it is hoped that zopiclone will prove less addictive than previous drugs of this type, it remains to be seen if this actually occurs in practice.
2. Patients taking courses of hypnotics may experience rebound insomnia when these are stopped, and careful counselling to reduce concern is often required.
3. Lower doses, e.g. half a tablet may be more appropriate in the elderly, who are very sensitive to sedative drugs.
4. Patients with liver impairment may also be very sensitive to zopiclone and require reduced dosage.
5. Since there is no evidence that zopiclone is safe in pregnancy it should be avoided in this situation. Also it is excreted in breast milk and should not be given to nursing mothers.
6. Gastrointestinal upsets have been reported and some patients have complained of a 'metallic' taste during treatment.

General note
Zopiclone tablets are stored at room temperature.

Z

SPECIAL NOTES

Note 1

Intravenous injection provides an important route of drug administration. It delivers the drug directly into the systemic circulation so hastening its onset of action and guarantees full absorption of the dose. It may be the preferred route of administration if an immediate pharmacological effect is required (e.g. a loading dose of phenytoin for rapid seizure control) or if slow or incomplete absorption from the gut or a peripheral site and first pass liver metabolism are to be avoided. More and more nurses outside Intensive Care Units are being trained to administer intravenous therapy to patients who already have venous access and many intravenous drugs, particularly antibiotics and anticancer agents, are being supplied in ready-to-use syringes, minibags and large volume infusions from centralized intravenous additive services (CIVAS) run by hospital pharmacy departments. Thus the nurse's role in administering as well as monitoring intravenous therapy is increasing. Some general principles and guidance are included in this section.

Method of intravenous administration
This varies according to the volume of the dose and the rate of drug administration. Intravenous (i.v.) drugs can be administered by rapid bolus injection (immediate delivery) or slow bolus injection (over 2–3 minutes or longer), or by rapid infusion (over 10–30 minutes for which low volume minibags are especially suitable) or by slow infusion (over 4–12 hours or longer). Continuous i.v. infusion (throughout each 24 hour period) is used if it is required to produce a constant level of the drug or when significant volumes of fluid are required. Precise control of the delivery rate can be achieved using a programmed delivery device such as a syringe pump or volumetric pump. The above considerations may have important implications for the effectiveness of the therapy and/or the toxicity of the drug in question and if instructions on the precise method of administration are not available advice must be sought. If doubt exists, check before proceeding. In the Table overleaf examples are given of the preferred method of delivery for some drugs in order to optimize therapy or limit toxicity.

Table 1.1
Preferred method of delivery

Drug	Preferred method	Comments
Amphotericin	Slow i.v. infusion (4–6 hours)	More rapid admin is associated with renal toxicity
Bleomycin	Rapid i.v. infusion (15–30 minutes)	Lung toxicity more common with i.v. bolus admin:
Gentamicin	Rapid i.v. bolus	High initial peak level required
Insulin	Continuous i.v. infusion	Continuous control in ketoacidosis required
Nitroprusside Sodium	Continuous i.v. infusion	Action so short, it is not maintained with intermittent injection
Ranitidine	Slow i.v. bolus	Bradycardia results if rapid admin
Vitamins B&C	Slow i.v. bolus or i.v. infusion	Likelihood of severe allergic reactions reduced

Displacement values

This describes the volume taken up by the dry powder in a vial when diluted. It is only relevant when using lyophilized (powder) vials. This figure indicates the additional volume of fluid a powdered medicine takes up after reconstitution. For example: the displacement value of amoxycillin is 0.2 ml/250 mg. Therefore when a 250 mg vial is reconstituted with 2ml diluent the final volume will be 2.2 ml. A 500 mg vial after reconstitution with 5ml diluent will have a final volume of 5.4 ml.

Displacement values are only important when less than a whole vial is prescribed e.g. commonly the case in paediatrics. Therefore, when calculating the volume required to be drawn up consideration must be given to the **actual** volume of fluid which is in the vial. For example: the displacement value of amoxycillin is 0.2 ml/250 mg. Therefore when a 250 mg vial is reconstituted with 2ml diluent the final volume will be 2.2 ml. If a dose of 125 mg is required, the volume of the injection should be 1.1 ml.

Nurse monitoring aspects of intravenous infusion fluid therapy

1. **Selection of the appropriate fluid:**   The most common fluids are
    0.9% sodium chloride (normal saline), 5% glucose (dextrose) and
    mixtures of glucose and sodium chloride (dextrose/saline). These
    solutions are termed 'isotonic' because they are compatible with body
    fluids, i.e. they mix with blood without damaging red blood cells and
    do not produce irritation (which is due to the fluid itself) at injection
    sites. Several other strengths of sodium chloride solutions and
    glucose solutions are used less often for more specialized
    applications; these are however not isotonic. It follows therefore that
    in a busy hospital ward where limited space results in the storage of
    different infusion fluids in the same area, there is always a possibility
    that the wrong bottle may be selected, particularly during an
    emergency situation. It is therefore important that the label attached
    to the bottle is carefully read and checked against the fluid prescription
    chart or checked separately by the doctor requesting that infusion
    fluid.

2. **Contamination by particles:**   During the manufacture of intra-
    venous infusion fluids, steps are taken to ensure their quality and
    sterility. While this minimizes contamination by foreign particles, the
    possibility that occasionally one or more bottles in each batch might
    be contaminated should not be overlooked. The nurse can provide
    an important final check by inverting the bottle and examining the
    solution in bright light. By this method even small particles can be
    spotted as they fall through the infusion fluid. (Particles which appear
    to rise through the solution are usually bubbles of air). Further visual
    examination of the fluid is important after the seal is punctured, when
    affixing the administration set and airway. On a few occasions
    extraneous particles may accidentally be forced into the solution.

3. **Contamination by bacteria and fungi:**   The contamination of
    infusion fluids by bacteria and fungi can produce severe and even
    fatal systemic infections. Contamination may be caused by:
    a. Incorrect sterilization as mentioned above.
    b. Following the introduction of microorganisms through a damaged
        container or a bad seal. If this occurs contaminated solutions
        may appear cloudy or turbid.
    c. Of particular importance to the nurse is the possibility of
        introducing microorganisms when puncturing the container while
        attaching the giving set or during the addition of drugs to the
        infusion fluid. This risk can be minimized by adequate aseptic
        techniques.

The nurse should always be alert to the possibility of bacteraemia or fungaemia occurring in patients receiving intravenous infusions and should always consider this as a possibility when patients receiving intravenous infusions develop fever or rigors. Should fever or rigor occur any infusion should be immediately stopped and the remaining solution retained for examination by both the bacteriology and pharmacy departments.

4. **Labelling:**   All intravenous infusions which have had drugs added to them, must immediately be labelled to indicate the name of the drug, the quantity added or final concentration in the infusion, the date and time prepared to ensure that all additives are used while they are still stable, the patient's name and the location (ward) and the time after which the infusion must not be used. Irrespective of stability considerations, no infusion prepared outside a purpose-built sterile environment should be used 24 hours after its preparation. This is necessary to limit the possibility of heavy microbial contamination.

Labelling is not required for single bolus injections which are administered immediately but it is if the drug is kept in the syringe for a prolonged period of time before administration.

5. **Incompatibility:**   This refers to an undesirable chemical or physical reaction between the drug and the solution in which it is administered, or between two or more drugs when mixed together. Incompatibility problems can also occur between the drug and the container in which it is administered. The following factors influence i.v. drug compatibility.

   a. **Drug concentration:**   Generally the higher the concentration, the greater the risk of incompatibility.

   b. **Duration in solution:**   Generally the longer the contact time between drugs and containers, the greater the risk of incompatibility.

   c. **Temperature:**   Lower temperatures usually preserve drug compatibility but this is not always the case.

   d. **pH:**   Adding drugs to solutions may result in a change of pH which in turn can affect their stability.

   e. **Light:**   Some solutions must be shielded from light to prevent chemical breakdown (photodegradation).

To avoid incompatibilities arising when two or more drugs are administered intravenously via the same access, a few millilitres of sodium chloride 0.9% injection should be used to flush the line or cannula before and after administration. This should also be performed for i.v. access in which heparin lock solution is used.

Parenteral nutrition, blood products, sodium bicarbonate and mannitol should not be used for intravenous drug administration, unless otherwise stated.

Finally, it is not reasonable to suggest that the nurse should remember every possible interaction between either two or more drugs in solutions or the drugs and the solutions themselves. In the list that follows, common problems with drugs and solutions are discussed and there is a section where the more common known interactions between drugs in fluids are listed. Should the nurse be faced with the problem of adding drugs to infusions which are not included in these lists, the information is usually readily available via the Pharmacy Department.

DIRECTIONS FOR THE ADMINISTRATION OF COMMON INJECTIONS

1. **Antibiotics**
   a. *Amoxycillin/Ampicillin:* These should preferably be Co-amoxiclav (Augmentin) administered by rapid i.v. infusion in a sodium chloride or glucose minibag. However if slow i.v. infusion is used, sodium chloride injection is preferred. Penicillins are less stable over prolonged periods in solutions of glucose or sodium lactate-containing solutions such as Hartmann's solution which may reduce the efficacy of the antibiotic.

   b. *Other penicillins*: As above

   c. *Cephalosporins*: These may be added to common infusion fluids, i.e. sodium chloride 0.9%, glucose 5%, dextrose/saline, etc. Rapid i.v. infusion via a minibag is generally preferred to prolonged i.v. infusion.

   d. *Cloxacillin*: As for other penicillins, see above.

   e. *Erythromycin*: This may be added to dextrose 5%, sodium chloride 0.9% or dextrose/saline mixtures. It is important that the injection be initially reconstituted to a 5% stock solution by adding 6 ml water for injection or dextrose 5% to each 300 mg vial.

   f. *Flucloxacillin*: As for other penicillins, see above.

   g. *Fusidic acid*: Must initially be reconstituted using the special buffer solution provided. Thereafter add to sodium chloride 0.9% or glucose 5% (but only if pH is above 5.5—check with the pharmacy) to a final concentration of 1 mg/ml i.e. 500 mg in 500 ml. Administer over 6 hours (2 hours if via a central venous catheter).

h. *Gentamicin*:   This drug is almost always given by intravenous bolus injection but may also be administered by rapid i.v. infusion in a saline or glucose minibag. It should never be mixed in the same syringe or minibag with a member of the penicillin or cephalosporin group with which nevertheless it is pharmacologically synergistic.

i. *Imipenem*:   Dilute to concentration of 500 mg in 500 ml in sodium chloride 0.9% or glucose 5% and administer over 30 minutes.

j. *Netilmicin*:   Administer as for gentamicin.

k. *Piperacillin*:   Dilute in 50 ml or 100 ml minibag containing saline, dextrose or dextrose/saline mixture. Compound sodium lactate (Hartmann's) solution may also be used. Administer over 20–30 minutes.

l. *Rifampicin*:   Reconstitute powder in vial with the solvent provided then dilute to 500 ml in saline, glucose or Ringers solution. Administer over 2-3 hours.

m. *Teicoplanin*:   After initial reconstitution of the vial with water for injection, dilute to 100 ml in sodium chloride 0.9%, glucose 5% or compound sodium lactate (Hartmann's) solution. Administer over 30 minutes.

n. *Tetracycline*:   Vials should be reconstituted with water for injection and added to dextrose 5%, sodium chloride 0.9% or dextrose/saline. The concentration of infusion must not exceed 0.05% and the rate of administration should not exceed 20 ml/minute and should, if possible, be administered within 12 hours.

o. *Vancomycin*:   Reconstitute 500 mg vial with 10 ml water for injection then dilute in 100 ml glucose 5% minibag. Administer over 60 minutes. Higher doses are further diluted and administered at a rate not exceeding 10 mg per minute. Continuous i.v. infusion may be considered.

2. **Aminophylline:**   This may be added to dextrose 5%, sodium chloride 0.9%, dextrose/saline or Hartmann's solution. A loading dose of 5 mg/kg may be administered over 20 minutes (if patient has not received oral theophylline previously). Maintenance doses of 1 mg/kg/hour are administered continuously.

3. **Chlorpromazine:**   Preferably given by intramuscular injection. If the intravenous route must be used, chlorpromazine may be administered in sodium chloride 0.9% injection. Do not add other drugs to the infusion fluid.

4. **Cytotoxic drugs:**   These drugs have a highly specialized use and the preferred method of intravenous administration may be critical and should be carefully checked in each case. Cytotoxic drugs are highly reactive chemically and should generally not be mixed together for ease of administration.

5. **Diazepam:**   Direct (slow) intravenous bolus injection is preferred. If necessary, an intravenous infusion containing up to a maximum of 40 mg in 500 ml of dextrose 5%, sodium chloride 0.9% or dextrose/saline solution may be given. Do not mix with any other drugs.

6. **Digoxin:**   This drug may be infused in 5% dextrose, 0.9% sodium chloride or dextrose/saline mixtures. A concentration of up to 1 mg in 500 ml may be used where appropriate. The total dosage depends on factors discussed under digoxin (q.v.).

7. **Frusemide:**   When high dose intravenous therapy is contemplated, the drug may be infused at a rate of 4 mg/minute in either sodium chloride 0.9%, Hartmann's solution or Ringer's solution. Other drugs should not be added to frusemide infusions.

8. **Heparin:**   This may be given by intravenous infusion in 5% dextrose, 0.9% sodium chloride or dextrose/saline mixtures.

9. **Hydrocortisone:**   100 mg, 500 mg and 1 g vials of hydrocortisone should be reconstituted with 2, 4 and 8 ml of water for injection respectively and these solutions may then be added to dextrose 5%, sodium chloride 0.9% or dextrose/saline mixtures to give a fluid concentration of 0.1% or less.

10. **Insulin:**   It is important to note that only soluble insulin should be given intravenously. This is compatible with 0.9% sodium chloride. A small proportion of the insulin may be inactivated by absorption on to the glass container.

11. **Isoprenaline:**   Should preferably be added to 5% dextrose. It should be diluted in a large volume of fluid according to manufacturers' instructions and must never be administered by bolus injection.

12. **Lignocaine:**   For infusion a 20% solution (200 mg in 1 ml) should be added to 500 ml of 5% dextrose or 0.9% sodium chloride or dextrose/saline mixtures or 5% laevulose. It is also compatible with dextran and Ringer's solution.

13. **Potassium chloride:**   Potassium chloride should be diluted in such a way that its maximum concentration in the infusion fluid is not greater than 20 mmol/l and a maximum infusion rate of 20 mmol/h is recommended. The total dose administered within any 24 hours period should not exceed 3 mmol/kg body weight. Potassium chloride solution may be added to dextrose 5%, sodium chloride 0.9%, dextrose/saline or Hartmann's solution.

14. **Vitamins** (*compound*):   The contents of each pair of ampoules should be added to dextrose 5%, sodium chloride 0.9% or dextrose/saline mixtures. It should not be mixed with other drugs in the infusion fluid.

INCOMPATIBILITIES OF COMMON DRUGS ARISING WHEN THEY ARE MIXED IN SYRINGES OR INFUSION FLUIDS

Drug	*Known Incompatibility*
Aminophylline	Erythromycin
	Cephalosporins
	Tetracyclines
	Penicillins
Calcium Salts (general)	Tetracyclines
Cephalosporins	Gentamicin
	Aminophylline
	Tetracyclines
	Erythromycin
	Heparin
	Hydrocortisone
Chloramphenicol	Erythromycin
	Tetracyclines
	Hydrocortisone
Erythromycin	Aminophylline
	Penicillins
	Heparin
	Chloramphenicol
	Cephalosporins
	Sodium salts
	Tetracyclines
Gentamicin	Penicillins
	Cephalosporins
	Heparin

Drug	Known Incompatibility
Heparin	Erythromycin Gentamicin Hydrocortisone Tetracyclines Penicillin Cephalosporins
Hydrocortisone	Heparin Chloramphenicol Penicillin Cephalosporins
Magnesium Sulphate	Tetracyclines
Penicillins	Gentamicin Aminophylline Erythromycin Heparin Hydrocortisone Tetracyclines
Tetracyclines	Aminophylline Calcium Salts Magnesium Salts Heparin Erythromycin Cephalosporins Penicillin Chloramphenicol

Note 2

INTRAVENOUS (PARENTERAL) FEEDING

INTRODUCTION

When food, even in its most basic form, cannot be taken by mouth, or if the intestinal absorption of food is seriously impaired, intravenous feeding becomes necessary to preserve life. Common situations in which this occurs include the immediate postoperative period of major surgery especially surgery to the bowel, as part of the intensive care of ventilated or comatose patients and in the treatment of persistent severe vomiting or malabsorption syndromes.

Actions and uses

Parenteral feeding should be designed to provide the patient with an adequate amount of all essential components of a diet. In the following scheme, quantities of the components necessary are quoted and the nurse should bear in mind that these are not the daily requirements of an average fit human being, but they are designed to give seriously ill patients who may, through previous prolonged ill-health or present multiple medical and surgical problems, require far more in the way of nutrition in order to prevent further physical deterioration. The essential components of any parenteral feeding regime are as follows:

1. **Amino acids:** Amino acids are a group of chemicals which are essential for production of protein. Almost every structure and functional component of the body requires protein. Amino acids in total comprise more than 20, but a number of these may be produced from other proteins and amino acids by the body itself. There are, however, eight amino acids which the body cannot produce and amino acid solutions are designed to provide both total protein requirements and also sufficient of these eight essential amino acids for the body's use. Many solutions of amino acids are available and these include: Vamin solutions, Aminoplex, Aminofusins, Freamine, Synthamins.

2. **Carbohydrate:** Carbohydrate in the normal diet is derived from various sugars and starches. The main function of carbohydrate is to provide a high energy source of calories. For intravenous parenteral nutrition, carbohydrates are available alone or in combination with amino acids. For parenteral feeding the simplest sugar, glucose, is available in varying concentrations including Glucose (Dextrose) 5%, Glucose (Dextrose) 10%, Glucose (Dextrose) 30%, Glucose (Dextrose) 50%.

3. **Fat:** Fat is another important source of energy and essential components necessary for bodily function. It is available as a suspension of fat globules in water and has a creamy, milk-like appearance. Available suspensions include Intralipid 10% and Intralipid 20%.

4. **Vitamins:** All the essential vitamins (see vitamin section) must be included in a parenteral feeding regime. They may be included in any regime either singly or by using compound solutions such as Pabrinex and they may be given either by intravenous bolus injection or intramuscular injection. It should be noted that vitamin D is not included in multiple preparations and should be given separately as required at intervals of approximately 1 month.

5. **Minerals:** Just as vitamins are necessary for many bodily functions, so are a number of minerals which are present in tiny, yet essential, quantities in the normal diet. These include sodium (Na), potassium (K), magnesium (Mg), zinc (Zn), calcium (Ca), iron (Fe), manganese (Mn), copper (Cu), fluoride (Fl), phosphate (PO_4). There are available preparations which contain all of these essential minerals and these preparations include:

   a. *Addamel:* A compound mineral supplement for injection which is added to Glucose mixtures

   b. *Ped-el:* A solution like Addamel which is appropriate for paediatric use

   c. *Addiphos:* A phosphate injection containing both sodium and potassium phosphate in solution.

6. **Alcohol:** Although alcohol itself is by no means a necessary part of the diet, it has been used frequently in the past as it is an excellent source of energy. There are, however, other suitable preparations available which are not associated with some of the side-effects found with alcohol solutions and it is sufficient that the nurse know that alcohol is occasionally included in these regimes, but is not absolutely essential.

Dosage

For seriously ill patients and in order to ensure that catabolism (break-down of the muscle and tissues of the body) does not occur, it is recommended that patients receive each day:

1. Sufficient amino acid to provide 15–20 g of nitrogen per day.
2. 2000–3000 kcal per day.
3. Two to three litres of fluid per day (the nurse should be careful to note that any patient with impaired renal function must have a strictly controlled fluid intake as discussed with the medical staff and the figure quoted is for patients with normal renal function).
4. Vitamin supplementation as required above.
5. Mineral supplementation as required above.

Method of administration

Two methods of administration are available:

1. **Total Parenteral Nutrition (TPN or 'Big Bag' Technique)**

   This involves adding the total daily feeding requirement to a single 2 or 3 litre capacity plastic bag and infusing the contents continuously over 12–24 hours. The technique has the advantage of being tailored to meet the needs of the individual and it is convenient and simple to use. Many hospitals are now capable of supplying a total parenteral nutritional programme including a domestic service to hospital outpatients who can be taught to administer their feeds overnight while sleeping. However, several important considerations exist:

   a. A TPN service requires the availability of a specialized pharma-ceutical unit within which a high standard of aseptic technique and manipulative skills are employed. The consequences of accidental contamination of intravenous feeds are potentially disastrous for the patient.

   b. TPN feeds are very expensive (up to £100 per bag or single daily feed) and since they are designed for individual patients the service requires close cooperation between pharmacist, doctor and nurse to avoid unnecessary waste. This is often ensured by the establishment of multidisciplinary teams through which feeding programmes are designed and requests for individual patients are approved.

   c. Concentrations of the various constituents are limited if it is intended to administer intravenous feeds via peripheral veins as a result of the potentially high irritant nature of concentrated solutions, and peripheral feeding should in any case only be carried out in the short-term, i.e. for a few days. Thus it is usual to prepare patients surgically for long-term feeding by insertion of a fine bore catheter into the great veins (vena cavae) or directly into the right atrium of the heart so that these highly concentrated solutions become rapidly diluted on administration. The catheter is usually channelled under the skin to a point distant from the point of intravenous access in order to limit the risk of entry of microorganisms into the venous site. Nevertheless catheter sepsis occasionally occurs and may necessitate removal of a central line.

d. It is important to stress that big bag feeds are intended for continuous (up to 24 hour) infusion and drip rates must be carefully checked throughout. Too rapid infusion of a 2 or 3 litre load can result, and has resulted, in precipitation of serious cardiac failure.

2. **Basic intravenous feeding systems**

    Individually tailored total parenteral nutritional support is not always possible, usually due to a lack of suitable facilities for its preparation, and a system which administers individual components of the regime must be devised. The following scheme is a simple example which delivers fluids simultaneously via a 'Y' connector along two separate lines:

    Line 1: 1 x 8 hour amino acid solution (500 ml), e.g. Vamin Glucose, followed by 1 x 8 hour fat emulsion (500 ml), e.g. Intralipid 20% followed by 1 x 8 hour amino acid solution (500 ml), e.g. Vamin Glucose.

    Line 2: 1 x 8 hour Glucose 30% (500 ml) repeated twice.

    Minerals and vitamins can be added to solutions as required and the entire regime will provide up to 3000 kcal of energy, 20 g or more of Nitrogen and 3 litres of fluid. There is sufficient choice among the various commercial amino acid solutions to allow flexibility in nitrogen administration.

Nurse monitoring

1. Peripheral intravenous sites should be examined regularly in order to detect early signs of irritancy, infection and phlebitis. The doctor should be alerted if pain and reddening of the area occurs.

2. Since patients receiving parenteral nutrition are invariably in poor physical state the consequences of systemic infection arising from catheter sepsis or entry of microorganisms at an inflamed peripheral

intravenous site are potentially disastrous. Nurses have an important role to play in ensuring that good aseptic technique is observed when setting up feeds and at bag changes and also in alerting the doctor to early signs of infection, increased temperature, rigors, etc. This is especially important when total parenteral nutrition is employed since contaminating pathogens have optimum conditions for rapid growth in such solutions. A cloudy appearance or turbidity in any feed solutions is an indication of possible contamination.

3. Prior to setting up an infusion of fat emulsion (Intralipid) the nurse should examine the consistency of the solution carefully. If fat globules in the solution have coalesced and produced a cream effect (similar to that seen on the surface of a bottle of milk) the solution should be discarded immediately.

4. It is a useful working rule to remember that all parenteral feeding solutions may contain, if examined under bright light, minute particles which if clearly visible point to contamination of the fluid and the need to discard it.

Note 3

Antibiotics (and also sulphonamides) are used for the prevention or treatment of infection by bacteria and to a lesser extent other organisms. When drugs of this type are discussed in the text, a number of terms are used, a knowledge of which is important in order to be able to understand the actions and uses of the drugs. These are as follows:

1. **Bacteriostatic:** Possessing an action which prevents the growth of bacterial microorganisms.

2. **Bactericidal:** Possessing an action which kills bacterial micro-organisms.

3. **Classification of bacterial microorganisms:** A bacteriologist by the name of Gram invented a staining technique whereby most common bacterial microorganisms fell into one of two groups, designated Gram-positive and Gram-negative on the results of the staining test. This has proved to be an immensely useful test in clinical practice, as many antibiotics seem to have spectrums of activity related to either one or the other group. These are listed below:

   a. **Gram-positive:**
      i. Cocci:
         Staphylococcus aureus
            other staphylococci
         Streptococcus viridans
         Streptococcus pyogenes
         Streptococcus faecalis
         Streptococcus bovis
         Streptococcus pneumoniae

      ii. Gram-positive bacilli:
         Bacillus anthracis
         Corynebacterium diphtheriae
         Listeria monocytogenes
         Clostridium tetani
         Clostridium welchii

b. **Gram-negative:**

   i. Cocci:
       Neisseria gonorrhoeae
       Neisseria meningitidis

   ii. Gram-negative bacilli:
       Haemophilus influenzae
       Klebsiella pneumonia
       E. coli
       Enterobacter species
       Proteus species
       Pseudomonas aeruginosa
       Pseudomonas pyocynaea

4. **Pathogen:**   This is a common term for a bacterial microorganism which produces infection.

5. **Strain:**   By using various staining and other techniques, major groups of pathogens such as staphylococci may be divided into sub-groups known as strains. This is useful in that differing strains of organisms can produce different patterns of disease and also have differing antibiotic sensitivity.

6. **Resistance:**   When antibiotics or sulphonamides are found to be ineffective against a particular microorganism, the microorganism is said to be resistant to the drug. Organisms have different means of acquiring resistance but such a discussion is beyond the scope of this text.

INFECTIONS CAUSED BY BACTERIA

Infection	Infecting microorganism (pathogen)
Bacteraemia or septicaemia	Coliforms Enterobacter species *Staphylococcus aureus* Streptococcus species
Bacterial meningitis	*Streptococcus pneumoniae* *Neisseria meningitidis*

N.B. — Various microorganisms may cause meningitis in neonates.

Endocarditis (acute)	*Staphylococcus aureus* *Streptococcus pyogenes* Gram-negative bacilli

(sub-acute)	Streptococcus species
	Staphylococcus epidermidis
	Gram-negative bacilli
Enteric fever	Salmonellae
Cholecystitis	Coliforms
	Streptococcus faecalis
	Salmonellae
Enterocolitis	*Staphylococcus aureus*
Food poisoning	Salmonellae
	Clostridium welchii
Gastroenteritis	Salmonellae (as for food poisoning)
	E. coli
Peritonitis	Mixed organisms commonly found in bowel including:
	Coliforms
	Proteus species
	Streptococcus faecali
	Clostridia
Peptic ulcer	*Helicobacter pylori*
Pseudomembranous colitis	*Clostridium dificile*
Impetigo	*Streptococcus pyogenes*
	Staphylococcus aureus
Postoperative wound infections	*Staphylococcus aureus*
	Coliforms
	Bacteroides (an anaerobe)
	Pseudomonas aeruginosa
Urinary tract	
i. Cystitis	Coliforms
	Proteus
	Streptococcus faecalis

N.B. — *Staphylococcus epidermidis* is often the cause of cystitis resulting from bladder catheterization

ii. Acute and chronic pyelonephritis	Gram-negative bacilli
Venereal disease	
i. Gonorrhoea	*Neisseria gonorrhoeae*
ii. Non-specific urethritis	Chlamydia
iii. Vaginitis	Normally fungal infection

Tuberculosis	*Mycobacterium tuberculosis*

Respiratory tract

   i. Exacerbation of chronic bronchitis   *Haemophilus influenzae*
Streptococcus pneumoniae

   ii. Pneumonia (previously healthy chest)   *Streptococcus pneumoniae*
Staphylococcus aureus

   iii. Pneumonia (previously unhealthy chest)   *Staphylococcus pneumoniae*
Staphylococcus aureus
Haemophilus influenzae

N.B. — Staphylococcus aureus infections commonly occur after respiratory viral infections, e.g. influenza

E.N.T.

   i. Tonsillitis   *Streptococcus pyogenes*

N.B. — Often caused by virus infection.

   ii. Otitis media   *Streptococcus pyogenes*
Streptococcus pneumoniae
Haemophilus influenzae
(infants)

   iii. Sinusitis   *Streptococcus pyogenes*
Streptococcus pneumoniae
Haemophilus influenzae
(infants)

Note 4

When a nursing mother ingests a drug, a proportion of that drug may appear in her breast milk. The actual amount of drug appearing depends on the type of drug, the amount ingested and its metabolism in the body. Although only small amounts of these drugs or their metabolites are excreted in breast milk they may still be relevant. Firstly, because the infants receiving these drugs are very small, so even small dosages can affect them. Secondly, young infants have immature liver and renal function and this can delay drug metabolism and therefore increase the drug's effect. It is obvious, therefore, that when drugs are given to a nursing mother a number of basic important principles must be adhered to by the doctor, and the nurse should be aware of them. They include:

1. Never prescribe a drug unless it is absolutely necessary.
2. Whenever possible use the safest alternative.
3. Use the lowest possible dose for the shortest possible time.
4. Ensure that the mother understands the dose regime and is aware of any recognisable effects on the baby.

The information available on the effect on babies of drugs given to mothers who are breast feeding is limited. A number of important groups, however, may be identified. These are:

1. **Drugs which can safely be given to nursing mothers:**
   Acetazolamide
   Aminoglycoside antibiotics
   Aminophylline slow
   Antacids
   Antidepressants, tricyclic
   Antihistamines
   Atenolol
   Baclofen
   Captopril
   Carbamazepine
   Cephalosporin antibiotics

Chloroquine
Cisapride
Codeine phosphate
Dextropropoxyphene (*in Distalgesic*)
Diclofenac
Digoxin
Disopyramide
Domperidone
Enalapril
Erythromycin
Ethambutol
Famotidine
Fenbufen
Fenoprofen
Fenoterol
Folic acid
Flurbiprofen
Fluvoxamine
Frusemide
Heparin
Hydroxychloroquine
Hyoscine
Ibuprofen
Insulin
Iron
Ketoprofen
Loperamide
Mefenamic acid
Methyldopa
Metoclopramide
Metronidazole (*avoid single high doses*)
Naproxen
Nefopam
Nifedipine
Nizatidine
Paracetamol
Penicillins
Pentazocine
Pethidine
Phenytoin
Piroxicam
Propranolol
Rifampicin

Rimiterol
Salbutamol
Sodium Valproate
Spironolactone
Terbutaline
Theophylline slow
Vitamins B complex and C
Warfarin

2. **Drugs which definitely should not be administered to nursing mothers:**
Aspirin (*regular dosage*)
Atropine (*in some gastrointestinal sedatives/antispasmodics*)
Belladonna (*as for Atropine*)
Carbimazole (*Neo-Mercazole*)
Danthron (*Dorbanex*)
Gold injection (*Myocrisin*)
Hyoscine (*as for Atropine*)
Hyoscyamine (*as for Atropine*)
Iodides
Meprobamate
Phenindione (*Dindevan*)
Reserpine (*Serpasil, Decaserpyl*)
Senna (*Senokot*)
Tetracyclines
Thiazide diuretics

It is worth also looking at this problem from another viewpoint and taking selected drug groups in turn:

1. **Anti-inflammatory and analgesic drugs:**

   a. None of the non-steroidal anti-inflammatory drugs is absolutely contraindicated.

   b. Breast milk concentration of opiates such as morphine and diamorphine are very low and unless the mother takes high doses there is negligible effect on the breast-fed baby. However, the infants appear to be particularly affected by the constipating action of these drugs.

   c. In high dosage salicylates given to the mother may cause skin rash and a bleeding tendency in the child.

d.   Gold injections given to the mother may produce skin rash in the infant.

2. **Anticoagulants:**
   a.   Phenindione has produced fatal haematoma in one infant.
   b.   Warfarin may safely be taken by nursing mothers.
   c.   Heparin, although excreted in breast milk, is inactivated in the infant's gastrointestinal tract and is therefore safe.

3. **Anti-infective agents:**
   a.   Sulphonamides if given to the mother may lead to jaundice in the infant. They are relatively contraindicated.
   b.   Penicillin and cephalosporin antibiotics may be given. Very few problems are likely to arise although diarrhoea and hypersensitivity reactions may occur.
   c.   Erythromycin, Ethambutol, Rifampicin and Metronidazole have safely been given to breast-feeding mothers.
   d.   Isoniazid enters breast milk in high concentration and produces restlessness and neuropathies. The drug should not be given unless prophylactic vitamin B_6, supplements are given to the child.
   e.   Chloramphenicol even in low doses can produce serious toxic effects in the infant and an alternative drug should be used, or if this is not possible breast feeding should be stopped.
   f.   Tetracyclines are not thought to be safe for administration to breast-feeding mothers as they may, via this route, affect the growth of long bones and stain teeth in infants.
   g.   Nitrofurantoin will accumulate in infants of breast-feeding mothers who receive this drug and, therefore, it should not be given.
   h.   Aminoglycoside antibiotics (Gentamicin, Kanamycin, Amikacin) are destroyed in the gastrointestinal tract of breast-fed infants and, therefore, are safe.

4. **Drugs acting on the central nervous system:**
   a.   Major tranquillizers of the Phenothiazine group (q.v.), Halo-peridol (q.v.) and Tricyclic antidepressant drugs (q.v.) may be safely used during the nursing period.
   b.   Of the benzodiazepines, Diazepam has been most widely studied and it is quite clear that the drug accumulates in breast-fed infants and may produce lethargy and weight loss. It also prolongs neonatal jaundice. It is, therefore, relatively contraindicated.

    c. Meprobamate produces high levels in breast milk and is contraindicated.

    d. Barbiturates are excreted in breast milk and cause drowsiness in the infant. They are therefore relatively contraindicated.

    e. Phenytoin has caused methaemoglobinaemia in one infant.

    f. Carbamazepine and sodium valproate appear safe but information is limited.

5. **Drugs acting on the cardiovascular system:**

    a. Diuretics suppress lactation by producing dehydration. There is also a risk of thrombocytopenia in the infant. Spironolactone, however, may be taken safely.

    b. There is no evidence that beta-blockers are harmful to the infant.

    c. Reserpine, a drug now rarely used, is relatively contraindicated because it produces nasal stuffiness and increased bronchial secretions in the infant.

    d. Methyldopa appears to be safe for administration to nursing mothers.

    e. Guanethidine does not appear to enter breast milk and is, therefore, safe for administration to nursing mothers.

    f. Digoxin enters breast milk in such low concentrations that it would appear safe for administration to breast-feeding mothers.

    g. Ergot and its derivatives used for the treatment of migraine are contraindicated as side-effects may be produced in the infant.

6. **Corticosteroids and other hormonal agents:**

    a. If drugs of this group are taken in physiological doses, i.e. replacement therapy, there is little risk to breast-fed infants. However, there is a potential risk of growth retardation if doses are higher than those of physiological replacement doses.

    b. The very low doses of oestrogens contained in most oral contraceptives present little risk to the breast-fed infant. However, oestrogens will tend to suppress lactation.

    c. Thyroxine and liothyronine are used to replace a physiological deficit and do not cause problems in the suckling infant. However, iodides and Carbimazole may produce goitre. Propylthiouracil appears to be useful in low dose, provided the circulating thyroid hormones in the baby are regularly checked.

    d. Of the oral hypoglycaemic drugs studied, only small amounts of Tolbutamide and Phenformin have been detected and these do not appear to affect the infant's blood glucose.

7. **Gastrointestinal drugs:**

   a. Anthraquinone laxatives such as Senna and Danthron (q.v.) can produce diarrhoea in breast-fed infants. Thus, non-absorbable bulk laxatives such as bran or Methylcellulose are preferable.

   b. Cimetidine, widely used for the treatment of peptic ulcer disease, is present in breast milk in high concentrations, Thus it is relatively contraindicated as long term effects of such exposure are not as yet known.

   c. Anticholinergic drugs do not appear to cause problems.

   d. Antacids do not appear to cause problems.

   e. Metoclopramide may be safely taken and may in fact increase milk flow.

   f. The anti-diarrhoeal preparation 'Lomotil' contains diphenoxylate and atropine, both of which could have profound effects on the breast-fed infant and is therefore contraindicated.

8. **Respiratory drugs:**

   a. Xanthine drugs, i.e. Aminophylline, Theophylline etc., when given to mothers may produce irritability, insomnia and fretfulness in the infant. In general, oral, slow-release xanthine preparations are less likely to produce this effect and, therefore, are relatively safer.

   b. Drugs taken by inhalation in asthma, chronic bronchitis such as beta agonists (Salbutamol, Terbutaline) and steroids Beclomethasone produce minimal blood levels and, therefore, appear safe.

9. **Vitamins and mineral supplements:**

   a. Fat soluble vitamins A and D, if taken in excess, may accumulate in the breast-fed infant and produce symptoms of hypervitaminosis.

   b. There are no such problems with water soluble vitamins (B complex and vitamin C).

   c. Iron preparations appear safe.

   d. Folate preparations appear safe.

   e. It is interesting to note that mothers who are thiamine deficient (i.e. have beri-beri) produce milk which is toxic to infants.

10. **Social factors:**

Nicotine and regular high alcohol consumption reduce milk flow. A high alcohol intake may also produce CNS depression and reduce clotting factor synthesis in the infant.

Note 5

OPHTHALMIC PREPARATIONS

INTRODUCTION

The following definitions are frequently encountered when dealing with ophthalmic preparations:

1. **Accommodation:**   The means by which the eye adapts for near or distant vision.

2. **Cycloplegia:**   Paralysis of accommodation.

3. **Myosis:** Constriction of the pupil (usually performed in clinical practice to facilitate drainage of ocular fluid in the treatment of glaucoma).

4. **Mydriasis:**   Dilatation of the pupil (usually performed to facilitate the examination of the interior of the eye).

Actions and uses

There are five major groups of ophthalmic preparations:

1. Those used to treat ophthalmic infection:

   a. Antibacterial drugs: Tetracycline, Chloramphenicol, Aminoglycosides, Sulphacetamide.

   b. Antiviral drugs: Idoxuridine, Vidarabine, Acyclovir.

These drugs are primarily to treat superficial infection of the eye and the surrounding structures.

2. To reduce inflammation and allergic inflammatory response. There are four groups of drugs useful for the treatment of inflammation and allergy:

   a. Corticosteroids, including Betamethasone, Dexamethasone, Hydrocortisone, Prednisolone

   b. Non-steroidal anti-inflammatory drugs, including Oxyphenbutazone, and Zinc Sulphate

   c. Antihistamines including Xylometazoline and Antazoline

   d. Sodium Cromoglycate.

The first two groups of drugs are used primarily for the treatment of inflammatory disorders, whereas the latter two are used for the treatment of allergic conditions.

3. **Drugs used in the management of glaucoma** (*raised intraocular pressure*):

    Glaucoma may be treated by oral administration of drugs (see Acetazolamide and Dichlorphenamide) or by topical applications which include: Adrenaline acid tartrate 0.5%, 1% and 2% (Simplene); Adrenaline (neutral) 1% (Eppy); Carbachol 3% (Isopto Carbachol); Demacarium 0.25% and 0.5% (Tosmelin); Ecthiopate 0.03%, 0.06%, 0.125% and 0.25% (Phospholine); Guanethidine 5.0% (Ismelin); Neostigmine 3% (Prostigmin); Physostigmine 1% (Eserine); Pilocarpine 1%, 2%, 3% and 4%; Timolol 0.25% and 0.5% (Timoptol).

4. **Drugs used to aid examination of the eye and operative techniques:**

    a. *Mydriatics and cycloplegics:* These drugs are used in the preoperative preparation of the eye, for refraction ophthalmoscopy and photography of the fundus. They include: Atropine sulphate 1% and 2%; Cyclopentolate 0.1%, 0.5% and 1%; Homatropine hydrobromide 1% and 2%; Hyoscine hydrobromide 0.2%; Phenylephrine 10%; Tropicamide 0.5% and 1%

    b. *Local anaesthetics:* These drugs are applied to the eye before minor ophthalmic surgery, prior to removal of foreign bodies and during other investigative procedures. They include: Amethocaine 0.5% and 1%; Cocaine (various strengths); Benoxinate 0.4%; Lignocaine 4%

    c. *Stains:* Staining the surface of the eye assists in the identification of corneal lesions and the presence of foreign bodies. Common stains are: Fluorescein sodium 2%, Rose Bengal 1%.

5. **In the treatment of anterior uveitis:**

    Mydriatics: e.g. Atropine sulphate 1% and 2%; Cyclopentolate 0.1%, 0.5% and 1%; Homatropine hydrobromide 1% and 2%; Hyoscine hydrobromide 0.2%.

Nurse monitoring

1. Most drugs available for direct application to the eye will come in the form of single dose units (minims) without an added bactericide, or as a multidose bottle, in which case they will have a bactericide and fungicide added. Multidose containers should be discarded after:

    a.   24 hours if used in an operating theatre.

    b.   1 week from the date of opening if used in a hospital ward.

    c.   4 weeks from the date of opening when used in domiciliary practice.

2.   It is always worth noting that to prevent cross-contamination from an infected eye to the other eye, in hospital use one bottle should be made available for the treatment of each eye, and should be labelled so that each bottle is applied to the appropriate eye.

Note 6

CHRONIC CANCER PAIN AND ITS CONTROL

Pain is a major sign or symptom of disease which can significantly compromise patient well-being and increase morbidity. Failure to appreciate its significance and so provide adequate pain control is widely recognised in many situations, in particular chronic pain associated with cancer.

Types of Pain

Pain may be defined as an unpleasant sensory and emotional experience associated with actual or potential tissue damage or described in terms of such damage. Chronic pain associated with cancer is quite distinct from the more commonly experienced acute pain. It may be difficult to describe or locate and is usually perceived by patients as an "endless" experience for which there is no adequate explanation. The different characteristics of acute and chronic pain can be summarized as follows:

Acute pain	Chronic pain
Transient intensity	Persistent, unvarying
Acts as a warning	Serves no useful purpose
Decreases	Tends to increase
Autonomic disturbance	Often no autonomic disturbance
Patient voices complaint	Often no complaint
Patient seeks help urgently	Often no help sought
Patient often anxious	Patient usually depressed

Types of Chronic Pain

This may have an important influence on its management. Three sub-divisions can be identified:

1. *Nociceptive pain:* In which there is stimulation of peripheral or visceral nociception or 'pain sensors' by noxious stimuli with information transferred centrally to the brain by an intact, normal functioning nervous system.

2. *Neurogenic pain:* Usually damage to the peripheral or central nervous system with interruption of nerve function e.g. post-herpetic neuralgia, as a result of damage to large nerve fibres by the shingles virus, or pain following trauma to a peripheral nerve. Neurogenic pain is often described as "burning" or "shooting" and may be associated with dysaesthesia (unpleasant sensation) and allodynia (pain from a stimulus which is not usually "painful").

3. *Psychogenic pain:* Psychological or psychiatric disturbance. This does not mean that the patient is not suffering pain and empathy, understanding, diversion and mood elevation are essential in addition to analgesic drug therapy.

Pain Assessment

Many pain-rating scales, questionnaires and other assessment criteria have been devised. Some are simple (e.g. linear analogue scale) while others are complex, extensive and demanding of patient and staff time and therefore are unworkable. In fact, pain is very subjective and pain tolerance varies widely between individuals so that it is difficult to uniformly apply good objective criteria in its assessment. Important points in assessing pain are as follows:

1. Believe the patient's reporting of pain. Objective parameters of acute pain such as tachycardia, sweating, pallor, or facial grimacing are helpful when present, but are often absent in chronic pain.

2. Sit, listen and reassure the patient that their pain can be controlled. Ask and observe. Do not wait for the patient to complain. Remember: patients with chronic pain do not always look as though they are "in pain".

3. Take a careful pain history including: duration, location and quality. Assess the effect of pain on the patient's mood and how it affects day-to-day activities. Does the pain interfere with sleeping, eating or movement?

4. Take a careful analgesic history including: present and past medication, response to analgesic therapy and the occurrence of side-effects.

5. If analgesics are indicated, regular and adequate dosage i.e. titrated against the individual's pain tolerance should be prescribed. The aim is to prevent recurrence of pain rather than to treat it after it arises and there is no place for "as required" analgesia, except to cover occasional breakthrough pain. Should this be frequently required it is a signal to increase regular analgesia.

6. **Set realistic goals. For example:**
    a. Achieve a pain-free, full night's sleep initially.
    b. Then maintain pain relief during the following day.
    c. Lastly, obtain freedom from pain on movement. May be difficult to achieve if there is skeletal instability, soft tissue inflammation, or infiltration by tumour.

7. Re-evaluate frequently (e.g. daily) using a pain scale/assessment tool where possible to determine success of treatment. Remember also that the increasing use of "as required" analgesics indicates the need for re-assessment of regular analgesia.

Prescribing Analgesia

Analgesic therapy of chronic pain should be prescribed according to three basic criteria, as follows:

1. **By mouth**
    Make adequate use of the oral route. It is frequently abandoned too soon. Remember that the sublingual route provides rapid onset of analgesia and avoids pre-systemic elimination by the liver (first pass metabolism).

2. **By the clock**
    The need for regular rather than 'prn' analgesia cannot be overemphasized. Most oral analgesics act for about 4 hours and should therefore be prescribed 4-hourly. Pain is increasingly difficult to control if frequent breakthrough is allowed to occur.

3. **By the ladder**
    The concept of an analgesic ladder, the steps of which represent analgesia of increasing strength, provides a helpful guide. If a single drug on one step does not control pain it is important to move up a step rather than persist with inadequate analgesic therapy.

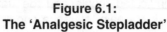

Figure 6.1:
The 'Analgesic Stepladder'

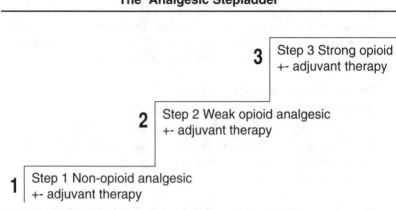

Note: The term "opioid" denotes a drug of the morphine family whether it be a low potency analgesic such as dihydrocodeine or a strongly analgesic drug such as diamorphine. Adjuvant therapy refers to the use of drugs other than recognised analgesics which may however modify the patient's response to pain. In particular this includes drugs for neurogenic pain (discussed later) and anti-emetics, laxatives, sedatives, etc.

Choice of Analgesic Drug

Step 1. Non-opioid analgesic, e.g. Paracetamol.

Step 2. Weak opioid, e.g. Dihydrocodeine or Co-proxamol.

Step 3. Strong opioid. Morphine is the standard oral agent. Diamorphine is usually the standard drug by subcutaneous injection.

While paracetamol, dihydrocodeine and co-proxamol are used in standard dosage, the required dose of morphine often varies and can be tailored to the individual by careful titration against response. Thus morphine is a "high ceiling" drug for which there is no maximum dosage.

Initial Prescription

When moving to Step 3 on the analgesic ladder it must not be assumed that dosage should initially be very low. For example, start with Morphine Mixture 4-hourly (e.g. 5–10mg, with lower doses for elderly or cachectic patients) then titrate the dose against the patient's pain tolerance. A suggested dosage increment scale is given in Figure 6.2.

Figure 6.2
Suggested morphine dosage incremental scale

300 mg etc

210 mg

180 mg

150 mg

120 mg

90 mg

60 mg

45 mg

30 mg

20 mg

15 mg

10 mg

5 mg

Once pain control has been achieved and the dosage stabilized, conversion to Sustained Release Morphine Sulphate tablets (e.g. MST Continus) is possible. To convert, calculate the total daily dose of oral morphine and give half this dose 12-hourly.

e.g. — Morphine HCl Mixture 30 mg 4-hourly = 180 mg in 24 hours = 90 mg MST Tablets 12-hourly

N.B. — Remember to give the first dose of MST together with the last dose of Morphine Mixture. This covers the period it takes for MST to achieve adequate morphine plasma levels (approximately 4 hours) and reduces the likelihood of breakthrough pain during this time.

Tolerance and Addiction

Addiction to morphine is rarely, if ever, seen in patients with advanced cancer. However, psychological dependence is often mistakenly inferred by the patient's "craving" for the few pain-free periods which may be achieved by inadequate analgesic therapy. Thus when patients regularly demand medication, rather than assume addiction a complete review of analgesic therapy would seem more appropriate. Tolerance to the analgesic effect of the opioids may develop after the first few months of treatment but is easily overcome by relatively small dosage increments.

There is evidence that a plateau is reached thereafter when effective analgesia can be maintained for longer periods at fixed dosage. Increased dosage may however be necessary where there is an increase in the level of pain due to an extension of the disease. Similarly, tolerance to narcotic-induced drowsiness and nausea rapidly occurs and is a useful phenomenon.

Alternatives to Oral Morphine

Drug/strength to 10mg oral morphine	Dose equiv:	Comments
Dextromoramide 5 mg tablet	5 mg	Sublingual—rapid onset/brief duration (2–3 hours). Useful for painful procedure (dressing change, bathing, etc) and for breakthrough pain
Phenazocine 5 mg tablets	2.5 mg	Oral or sublingual 4–6 hourly. Less nausea and constipation than with morphine
Rectal morphine	15 mg 30 mg supps:	Use oral morphine dose as a guide. Insert 4-hourly and titrate against pain tolerance

Parenteral Analgesic Therapy

Diamorphine is now frequently administered by continuous subcutaneous infusion (CSI). Subcutaneous injections are more comfortable for patients and are easily administered, especially to patients with poor veins or little muscle bulk. Continuous infusion provides regular analgesia without the discomfort of frequent injections and the dose is readily titrated against the individual's pain tolerance and within narrow therapeutic limits (i.e. any high peak/low trough effect is eliminated). It is also cost effective in terms of nursing time and the overall use of disposables. Modern syringe drivers are relatively inexpensive, non-bulky and readily portable.

When is parenteral therapy required?

CSI is not a universal method of delivering analgesia and it does not replace the oral or sublingual routes. It is an alternative which is available should these first line routes of administration become impractical or impossible. It has been mistakenly assumed in the past that injections are necessary for all patients with severe pain though, in fact, oral analgesics are equally effective in equipotent dosage.

Subcutaneous diamorphine should however be considered in the following situations:

1. Where patients can no longer tolerate oral therapy due to nausea, vomiting, or dysphagia

2. Where patients are very drowsy, comatose or semi-comatose.

3. Where patients experience adverse effects related to high peak levels soon after dosing (drowsiness, nausea, hallucinations, etc.) and/orbreakthrough pain before the next dose, i.e. to smooth out a high peak/low trough profile.

4. For patients whose analgesic requirements would involve the use of excessive numbers of tablets.

5. For patients at home, to facilitate the supervision of regular parenteral analgesia. This is easily managed by the community nurse visiting on a daily basis.

The above does not cover all contingencies and there may be other situations where CSI is considered.

The possibility of re-establishing patients on oral therapy should be considered once an acute problem necessitating parenteral dosing has been resolved. It is recognized that some derive great psychological benefit from syringe drivers and may be reluctant to return to oral therapy. This is not a sign of drug dependence: it is more likely to indicate the efficacy of the subcutaneous route coupled with a fear of recurring severe pain.

The Role of Diamorphine

As hydrochloride, diamorphine is fifteen times more soluble than morphine so that very small volumes can be injected at any dosage level. For example, 120 mg diamorphine can be administered in as little as 0.2 ml water and most single doses are soluble in less than 0.1 ml. With morphine, on the other hand, dosage may become a limiting factor due to the volume required to be administered at higher dosage.

Diamorphine is also widely preferred to morphine because of its more favourable pharmacokinetics and useful sedative properties. Although it is eventually converted to morphine its rate of distribution to the tissues (as 6–0-acetylmorphine) is much more rapid so that its onset of action is faster, and more intense, albeit slightly briefer. The potency ratio of diamorphine to morphine is 2:3 i.e. 2 mg diamorphine has the analgesic potency of 3 ml morphine.

Dosage of Diamorphine by CSI

For any patient, the diamorphine requirement is only established by careful titration of dose against the individual's pain tolerance.

When transferring from oral morphine the '3:2:1 Rule' (below) is a useful guide:

$$3 \text{ mg oral} \quad = \quad 2 \text{ mg oral} \quad = \quad 1 \text{ mg s.c.}$$

morphine   diamorphine   diamorphine

Therefore, one-third of the total daily dose of oral morphine is used initially as a guide.

Some examples are given below.

Table 6.3:
Total daily dose (mg)

Oral morphine	Subcutaneous diamorphine for breakthrough pain*	Dose of s.c. diamorphine
90	30	5
120	40	5
150	50	10
180	60	10
240	80	15
300	100	20

*It is good practice to prescribe additional bolus s.c. doses of diamorphine, approximately 1/6th of the total daily dose, 3-hourly prn for breakthrough pain. In this way effective pain control can be maintained even if, for any reason, pain increases e.g. as a result of extension of the disease itself or worsening of other signs or symptoms. Regular need for additional doses is a signal that total analgesic therapy should be reviewed. Also, remember to give a stat s.c. bolus "loading" dose (1/6th of the 24-hour dose) when setting up a syringe driver.

Stability of admixtures for subcutaneous infusion

Mixtures of diamorphine and various adjuvant drugs have been administered in day-to-day practice in response to patient need although extensive stability data are generally lacking. Nevertheless experience has shown that few, if any, problems arise if attention is paid to the following:

1. Drug combinations should be used within 24 hours of admixture.
2. Visual inspection of the mixture to detect signs of flocculation or precipitation, particularly when higher doses of diamorphine are used, is essential.

Adverse effects of diamorphine administered by CSI

This is generally a well tolerated method of administering analgesia. In a proportion of patients however, usually those receiving higher doses of diamorphine, the appearance of small areas of redness, induration and swelling at the injection site has been noted, often necessitating re-siting of the needle. Biopsies show formation of sterile granulomas and exclude an infective cause. It seems likely therefore that the reaction is due to some property of the solution itself (chemical irritancy, pH, osmolarity, etc.) or a degradation product, or perhaps to the needle in situ. Experience has shown that 1,500 i.u. hyaluronidase added to the syringe will reduce the reaction, presumably by hastening removal of the drug from its site of administration. So far chemical incompatibility between hyaluronidase and other syringe contents has not been noted. An alternative method is to infuse the mixture via a 22 gauge blue (e.g. Venflon) i.v. cannula which is sited subcutaneously but it is important to note that these may "kink" and interrupt the flow of drug.

Additional Therapy

1. *Treatment of neurogenic pain*
    a. Pain due to nerve destruction i.e. 'burning' pain or superficial hyperaesthesia.

A tricyclic or related antidepressant e.g. **amitriptyline** (dose: up to 75 mg daily, but start with 25 mg at night for elderly subjects) may be useful in relieving the "burning" element of this type of pain. Sedation and anticholinergic side-effects (blurred vision, dry mouth, etc) may limit its usefulness.

    b. Pain due to nerve compression or infiltration by tumour.

An anticonvulsant e.g. **sodium valproate** (dose: 200 mg tid), may be useful in relieving the 'stabbing' or 'shooting' element.

    c.   Nerve compression pain, headache due to raised intracranial pressure, or pain associated with stretched liver capsule.

A corticosteroid e.g. **dexamethasone** (dose: 2–4 mg tid for stretched liver capsule: 16 mg daily, or higher dose if necessary, for raised intracranial pressure).

    d.   Pain associated with tenesmus.

A phenothiazine e.g. **chlorpromazine** (dose: 25–50 mg tid).

2.   *Treatment of other types of pain.*

    a.   Metastatic bone pain.

Radiotherapy is first line treatment but the inflammatory component of this pain may respond to a non-steroidal anti-inflammatory drug (NSAID) also. Common examples of NSAIDs include **naproxen** 500 mg bd, **diclofenac** 50 mg bd, **ketoprofen** 100 mg bd and **indomethacin** 50 mg tid (suggested doses only; slow-release forms also exist).

    b.   Pain associated with smooth muscle spasm.

The anticholinergic, antispasmodic **hyoscine butylbromide** (dose: 20 mg qid) may relieve colicky pain in the bowel and ureter.

    c.   Pain associated with spinal infiltration and skeletal muscle spasm.

Baclofen, an antispasmodic which inhibits reflex voluntary muscle spasm may be tried. The dose is established by careful titration from a starting dose of 5 mg tid gradually increased (every 3 days) up to a maximum of 20 mg tid, until control is achieved.

    d.   Pain associated with soft tissue infection.

Cellulitis is treated with an appropriate antibiotic e.g. oral **flucloxacillin** 250 mg qid, **clindamycin** 300 mg qid or **co-amoxiclav** 2 tablets tid (parenteral benzylpenicillin or flucloxacillin may be required).

Note 7

HIV AND THE ACQUIRED IMMUNE DEFICIENCY SYNDROME (AIDS)

INTRODUCTION

Since the first case of AIDS was described in 1981 in America the disease, as anticipated, has spread rapidly throughout communities worldwide but actual numbers of HIV positive subjects in the U.K. and deaths from AIDS have fallen far short of those predicted at the outset. This has probably been due, at least in part, to the widespread publication of advice and warnings on HIV transmission, to the introduction of other initiatives such as needle exchange programmes in the community and "safe sex" promotion and to the advances which have been made in patient care which have improved survival. However some major issues remain unresolved—it is still uncertain what the implications of being identified as a carrier of the HIV virus are in terms of the likelihood of developing the various clinical manifestations, and of survival overall and although major routes of transmission have been defined, the true incidence of heterosexual spread and occupational spread remain unknown. Importantly, there is still no commercial vaccine against the disease available although active research continues.

Nurses have become more and more involved in communicating with the public on issues related to AIDS and it is important to remember that what we may be learning about the disease today may change in the very near future. It therefore remains the responsibility of all health care professionals to try to maintain an up-to-date knowledge of HIV/AIDS so that they may effectively execute their role of communication with and education of the public.

Below are summarized some of the most important aspects of the disease from the nurses' points of view.

NURSE MONITORING

1. Transmission of the disease

The four main ways of contracting the disease are:

    a. Sexual intercourse (anal, oral and vaginal).

    b. Contaminated needles (intravenous drug abuse, injections, needlestick injuries).

    c. Transmission from mother to child (*in utero*, at birth, and possibly via breast milk).

    d. Organ/tissue donations (semen, kidneys, skin, bone marrow, corneas, heart valves etc.).

Since a test for the carrier state has been developed, the risk of receiving a blood transfusion containing infected blood has been much reduced. However, as there is a latent period of some weeks between infection and development of antibodies in the blood, there is still a theoretical, if minimal, risk of contracting the disease by blood transfusion.

Whereas in the early stages of the disease transmission was mainly between homosexual sexual partners, the spread of the disease into the intravenous drug abusing population has led to an increase in female cases. As it is possible for a male to contract the disease from an infected female and a female from an infected male, further spread into the heterosexual population may be anticipated.

It should be noted that it is currently considered safe to share washing equipment (including swimming pools), eating and drinking utensils and toilet facilities with infected individuals.

2. Clinical manifestations

    a. Following infection with HIV there is a lag or latent period before symptoms develop. The exact time course is not yet clear—estimates range from periods of up to 1 year to very much longer. The percentage of people who, after becoming HIV positive, subsequently develop the disease and eventually die has not yet been accurately assessed.

    b. The full-blown disease is caused by a virus-induced cellular immune deficiency and as a result, multiple and variable infections and cancers may occur. It is in the prevention and treatment of these that major advances have been made.

Some patients have developed symptoms of the syndrome but without occurrence of opportunistic infection, and this is known as AIDS-related complex (ARC). In other patients the only symptom may be a persistent generalized lymphadenopathy (PGL). It is currently considered that patients with both ARC and PGL are likely eventually to develop the full-blown disease syndrome.

3. Drugs used in HIV patients

Since HIV causes a gradual destruction of the immune system characterized by depletion of CD4 lymphocytes, the patient becomes susceptible to opportunistic infections and certain neoplastic disorders. HIV also infects the central nervous system and causes a variable loss of neuronal tissue. Measurement of the CD4 lymphocyte count (normally 0.5–1.0 x 10^9/litre) helps to select patients who will benefit from zidovudine and newer antiviral drugs and allows prediction of the opportunistic infections which are likely to occur. The combination of antiviral therapy and appropriate antimicrobial prophylactic regimens has revolutionized the management of HIV over the past five years. The major benefits to the patient include prolonged survival and reduction in the number of days spent in hospital.

a. *Antiviral drugs*

Zidovudine continues to be the antiviral drug of first choice. It is indicated for the following groups:

i. Asymptomatic HIV infection with a CD4 lymphocyte count of less than 0.5 x 10^9 and falling, although some specialists argue that treatment should be delayed until there is clear evidence of disease progression.

ii. CD4 lymphocyte count of less than 0.5 x 10^9 accompanied by HIV related symptoms.

iii. HIV related thrombocytopenia.

iv. HIV dementia where much higher than normal doses are used.

Newer antiviral drugs, which should be commercially available at the time of publication of this edition, include **didanosine** (ddI) and **zalcitabine** (ddC). Their action is similar to that of zidovudine with which they are, at present, given in combination in order to limit the development of resistance. Neither drug produces the bone marrow suppression with which zidovudine is associated but both may cause a painful peripheral neuropathy and didanosine therapy carries the additional risk of acute pancreatitis.

b. *Prophylactic antimicrobial agents*

These are indicated when either the CD4 lymphocyte count falls below a predetermined value or when the patient has suffered an acute opportunistic infection and needs long-term secondary prevention to avoid relapses. They are intended as life-long therapies and should not be discontinued.

i. CD4 count less than 0.2 x 10^9/litre

Pneumocystis carinii pneumonia (PCP) prophylaxis should be started. **Co-trimoxazole** in a single daily dose of two tablets taken on three days per week or a similar sulphonamide-containing combination (e.g. **Fansidar**, taken as a single weekly dose of one tablet) is indicated. These drugs also prevent the occurrence of other life-threatening infections such as cerebral toxoplasmosis and certain gastrointestinal infections. About 5–10% of patients who develop allergy to sulphonamide (mainly skin rashes) may receive instead various combinations of **dapsone** and/or **pyrimethamine** and/or **trimethoprim**. Nebulized **pentamidine** (administered once per month) has fallen from favour because there is little evidence that it is any better and it is expensive and requires to be given via specialized equipment under close supervision.

Oesophageal candidiasis can be prevented by daily dosing with the antifungal drugs **fluconazole, itraconazole** or **ketoconazole** which, in order to limit development of resistance, may be given in turn on a rotational basis.

ii. CD4 count less than 0.1 x 10^9/litre.

Cryptococcal meningitis prophylaxis should be started using high dose **fluconazole**, 200 mg daily. Oral absorption and/or penetration into the CSF of itraconazole and ketoconazole is however unreliable in patients with this degree of immunodeficiency.

iii. Use of **acyclovir** when CD4 count less than 0.2 x 10^9/litre.

Acyclovir has been tried in a variety of dosages e.g. 800 mg twice daily, to improve survival, with mixed results. It is effective in preventing infections caused by the Herpes simplex and Herpes zoster viruses and it also appears to control oral hairy leukoplakia though the mechanism for this is uncertain.

c. *Treatment of opportunistic infections.*

Major opportunistic infections which may arise despite prophylactic measures and which are treated under specialist supervision include the following.

i. Acute pneumocystis pneumonia.

High dose **co-trimoxazole** with up to 16 tablets administered daily is required. The addition of **prednisolone** (e.g. 60 mg daily) further dramatically reduces mortality during the acute illness by preventing respiratory failure and also reduces pulmonary fibrosis during recovery.

The optimum length of treatment is unclear but usually the patient can revert to prophylactic co-trimoxazole (see above) after three weeks.

ii.   CMV (cytomegalovirus) infection.

Ganciclovir is a more effective yet more toxic analogue of acyclovir for use in CMV infection. It is administered by i.v. infusion in 100 ml sodium chloride 0.9% or glucose 5% over 1 hour: initially in a dose of 5 mg/kg twice daily for 2-3 weeks, then once daily to prevent relapse. Neutropenia, especially in patients already taking zidovudine, is a major risk with this drug. **Foscarnet** is an alternative which is administered in a loading dose of 20 mg/kg followed by continuous infusion of up to 200 mg/kg/day in 500 ml to 1 litre of dextrose 5% **only.**

d.   *Treatment of malignancies.*

The management of HIV related **Kaposi's sarcoma** and **lymphomas** is a specialist topic involving cytotoxic chemotherapy. Lymphomas are largely resistant to chemotherapy however, unless the CD4 count is $> 0.2 \times 10^9$/litre i.e. only when there is some functional immunity.

e.   *HIV dementia.*

The incidence of this serious complication has been increasing as the doses of zidovudine have fallen and there is some concern that the current low doses used (e.g. 500 mg daily) may be insufficient to produce adequate concentrations of zidovudine in the central nervous system.

4.   **Nursing the patient**

a.   As most patients with AIDS suffer symptoms of the secondary manifestations, they require considerable nursing care and support for their infections and cancers. The nurse may make a major contribution towards the well-being of the patients by providing excellent quality nursing care and interpersonal skills.

b.   All nurses working within the hospital environment should be aware of local policies for handling blood, body fluids and materials contaminated with the AIDS virus. Otherwise it should be pointed out that effective guidelines for dealing with the Hepatitis B virus should also adequately protect against HIV. Briefly the following guidelines may be used:

i.   Special clothing need not be worn routinely. Gowns, gloves and masks are necessary when carrying out invasive procedures or when nursing patients requiring protection against infection due to immunosuppression.

ii.   It is advisable for nurses to wear gloves when handling blood and body fluids. As many carriers of the AIDS virus are as yet undetected, the need to wear gloves when handling blood should be extended to handling all blood specimens from all patients.

iii. It is sensible for the nurse to cover any cuts or abrasions, particularly on exposed areas on the hands and face.

iv. The AIDS virus cannot survive for long outside the body and is very sensitive to sodium hypochlorite disinfectants.

Hypochlorite (or more correctly hypochlorous acid) is the disinfectant which is present in household bleaches and 'Milton' and 'Chloros' solutions. For the sake of the nurse, her colleagues and other patients, spillages of potentially infective body fluids should be immediately dealt with using one of these fluids.

Chloros is a simple solution of hypochlorite containing 10% by weight in volume, w/v (10 g in 100 ml). The strength is frequently described in terms of 'available chlorine' using the units 'parts per million' or ppm. A 10% solution contains 100 000 ppm of available chlorine and it should be noted that at this concentration it is corrosive and must be handled with extreme care; avoid skin and, particularly, eye contamination; wash off immediately with copious amounts of tap water if this occurs. Chloros solution is freshly diluted ten times (1 in 10) to produce a 1% solution (containing 10, 000 ppm) for general large surface disinfection, e.g. floors and walls, beds, furniture, etc.

Milton is a stabilized hypochlorite solution (it contains sodium chloride which reduces the release of chlorine, thereby stabilising the solution) which is considerably more expensive than Chloros but provides hypochlorite in a ready to use 1% solution (10 000 ppm). It does not therefore present the same handling hazard as Chloros. Note also that double strength Milton is available (2% or 20 000 ppm) and requires 50/50 dilution before use. Milton is used without dilution as a disinfectant for small surfaces, e.g. benches, trolleys, soaking glassware, etc. and for treating blood spills. It should be poured gently onto blood spills and kept in contact for at least 30 minutes before wiping off. Glassware should be soaked in solution for 2-3 hours or even overnight.

Metal instruments and equipment containing rubber connecting pieces may be chemically damaged by treatment with sodium hypochlorite, so an alternative disinfectant is required. Activated glutaraldehyde (e.g. Cidex), which disinfects by releasing formaldehyde, is a suitable alternative to hypochlorite in such situations. Glutaraldehyde is supplied as a solution which becomes active after the addition of a second chemical; the container should be consulted for details on method of preparation and use.

c. Confidentiality: as with all diseases, confidentiality should be maintained at all times. However, considering the highly emotive and difficult issues that face HIV positive patients from the point of view of their domestic circumstance, their personal relationships and their employment, the nurse should establish with the patient the identity of those who know their diagnosis and to identify who may or may not be informed of the diagnosis. Further, case records which contain information of the diagnosis should be kept with great care.

5. **Prevention**

a. Since there is no effective treatment or immunization available, considerable importance must be placed on prevention of the disease and the nurse, as a health care professional, should familiarize herself with the advice given in Government Health Department and other bodies' pamphlets and educational programmes.

    Considerable publicity has been given to the importance of minimizing sexual contact, particularly with 'at risk' sub-groups of the population and to the use of barrier contraceptives (condoms).

b. Very few cases of contraction of the disease by health care professionals have been recorded. To give an example, if a nurse was subject to a needle-stick injury by blood infected by both Hepatitis antigen and HIV there would be a considerably larger risk of developing Hepatitis than AIDS. However, a small risk remains and therefore careful and vigilant adherence to the basic principles of avoiding contact with infected blood and blood products should prevent occupational exposure.

c. As mentioned above, avoidance of occupational exposure and spread to other patients by the appropriate treatment of areas contaminated by spilled blood or body fluids is highly important.

APPENDICES

Appendix 1

THE SECURITY AND ADMINISTRATION OF MEDICINES IN HOSPITAL

The nurse should be familiar with a few important general points related to the security of medicines in the ward.

1. *All* medicines should be locked up to prevent access by unauthorized persons. This is particularly important where there is freedom of movement for patients in the ward area.
2. Special considerations apply to controlled drugs which are covered by the Misuse of Drugs Act, 1971—they are designated M.D.A. or C.D. These drugs usually have a powerful addictive potential and are particularly liable to misuse or abuse. The following points are important with regard to the storage and administration of controlled drugs.
   a. They should be stored on the ward in a locked cupboard within a locked cupboard and the keys held by the ward sister or nurse-in-charge.
   b. They may *only* be supplied against an order bearing the signature of the ward sister or the nurse-in-charge. For this purpose a special controlled drugs order book is available. When administering to the patient, two nurses, one of whom must be state-registered, check the drug, then an appropriate entry is made in the controlled drugs record book. This entry indicates date and time of administration; the patient's name; the amount given; the amount discarded (if any) and the balance remaining in stock. The entry is made at the time of administration and is witnessed by the second nurse.
   c. The controlled drugs record book indicates the balance remaining in stock of individual preparations and these amounts should be checked regularly against the actual stock in the controlled drugs cupboard.
   d. When checking the amounts of controlled drugs remaining in stock, the nurse should pay particular attention to expiry dates whenever they appear on the label.

e. A hospital pharmacist or ward pharmacist should carry out regular independent checks of controlled drugs against the controlled drugs record book. In addition he/she will take charge of the removal or destruction of out-of-date medicines and supervise the record book entry.

3. Prescription Only Medicines (designated P.O.M.) is a term which indicates that the medicine can only be supplied by the pharmacy on the written order of the ward sister or nurse-in-charge. These drugs must be kept in a locked cupboard although the very strict regulations for controlled drugs (see above) do not apply. The term 'Prescription Only' indicates the need for a doctor's prescription before such medicines are supplied to patients in the community.

4. Oral medicines, injections, ointment, creams and lotions and eye preparations should each be stored in separate areas to avoid confusion when selecting drugs. *Note* that disinfectants must be stored in a separate area away from all medicines.

The Pharmacist should advise on any matter relating to the security and administration of medicines in the ward.

Appendix 2

METRIC WEIGHTS AND OTHER MEASURES

In recent years the introduction of metrication into medical practice has altered the ways in which drug dosages and concentrations, patient data (including height, weight and body surface area), drug levels in the body and other measurements are expressed. The following are those units of measurements which the nurse will commonly encounter in everyday practice.

1. **Weight.** The unit of weight is the kilogram (kg). This is made up of 1000 grams (g) and each gram is composed of 1000 milligrams (mg). Each milligram in turn is composed of 1000 micrograms (μg or mcg)— hence, 1 kg = 1000 g; 1 g = 1000 mg; 1 mg = 1000 μg or mcg. When converting from or to the imperial system 1 kg = 2.2 lb. N.B. Whenever drugs are prescribed in microgram dosages it is good practice to write the units in full i.e., digoxin 250 micrograms, as the use of the contracted terms μg or mcg may in practice be mistaken for mg and as this dose is one thousand times greater, disastrous consequences may follow.

   Drug dosages are often described in terms of unit dose per kg of body weight i.e. mg/kg, μg/kg, etc. This method of dosage is frequently used in paediatric medicine and allows doses to be tailored to the individual patient's size.

2. **Volume.** The unit of volume is the litre which is denoted by the symbol 'l'. One litre comprises 1000 millilitres (ml). Occasionally the term decilitre (dl) is used. 1 l = 10 dl; l dl = 100 ml and 1 l = 1000 ml. When converting from or to the imperial system 1 l = 35.2 fluid ounces (fl oz) or 1 ml = 0.0352 fl oz. The symbols 'l' or 'ml' account for almost all measurements expressed in unit volume for the prescription and administration of drugs.

3. **Concentration.** When expressing concentration or dosages of a medicine in liquid form, several methods are available:

   a. **Unit weight per unit volume:** This describes the unit of weight of a drug contained in unit volume, e.g. 1 mg in 1 ml; 2 mg in 1 l; 40 mg in 2 ml; etc. Examples of drugs in common use expressed in these terms: diazepam injection 10 mg in 1 ml; chloral hydrate mixture 1 g in 10 ml; penicillin suspension 250 mg in 5 ml.

b. **Percentage (weight in volume):** This describes the weight of a drug expressed in grams (g) which is contained in 100 ml or 1 dl of solution. Common examples are: lignocaine hydrochloride injection 2%: this contains 2 g in each 100 ml of solution or 0.2 g (200 mg) in each 10 ml of solution or 0.02 g (20 mg) in each 1 ml of solution, etc. Calcium gluconate injection 10%: this contains 10 g in each 100 ml of solution or 1 g in each 10 ml or 0.1 g (100 mg) in each 1 ml, etc.

c. **Percentage (weight in weight):** This describes the weight of a drug expressed in grams (g) which is contained in 100 g of a solid or semi-solid medicament, e.g. ointments and creams. Examples are: Fucidin ointment 2% which contains 2 g of fusidic acid in each 100 g of ointment; Betnovate cream 25% in Aqueous cream which contains 25 g Betnovate cream mixed with 75 g of Aqueous cream (overall weight 100 g).

d. **Volumes containing '1 part':** A few liquids and to a lesser extent gases, particularly those containing drugs in very low concentrations, are often described as containing 1 part per 'x' units of volume. For liquids 'parts' are equivalent to grams and volume to millilitres, e.g. adrenaline injection 1 in 1000 which contains 1 g in 1000 ml or expressed as a percentage (w/v): 0.1%.

e. **Molar concentration:** Only very occasionally are drugs in liquid form expressed in molar concentration. The mole is the molecular weight of a drug expressed in grams and a one molar (1 M) solution contains this weight dissolved in each litre. More often the term millimole (mmol) is used to describe a medicinal product. 1000 mmol = 1 mole, e.g. potassium chloride solution 15 mmol in 10 ml indicates a solution containing the molecular weight of potassium chloride in milligrams x 15 dissolved in 10 ml of solution. Molar concentrations are most commonly seen in the results of biochemical investigations.

4. **Body height and surface area.** Occasionally drug doses are expressed in terms of microgram, milligram or gram per unit of body surface area. This is frequently the case where precise dosages tailored to individual patient's needs are required. Typical examples may be seen in cytotoxic chemotherapy or in drugs used in paediatric problems. Body surface area is expressed as square metres or m^2 and drug dosages as units/m^2 or units per square metre. Examples are: cytarabine injection 100 mg/m^2 (q.v.); dacarbazine injection 250 mg/m^2 (q.v.). The surface area is calculated from the patient's body weight (in kilograms, kg) and height (in centimetres, cm), as follows:

BODY SURFACE AREA OF CHILDREN
NOMOGRAM FOR DETERMINATION OF BODY SURFACE AREA FROM HEIGHT AND WEIGHT

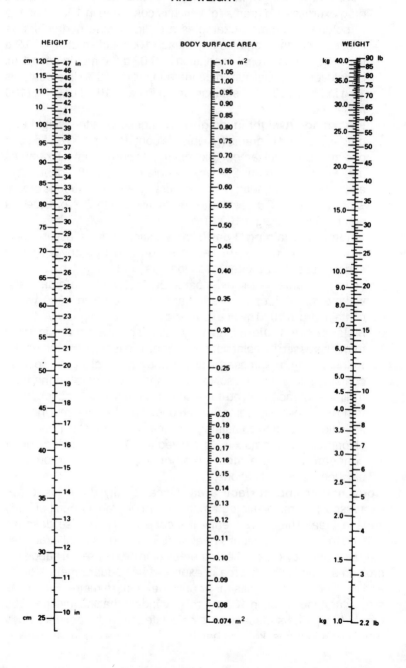

BODY SURFACE AREA OF ADULTS
NOMOGRAM FOR DETERMINATION OF BODY SURFACE AREA FROM HEIGHT AND WEIGHT

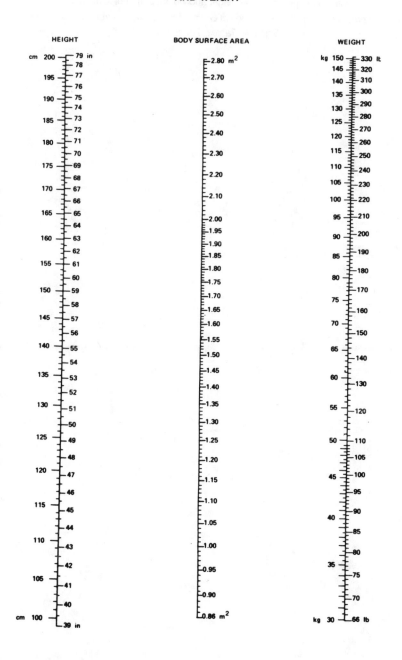

INSTRUCTIONS FOR USE OF TABLE

With a ruler join the points corresponding height and weight. The surface area is then determined by the point at which the central perpendicular line is crossed by the line joining the points on the height and weight perpendicular lines.

(Table reproduced with kind permission of Geigy Pharmaceuticals from Documenta Geigy Scientific Tables, 7th edn. 1970.)

DRUG UPDATE
(arranged alphabetically by approved name)

CISAPRIDE (Alimix, Prepulsid)

Presentation

Tablets—10 mg

Suspension—5 mg in 5 ml

Actions and uses

This drug is often described as a gastrointestinal prokinetic. It is so called because it stimulates gut motility throughout the gastrointestinal tract, from mouth to anus. The precise mechanism of action is not clearly understood. Although cisapride is chemically related to domperidone and metoclopramide, it appears to have a unique action which is related, at least in part, to facilitation of the release or subsequent action of the neurotransmitter substance acetylcholine in the gastrointestinal tract. Cisapride has several uses in practice:

1. It stimulates oesophageal transit and is used therefore in disorders associated with reduced oesophageal motility.
2. It stimulates upper gastrointestinal motility and so increases gastric emptying and is used in the treatment of reflux oesophagitis, gastric stasis and non-ulcer dyspepsia.
3. Its action in the upper gastrointestinal tract, together with a possible inhibitory action on the chemoreceptor trigger zone, make it a useful anti-emetic.
4. Its stimulant action in the colon has led to its use as a laxative.

Dosage

Adults: 10 mg taken two, three or four times a day. A single bedtime dose of 20 mg may be used to treat heartburn.

Children (including neonates) with gastro-oesophageal reflux disorders: 0.1–0.3 mg/kg three times daily.

Nurse monitoring

1. This drug is generally well tolerated but a few problems related to an unwanted increase in gut motility may arise. These include diarrhoea, abdominal cramps and borborygmi.

2. Cisapride should be avoided in those with gastrointestinal obstruction or perforation. It is also contraindicated in pregnancy.
3. Since cisapride increases the rate of gastric emptying it may increase the rate of absorption and so enhance the action of other drugs. It has so far been shown to potentiate the action of warfarin and close monitoring of anticoagulant control is advised.

General note

Cisapride tablets and suspension are stored at room temperature.

FLUCONAZOLE (Diflucan)

Presentation

Capsules—50 mg, 150 mg, 200 mg

Oral suspension—50 mg in 5 ml
200 mg in 5 ml

Injection—50 mg in 25 ml
200 mg in 100 ml

Actions and uses

Fluconazole (like itraconazole) is a member of the triazole group of antifungals which selectively inhibit fungal synthesis of ergosterol, an essential component of the cell wall. Thus leakage of cell contents and eventual death of the fungus follow. In practice fluconazole is used for:

1. Treatment of acute and recurring vaginal candida infection.
2. Oral candidiasis and oropharyngeal and oesophageal candidiasis.
3. Bronchopulmonary candida infections.
4. Systemic candidiasis.
5. *Tinea pedis, tinea corporis, tinea cruris,* tinnea versicolor and dermal candida infections.
6. Cryptococcal infection including meningitis and pulmonary and cutaneous infections.
7. Urinary candidiasis.
8. Prevention of opportunistic fungal infections in immunocompromised patients.

Dosage

Adults:

1. Vaginal candidiasis: Oral 150 mg single dose.

2. Mucosal candidiasis: Oral 50 mg once daily for 1–2 weeks.
3. Denture-related candida infection: Oral 50 mg once daily for 2 weeks in combination with oral antiseptic use.
4. Systemic (disseminated) candida infection: 400 mg initially then 200–400 mg once daily until clinical recovery. May require treatment for 2 months or longer in cryptococcal meningitis infection. Intravenous therapy in acutely ill patients.
5. Prevention of relapse of crypto-coccal meningitis in AIDS patients: 100–200 mg orally once daily may be administered indefinitely.
6. Prevention of fungal infections in 'at risk' or immunocompromised groups: 50–100 mg once daily orally.
7. Tinea and dermal candida infections: 50 mg once daily orally for up to 6 weeks.
Children:
1. Daily doses of up to 12 mg/kg have been administered with a maximum 400 mg/day but experi-ence in children is generally limited.

Nurse monitoring
1. The only common side-effect of this drug is mild gastrointestinal upset (discomfort, nausea, diarrhoea, etc).
2. Since fluconazole is excreted mainly unchanged in the urine the dosage interval should be prolonged to 48 and 72 hourly in patients with moderate and severe renal impairment. Patients on haemodialysis should receive their daily dose immediately after dialysis is completed.
3. Fluconazole potentiates warfarin and the oral hypoglycaemic (antidiabetic) drugs (chlorpropa-mide. glibenclamide, etc). Close monitoring is therefore required to detect any increased bleeding or the development of hypoglycae-mia in patients on warfarin and oral antidiabetic drugs respectively.

4. Concurrent use with phenytoin may lead to accumulation and phenytoin intoxication.
5. Fluconazole significantly increased serum levels of cyclosporim in patients who had undergone renal transplantation.

General notes
1. Fluconazole capsules, oral suspension and injection solution are all stored at room tempera-ture.
2. Once reconstituted, the oral suspension should be refrigerated if possible and used within 2 weeks.
3. Injection solution is administered intravenously undiluted but, if required, it can be mixed with common solutions containing sodium chloride and glucose.

GANCICLOVIR (Cymevene)

Presentation
Injection—vial containing 500 mg powder
Actions and uses
Ganciclovir is an antiviral drug which, like acyclovir, inhibits DNA synthesis. It is however much more active than acyclovir and, in particular, is effective in the treatment of cytomegalovirus (CMV) infections including retinitis. This is reflected in its common adverse effects on rapidly dividing normal cells to the extent that ganciclovir is reserved for the treatment of severe or life-threatening (or sight-threatening) viral infections, especially in the immunocompromised host.
Dosage
1. Treatment of CMV infections: initially, 5 mg/kg every 12 hours for a period of 2–3 weeks. Long-term maintenance treatment for patients at risk of relapse may be administered at a dose of 6 mg/kg/day on 5 days/week, or 5 mg/kg/day on 7 days/week. Re-introduction of the high initial dose may be necessary if there is progressive CMV retinitis.

2. Prevention of CMV infection: initially, 5 mg/kg every 12 hours for 1–2 weeks. Maintenance treatment is then given as above.
Initial doses must be reduced in patients with renal failure. Check with pharmacy.

Nurse monitoring
1. Ganciclovir has notable toxicity. Bone marrow suppression with neutropenia and thrombocytopenia is particularly common and if severe requires dosage reduction.
2. Anaemia, fever, skin rashes and liver dysfunction are reported in about 2% of patients.
3. Other reported adverse effects include alopecia, pruritis, fluctuations in blood pressure, cardiac arrhythmias, ataxia, sleep disturbances, confusion, tremor, and psychosis.
4. Nausea, vomiting, gut pain and bloody diarrhoea may prove troublesome. Haematuria is also reported.
5. Retinal detachment is reported in AIDS patients treated for CMV retinitis.

General notes
1. Vials of ganciclovir must be handled with caution as for cytotoxic drugs. Skin contact, inhalation or ingestion must be avoided.
2. Each vial is reconstituted with 10 ml water for injection (without preservative).
3. Reconstituted vials are then stable for 12 hours at room temperature and must not be refrigerated.
4. The drug is administered by intravenous infusion over 1 hour in 100 ml sodium chloride 0.9% or glucose 5%.

ITRACONAZOLE (Sporanox)
Presentation
Capsules—100 mg
Actions and uses
Itraconazole (like fluconazole) is a member of the triazole group of antifungals which selectively inhibit fungal synthesis of ergosterol, an essential component of the cell wall. Thus leakage of cell contents and eventual death of the fungus follow. In practice itraconazole is used for:
1. Vulvovaginal candidiasis.
2. *Pityriasis versicolor.*
3. Dermatophytic infection e.g. due to Trichophyton spp, Microsporum spp, including *tinea pedis, tinea cruris* and *tinea corporis.*
4. Oropharyngeal candidiasis.
5. Aspergillus infection of the lung.
Dosage
Adults:
1. Vulvovaginal candidiasis: 200 mg 12-hourly for a single day.
2. *Pityriasis versicolor.* 200 mg once daily for 7 days.
3. *Tinea corporis* and *tinea cruris*: 100 mg once daily for 2 weeks.
4. *Tinea pedis, tinea manuum*: 100 mg once daily for 1 month.
5. Oropharyngeal candidiasis: 100 mg once daily (200 mg if immunocompromised) for 2 weeks.
6. Much higher doses are used under specialist supervision for serious aspergillus infection of the lung.

Nurse monitoring
1. The only common side-effects of this drug are mild gastrointestinal upset (discomfort, nausea, diarrhoea, etc), headache and dizziness.
2. Rare cases of hepatitis and cholestatic jaundice have been reported.
3. Itraconazole potentiates warfarin and close monitoring of clotting time is important in anticoagulated subjects.
4. Concurrent use with phenytoin may lead to accumulation of itraconazole.
5. Concurrent use with cimetidine, ranitidine, omeprazole and related drugs may impair the absorption of itraconaziole.

General note
Itraconazole capsules are stored at room temperature and protected from light.

PIPERACILLIN (Pipril)

(See also Note 3, p. 362)

Presentation

Injection—1 g, 2 g and 4 g vials

Actions and uses

This is a broad spectrum antibiotic of the penicillin group which however has notable activity against Gram-negative bacilli, in particular *Pseudomonas aeruginosa*. This has led to its description as an anti-pseudomonal penicillin. Piperacillin is used as follows:

1. In the treatment of severe infections when broad spectrum antibacterial therapy is required, often in combination with other antibiotics such as gentamicin.
2. It is especially useful in neutropenic patients and in other situations in which there is a major risk of infection e.g. cystic fibrosis.
3. It is occasionally used for surgical prophylaxis.

Dosage

Adults and children: Although lower doses may be used for less severe infections, this drug is generally administered in a dose 200–300 mg/kg/day in 3–4 divided doses. Adults with life-threatening infections may receive up to 16 g daily.

Nurse monitoring

1. Since piperacillin is chemically related to the penicillins, cross-hypersensitivity can be anticipated in those with known penicillin allergy.
2. High doses are administered by intravenous infusion. Local irritancy is likely if extravasation occurs and injection sites should be carefully monitored.
3. Dosage reduction is required in patients with renal impairment. Seek advice from the pharmacist.

General notes

1. Piperacillin injection vials are stored at room temperature.
2. Each vial should be reconstituted with 5–10 ml water for injection.

Further dilution in 50–100 ml sodium chloride 0.9%, glucose 5%, or glucose/saline injection and administration over 15–20 minutes is generally recommended.

3. Low doses e. g. 1–2 g can be administered mixed with lignocaine 1% by the intramuscular route.
4. Reconstituted vials are stable for up to 24 hours at room temperature or 48 hours under refrigeration.

TEICOPLANIN (Targocid)

Presentation

Injection—200 mg, 400 mg vials

Actions and uses

Teicoplanin, like vancomycin, is a member of the glycopeptide group of antibiotics. Its uses are therefore very similar to those of vancomycin i.e. treatment of severe or resistant staphylococcal infection of the respiratory tract, skin, soft tissue and bone; septicaemia; and endocarditis. It is generally much better tolerated than vancomycin, can be administered by a variety of routes and has a notably long duration of action which allows for once daily dosage.

Note: Vancomycin is still specifically indicated for the treatment of pseudomembranous colitis associated with the organism *Clostridium difficile*.

Dosage

Teicoplanin may be administered by intramuscular or intravenous bolus injection or by intravenous infusion.

Adults: Severe infection: a loading dose of 400 mg 12-hourly for three doses may be followed by 400 mg once daily maintenance therapy. Maintenance doses of up to 12 mg/kg/day may be required in severely ill or burns patients. Half the above dose may be used in less severe infections in which the intramuscular route can also be used.

Children: 10 mg/kg 12-hourly for three (loading) doses followed by 10 mg/kg/day maintenance therapy.
In less severe infections the maintenance dose can be reduced to 6 mg/kg/day.

Nurse monitoring

1. Unlike vancomycin, injection of this drug is rarely associated with local injection site redness and pain.
2. Allergic skin rashes, fever, pruritis, and wheezing may occur.
3. Gastrointestinal upsets include nausea, vomiting and diarrhoea.
4. Occasionally a reduction in white blood cells and platelets can develop in patients receiving high dose therapy.

---

5. Teicoplanin may produce dizziness and headache but much less so than vancomycin.
6. Minor adjustment in dosage may be required after a few days of treatment in patients with renal impairment. Seek advice from the pharmacy.

General notes

1. Unopened vials may be stored at room temperature.
2. Reconstitute each vial with the ampoule of water for injection provided and allow any foaming to subside before use.
3. Reconstituted vials may be stored for up to 24 hours in a refrigerator.
4. For intravenous infusion the vial contents are further diluted in sodium chloride 0.9% or glucose 5% injection 100 ml and administered over 30 minutes.

DRUG INDEXES

Index 1 Drugs by approved and group name

Drugs appear in the text under their official British or approved name. It should be noted that, with few exceptions, doctors are encouraged to use this title whenever prescribing.

Index 2 Drugs by proprietary and other common names

Axid (Ulcer healing agent) see Nizatidine
Azactam (Antibiotic) see Aztreonam

Bactrim (Antibacterial) see
Co-Trimoxazole
Banocide (Anthelmintic) see
Diethylcarbamazine
Baxan (Antibiotic) see Cefadroxil
Baycaron (Diuretic) see Mefruside
Beconase (Corticosteroid) see
Beclomethasone
Becotide (Corticosteroid) see
Beclomethasone
Belladonna (Antimuscarinic,
anticholinergic) see Atropine
Benemid (Urate lowering drug and
penicillin potentiator) see Probenecid
Benoral (Analgesic) see Benorylate
Berotec (Bronchodilator) see Fenoterol
Beta-Cardone (Beta-blocker) see Sotalol
Betaloc (Beta-blocker) see Metoprolol
Betnelan (Corticosteroid) see
Betamethasone
Betnesol (Corticosteroid) see
Betamethasone
Betnovate (Corticosteroid) see
Betamethasone
Betoptic (Beta-blocker) see Betaxolol
Bextasol (Corticosteroid) see
Betamethasone
Bezalip (Lipid lowering agent) see
Bezafibrate
BiCNU (Cytotoxic agent) see Carmustine
Binovum (Contraceptive) see
Contraceptives, Oral
Biogastrone (Ulcer healing agent) see
Carbenoxolone
Blocadren (Beta-blocker) see Timolol
Bolvidon (Antidepressant) see Mianserin
Bradilan (Peripheral vasodilator: see
Nicofuranose
Bretylate (Antidysrhythmic) see Bretylium
Brevibloc (Beta-blocker) see Esmolol
Brevinor (Contraceptive) see
Contraceptives, Oral
Bricanyl (Bronchodilator) see Terbutaline
Brietal (Barbiturate) see Methohexitone
Britiazim (Calcium antagonist) see
Diltiazem
Bronchodil (Bronchodilator) see
Reproterol
Brufen (Anti-inflammatory agent) see
Ibuprofen
Buccastem (Phenothiazine) see
Prochlorperazine
Burinex (Diuretic) see Bumetanide

Buscopan (Antispasmodic) see
Hyoscine-N-Butylbromide
Buspar (Anxiolytic/Antidepressant) see
Buspirone

Cafergot (Vasoconstrictor) see
Ergotamine
Calciparine (Anticoagulant) see Heparin
Calcitare (Thyroid hormone) see
Calcitonin
Calpol (Analgesic) see Paracetamol
Calsynar (Thyroid hormone) see
Salcatonin
Camcolit (Antidepressant) see Lithium
Carbonate
Canesten (Antifungal) see Clotrimazole
Capastat (Antitubercule) see
Capreomycin
Capoten (Antihypertensive) see Captopril
Carace (Antihypertensive) see Lisinopril
Cardene (Anti-anginal/Hypotensive) see
Nicardipine
Catapres (Antihypertensive) see
Clonidine
Caved-S (Ulcer healing agent) see
Deglycyrrhizinised Liquorice
CCNU (Cytotoxic agent) see Lomustine
Cedocard (Anti-anginal) see Isosorbide
Dinitrate
Cefizox (Antibiotic) see Ceftizoxime
Celectol (Beta-blocker) see Celiprolol
Celbenin (Antibiotic) see Methicillin
Celevac (Laxative) see Methylcellulose
Ceporex (Antibiotic) see Cephalexin
Cerubidin (Cytotoxic agent) see
Daunorubicin
Cesamet (Anti-emetic) see Nabilone
Chendol (Gallstone dissolving agent) see
Chenodeoxycholic Acid
Chloromycetin (Antibiotic) see
Chloramphenicol
Choledyl (Bronchodilator) see Chorine
Theophyllinate
Cidomycin (Antibiotic) see Gentamicin
Ciproxin (Antibiotic) see Ciprofloxacin
Citanest (Local anaesthetic) see
Prilocaine
Claforan (Antibiotic) see Cefotaxime
Clexane (Heparin-like anticoagulant) see
Enoxaparin
Clinoril (Anti-inflammatory agent) see
Sulindac
Clomid (Anti-oestrogen) see Clomiphene
Clopixol (Tranquillizer) see Clopenthixol
Cogentin (Anticholinergic) see
Benztropine

Colofac (Antispasmodic) see Mebeverine
Comprecin (Antibiotic) see Enoxacin
Co-beneldopa (Antiparkinson drug) see Madopar
Co-careldopa (Antiparkinson drug) see Sinemet
Concordin (Antidepressant) see Protriptyline
Conova 30 (Contraceptive) see Contraceptives, Oral
Convulex (Anticonvulsant) see Valproic acid
Coracten (Calcium antagonist) see Nifedipine
Cordarone X (Antidysrthythmic) see Amiodarone
Cordilox (Anti-anginal and antidysrhythmic agent) see Verapamil
Corgard (Beta-blocker) see Nadolol
Coro-Nitro (Anti-anginal) see Glyceryl Trinitrate
Cortelan (Corticosteroid) see Cortisone
Cortistab (Corticosteroid) see Cortisone
Cortisyl (Corticosteroid) see Cortisone
Corwin (Beta-blocker/beta-agonist) see Xamoterol
Cosmegen Lyovac (Cytotoxic agent) see Actinomycin D
Coversyl (Antihypertensive) see Perindopril
Cream of Magnesia (Antacid) see Magnesium Hydroxide
Creon (Pancreatic enzyme) see Pancreatin
Crystapen G (Antibiotic) see Benzylpenicillin
Cyclogest (Progestational hormone) see Progesterone
Cyclo-Progynova (Hormone replacement therapy) see Oestradiol Valerate
Cyklokapron (Antifibrinolytic agent) see Tranexamic acid
Cymevene (Antiviral agent) see Ganciclovis, Drug Update section, p. 401
Cyprostat (Anti-androgen) see Cyproterone Acetate
Cytacon (Vitamin) see Cyanocobalamin
Cytamen (Vitamin) see Cyanocobalamin
Cytosar (Cytotoxic agent) see Cytarabine
Cytosine Arabinoside (Cytotoxic agent) see Cytarabine

Dactinomycin (Cytotoxic agent) see Actinomycin D
Daktarin (Anti-fungal) see Miconazole
Dalacin-C (Antibiotic) see Clindamycin
Dalmane (Hypnotic) see Flurazepam
Danaparoid (Heparin-like anticoagulant) see Low molecular weight heparin
Danol (Steroid blocker) see Danazol
Daonil (Hypoglycaemic agent) see Glibenclamide
Daranide (Carbonic anhydrase inhibitor) see Dichlorophenamide
Daraprim (Antimalarial) see Pyrimethamine
DDAVP (Antidiuretic hormone analogue) see Desmopressin
Deca-Durabolin (Anabolic steroid) see Nandrolone
Decadron (Corticosteroid) see Dexamethasone
Declinax (Antihypertensive) see Debrisoquine
Decortisyl (Corticosteroid) see Prednisone
Deltacortone (Corticosteroid) see Prednisone
Deltacortril (Corticosteroid) see Prednisolone
Deltaparin (Heparin-like anticoagulant) see Low molecular weight heparin
Demethylchlortetracycline (Antibiotic) see Demeclocycline
Dendrid (Antiviral agent) see Idoxuridine
De-Nol (Ulcer healing agent) see Tri-Potassium Di-Citrato Bismuthate
Depixol (Tranquillizer) see Flupenthixol
Depo-Medrone (Corticosteroid) see Methylprednisolone
Depo-Provera (Progestational hormone) see Medroxyprogesterone Acetate
Dermovate (Corticosteroid) see Clobetasol
Deseril (Antiserotonin agent) see Methysergide
Destolit (Gallstone dissolving agent) see Ursodeoxycholic Acid
Dexamphetamine (CNS stimulant) see Amphetamines and Related Drugs
Dexedrine (CNS stimulant) see Amphetamines and Related Drugs
DF 118 (Analgesic) see Dihydrocodeine
Diabenese (Hypoglycaemic agent) see Chlorpropamide
Diamicron (Hypoglycaemic agent) see Gliclazide

Diamox (Carbonic anhydrase inhibitor) see Acetazolamide
Diazemuls (Tranquillizer) see Diazepam
Dibenyline (Vasodilator) see Phenoxybenzamine
Dibromomannitol (Cytotoxic agent) see Mitobronitol
Diconal (Narcotic analgesic) see Dipipanone
Didronel (Bisphosphonate) see Etidronate
Difuclan (Antifungal) see Fluconazole, Drug Update section, p. 401
Dimotane (Antihistamine) see Brompheniramine
Dindevan (Anticoagulant) see Phenindione
Dinoprost (Prostaglandin) see Prostaglandin F_2 Alpha
Dinoprostone (Prostaglandin) see Prostaglandin E_2
Dioctyl Medo (Laxative) see Docusate Sodium
Disalcid (Anti-inflammatory) see Salsalate
Disipal (Anticholinergic) see Orphenadrine
Disprol (Analgesic) see Paracetamol
Distaclor (Antibiotic) see Cefaclor
Distalgesic (Analgesic) see Dextropropoxyphene
Distamine (Antirheumatic and heavy metal poison antidote) see Penicillamine
Diurexan (Diuretic) see Xipamide
Dixarit (Migraine prophylactic) see Clonidine
DNase (DNA specific enzyme) see Dornase alfa
Dobutrex (Cardiac stimulant) see Dobutamine
Dolobid (Analgesic) see Diflunisal
Doloxene (Analgesic) see Dextropropoxyphene
Dopram (Respiratory stimulant) see Doxapram
Dorbanex (Laxative) see Danthron
Dovonex (Vitamin D analogue) see Calcipotriol
Dramamine (Antihistamine) see Dimenhydrinate
DTIC (Cytotoxic agent) see Dacarbazine
Dulcolax (Laxative) see Bisacodyl
Duphalac (Laxative) see Lactulose
Duphaston (Progestational hormone) see Dydrogesterone

Durabolin (Anabolic steroid) see Nandrolone
Duromine (Appetite suppressant) see Phentermine
Dyazide (Diuretic) see Triamterene
Dyspamet (Ulcer healing agent) see Cimetidine
Dytac (Diuretic) see Triamterene
Dytide (Diuretic) see Triamterene

Ecostatin (Anti-fungal) see Econazole
Edecrin (Diuretic) see Ethacrynic Acid
Efcortelan (Corticosteroid) see Hydrocortisone
Efcortesol (Corticosteroid) see Hydrocortisone
Efudix (Cytotoxic) see Fluorouracil
Elantan (Anti-anginal agent) see Isosorbide Mononitrate
Eldepryl (Anti-Parkinson agent) see Selegiline
Eldisine (Cytotoxic agent) see Vindesine
Eltroxin (Thyroid hormone) see Thyroxine
Emcor (Beta-blocker) see Bisoprolol
Emeside (Anticonvulsant) see Ethosuximide
Emflex (Anti-inflammatory) see Acemetacin
Eminase (Thrombolytic drug) see Anistreplase
Endoxana (Cytotoxic agent) see Cyclophosphamide
Enoxaparin (Heparin-like anticoagulant) see Low molecular weight heparin
Epanutin (Anticonvulsant and Antidysrhythmic agent) see Phenytoin
Ephynal (Vitamin) see Vitamin E
Epilim (Anticonvulsant) see Sodium Valproate
Eppy (Sympathetic hormone) see Adrenaline
Eprex (Erythropoietin) see Epoetin
Equanil (Tranquillizer) see Meprobarnate
Eradicin (Antibiotic) see Acrosoxacin
Erymax (Antibiotic) see Erythromycin
Erythrocin (Antibiotic) see Erythromycin
Esbatal (Antihypertensive) see Bethanidine
Estracyt (Cytotoxic agent) see Estramustine
Estraderm (Oestrogen) see Oestradiol
Eudemine (Antihypertensive) see Diazoxide

Euglucon (Hypoglycaemic) see
  Glibenclamide
Eugynon (Contraceptive) see
  Contraceptives, Oral
Euhypnos (Hypnotic) see Temazepam
Eumovate (Corticosteroid) see
  Clobetasone
Evadyne (Antidepressant) see
  Butriptyline
Exirel (Bronchodilator) see Pirbuterol

Fabahistin (Antihistamine) see
  Mebhydrolin
Fabrol (Mucolytic agent) see
  Acetylcysteine
Famvir (Antiviral) see Famociclavir
Fasigyn (Antibiotic) see Tinidazole
Faverin (Antidepressant) see
  Fluvoxamine
Fe Cap Folic (Iron and vitamin) see
  Ferrous Sulphate
Fefol (Iron salt) see Ferrous Sulphate
Fefol Vit (Iron and vitamins) see Ferrous
  Sulphate
Fefol Z (Iron and zinc) see Ferrous
  Sulphate
Feldene (Anti-inflammatory agent) see
  Piroxicam
Femodene (Contraceptive) see
  Contraceptives, Oral
Femulen (Contraceptive) see
  Contraceptives, Oral
Fenopron (Anti-inflammatory agent) see
  Fenoprofen
Fentazin (Phenothiazine) see
  Perphenazine
Feospan (Iron salt) see Ferrous Sulphate
Ferfolic (Iron and vitamin) see Ferrous
  Gluconate
Fergluvite (Iron and vitamins) see
  Ferrous Gluconate
Fergon (Iron salt) see Ferrous Gluconate
Ferrocap (Iron salt) see Ferrous
  Fumarate
Ferrocap-F 350 (Iron and vitamin) see
  Ferrous Fumarate
Ferrograd C (Iron and vitamin) see
  Ferrous Sulphate
Ferrograd Folic (Iron and vitamin) see
  Ferrous Sulphate
Ferro-Gradumet (Iron salt) see Ferrous
  Sulphate
Ferromyn (Iron salt) see Ferrous
  Succinate
Ferromyn B (Iron and vitamin) see
  Ferrous Succinate

Ferromyn S (Iron salt) see Ferrous
  Succinate
Ferromyn S Folic (Iron and vitamin) see
  Ferrous Succinate
Fersaday (Iron and vitamin) see Ferrous
  Fumarate
Fersamal (Iron salt) see Ferrous
  Fumarate
Fesovit Z (Iron, vitamins and zinc) see
  Ferrous Sulphate
5-Fluorouracil (Cytotoxic) see
  Fluorouracil
5-FU (Cytotoxic) see Fluorouracil
Flagyl (Antibiotic) see Metronidazole
Flixotide (Corticosteroid) see Fluticasone
Florinef (Corticosteroid) see
  Fludrocortisone
Floxapen (Antibiotic) see Flucloxacillin
Fluanxol (Tranquillizer) see Flupenthixol
Folex 350 (Iron and vitamin) see Ferrous
  Fumarate
Folicin (Iron and vitamin) see Ferrous
  Sulphate
Fortum (Antibiotic) see Ceftazidime
Fragmin (Heparin-like anticoagulant) see
  Low molecular weight heparin
Frisium (Tranquillizer) see Clobazam
Froben (Anti-inflammatory agent) see
  Flurbiprofen
Fucidin (Antibiotic) see Fusidic
  Acid/Sodium Fusidate
Fulcin (Anti-fungal) see Griseofulvin
Fungilin (Anti-fungal) see Amphotericin B
Fungizone (Anti-fungal) see
  Amphotericin B
Furadantin (Antibacterial) see
  Nitrofurantoin
Fybogel (Laxative) see Ispaghula

Gamanil (Antidepressant) see
  Lofepramine
Gastrocote (Antacid) see Alginic Acid
Gastrozepin (Ulcer-healing agent) see
  Pirenzepine
Gaviscon (Antacid) see Alginic Acid
Genticin (Antibiotic) see Gentamicin
Gestanin (Progestational hormone) see
  Allyloestrenol
Glauline (Beta-blocker) see Metipranolol
Glibenese (Hypoglycaemic agent) see
  Glipizide
Globin Insulin (Insulin) see Insulin
Glucobay (Starch blocker) see
  Acarbose
Glucophage (Hypoglycaemic agent) see
  Metformin

Glurenorm (Hypoglycaemia agent) see
   Gliquidone
Glypressin (Haemostatic) see Terlipressin
Gopten (Antihypertensive) see
   Trandolapril
Grisovin (Anti-fungal) see Griseofulvin

Haelan (Corticosteroid) see
   Flurandrenolone
Halciderm (Corticosteroid) see
   Halcinonide
Halcort (Corticosteroid) see Halcinonide
Haldol (Tranquillizer) see Haloperidol
Harmogen (Oestrogen) see Piperazine
   Oestrone Sulphate
Hemabate (Prostaglandin) see
   Carboprost
Heminevrin (Sedative) see
   Chlormethiazole
Hep-flush (Anticoagulant) see Heparin
Heplok (Anticoagulant) see Heparin
Hepsal (Anticoagulant) see Heparin
Heroin (Narcotic analgesic) see
   Diamorphine
Herpid (Antiviral agent) see Idoxuridine
Hexopal (Peripheral vasodilator) see
   Inositol Nicotinate
Hismanal (Antihistamine) see Astemizole
Histryl (Antihistamine) see
   Diphenylpyraline
Humulin (Insulin) see Insulin
Hyalase (Enzyme) see Hyaluronidase
Hydrenox (Diuretic) see
   Hydroflumethiazide
Hydrocortone (Corticosteroid) see
   Hydrocortisone
Hydrosaluric (Diuretic) see
   Hydrochlorothiazide
Hygroton (Diuretic) see Chlorthalidone
Hyoscine (Antimuscarinic,
   anticholinergic) see Atropine
Hypovase (Antihypertensive) see
   Prazosin
Hypurin Isophane (Insulin) see Insulin
Hypurin Lente (Insulin) see Insulin
Hypurin Neutral (Insulin) see Insulin
Hypurin Protamine Zinc (Insulin) see
   Insulin
Hytrin (Antihypertensive) see
   Terazosin
Ilosone (Antibiotic) see Erythromycin
Ilotycin (Antibiotic) see Erythromycin
Imdur (Anti-anginal) see Isosorbide
   Mononitrate
Imigran (Anti-migraine drug) see
   Sumatriptan

Imodium (Anti-diarrhoeal) see
   Loperamide
Imperacin (Antibiotic) see
   Oxytetracycline
Imtak (Anti-anginal) see Isosorbide
   Dinitrate
Imuran (Immunosuppressant) see
   Azathioprine
Inderal (Beta-blocker) see Propranolol
Indocid (Anti-inflammatory agent) see
   Indomethacin
Initard (Insulin) see Insulin
Innohep (Heparin-like anticoagulant) see
   Low molecular weight heparin
Innovace (Antihypertensive) see
   Enalapril
Insulatard MC (Insulin) see Insulin
Intal (Anti-allergic agent) see Sodium
   Cromoglycate
Intraval (Barbiturate) see Thiopentone
Intron-A (Antiviral/Antitumour) see
   Interferon
Intropin (Cardiac stimulant) see
   Dopamine
Ionamin (Appetite suppressant) see
   Phentermine
Ipral (Antibacterial) see Trimethoprim
Ismelin (Antihypertensive) see
   Guanethidine
Ismo (Anti-anginal agent) see Isosorbide
   Mononitrate
Isogel (Laxative) see Ispaghula
Isoket (Anti-anginal) see Isosorbide
   Dinitrate
Isophane NPH (Insulin) see Insulin
Isordil (Anti-anginal) see Isosorbide
   Dinitrate
Istin (Calcium antagonist) see Amlodipine

Jectofer (Iron salt) see Iron (Parenteral)

Kabikinase (Fibrinolytic agent) see
   Streptokinase
Kefadol (Antibiotic) see Cefamandole
Keflex (Antibiotic) see Cephalexin
Keflin (Antibiotic) see Cephalothin
Kefzol (Antibiotic) see Cephazolin
Kemadrin (Anticholinergic) see
   Procyclidine
Kenalog (Corticosteroid) see
   Triamcinolone
Kerlone (Beta-blocker) see Betaxolol
Kinidin (Antidysrhythmic agent) see
   Quinidine
Klaricid (Antibiotic) see Clarithromycin

Konakion (Vitamin) see Vitamin K
Kytril (Anti-emetic) see Granisetron

Lamictal (Anticonvulsant) see
   Lamotrigine
Lamisil (Antifungal) see Terbinafine
Lanoxin (Cardiac stimulant) see Digoxin
Lanvis (Cytotoxic agent) see Thioguanine
Largactil (Phenothiazine) see
   Chlorpromazine
Larodopa (Anti-Parkinson agent) see
   Levodopa
Lasix (Diuretic) see Frusemide
Lasma (Bronchodilator) see Theophylline
Laxoberal (Laxative) see Sodium
   Picosulphate
Ledercort (Corticosteroid) see
   Triamcinolone
Lederfen (Anti-Parkinson agent) see
   Fenbufen
Ledermycin (Antibiotic) see
   Demeclocycline
Lederspan (Corticosteroid) see
   Triamcinolone
Lentard MC (Insulin) see Insulin
Lentaron (Cytotoxic agent) see
   Formestane
Lente Insulin (Insulin) see Insulin
Leukeran (Cytotoxic agent) see
   Chlorambucil
Lexotan (Benzodiazepine) see
   Bromazepam
Librium (Tranquillizer) see
   Chlordiazepoxide
Lidothesin (Local anaesthetic) see
   Lignocaine
Lignostab (Local anaesthetic) see
   Lignocaine
Lioresal (Anti-spastic agent) see
   Baclofen
Li-Liquid (Antidepressant) see Lithium
Lipostat (Lipid-lowering agent) see
   Pravastatin
Litarex (Antidepressant) see Lithium
Lodine (Anti-inflammatory agent) see
   Etodolac
Loestrin (Contraceptive) see
   Contraceptives, Oral
Logiparin (Heparin-like anticoagulant)
   see Low molecular weight heparin
Logynon (Contraceptive) see
   Contraceptives, Oral
Lomotil (Anti-diarrhoeal) see
   Diphenoxylate
Lopid (Lipid lowering agent) see
   Gemfibrozil

Loron (Bisphosphonate) see Clodronate
Losec (Ulcer healing agent) see
   Omeprazole
Ludiomil (Antidepressant) see
   Maprotiline
Lurselle (Lipid lowering agent) see
   Probucol

Macrodantin (Antibacterial) see
   Nitrofurantoin
Madopar (Anti-Parkinson agent) see
   Madopar
m-AMSA (Cytotoxic agent) see
   Amsacrine
Manerix (Antidepressant) see
   Moclobemide
Marcaine (Local anaesthetic) see
   Bupivacaine
Marevan (Anticoagulant) see Warfarin
Marplan (Antidepressant) see
   Isocarboxazid
Marvelon (Contraceptive) see
   Contraceptives, Oral
Maxepa (Fish Oils) see Maxepa
Maxolon (Gastric emptier and
   anti-emetic) see Metoclopramide
Medrone (Corticosteroid) see
   Methylprednisolone
Mefoxin (Antibiotic) see Cefoxitin
Megace (Progestogen) see Megestrol
   Acetate
Melleril (Phenothiazine) see Thioridazine
Menophase (Oestrogen) see Mestranol
Meptid (Analgesic) see Meptazinol
Merbentyl (Antispasmodic) see
   Dicyclomine
Mercilon (Contraceptive) see
   Contraceptives, Oral
Mestinon (Anticholinesterase) see
   Pyridostigmine
Metenix (Diuretic) see Metolazone
Metopirone (Steroid inhibitor) see
   Metyrapone
Metosyn (Corticosteroid) see
   Fluocinonide
Mexitil (Antidysrhythmic agent) see
   Mexiletine
Miacalcic (Thyroid hormone) see
   Salcatonin
Microgynon 30 (Contraceptive) see
   Contraceptives, Oral
Micronor (Contraceptive) see
   Contraceptives, Oral
Microval (Contraceptive) see
   Contraceptives, Oral
Midamor (Diuretic) see Amiloride

Migril (Vasoconstrictor) see
  Ergotamine
Milk of Magnesia (Antacid) see
  Magnesium Hydroxide
Minihep (Anticoagulant) see Heparin
Minocin (Antibiotic) see Minocycline
Minodiab (Hypoglycaemic) see
  Glipizide
Mintezol (Anthelmintic) see
  Thiabendazole
Minulet (Contraceptive) see
  Contraceptives, Oral
Mixtard Insulin (Insulin) see Insulin
Modecate (Phenothiazine) see
  Fluphenazine
Moditen (Phenothiazine) see
  Fluphenazine
Modrasone (Corticosteroid) see
  Alclometasone
Modrenal (Steroid inhibitor) see
  Trilostone
Mogadon (Hypnotic) see Nitrazepam
Molipaxin (Antidepressant) see
  Trazidone
Monacor (Beta-blocker) see Bisoprolol
Monaspor (Antibiotic) see Cefsulodin
Monit (Anti-anginal agent) see Isosorbide
  Mononitrate
Mono-Cedocard (Anti-anginal agent) see
  Isosorbide Mononitrate
Monoparin (Anticoagulant) see Heparin
Monotard MC (Insulin) see Insulin
Motilium (Anti-emetic) see Domperidone
MST Continus (Analgesic) see Morphine
Mucaine (Antacid with local anaesthetic)
  see Oxethazine
Multiparin (Anticoagulant) see Heparin
Myambutol (Antitubercule) see
  Ethambutol
Mycardol (Anti-anginal) see
  Pentaerythritol Tetranitrate
Myelobromol (Cytotoxic agent) see
  Mitobronitol
Myleran (Cytotoxic agent) see Busulphan
Myocrisin (Gold salt) see Sodium
  Aurothiomalate
Myotonine (Sympathomimetic) see
  Bethanechol
Mysoline (Anticonvulsant) see Primidone

Nacton (Anticholinergic) see Poldine
  Sulphate
Nalcrom (Anti-allergic agent) see Sodium
  Cromoglycate
Napratec (Anti-inflammatory agent) see
  Naproxen

Naprosyn (Anti-inflammatory agent) see
  Naproxen
Nardil (Antidepressant) see Phenelzine
Narphen (Narcotic analgesic) see
  Phenazocine
Natrilix (Antihypertensive) see
  Indapamide
Natulan (Cytotoxic agent) see
  Procarbazine
Navoban (Anti-emetic) see Tropisetron
Navidrex (Diuretic) see Cyclopenthiazide
Nebcin (Antibiotic) see Tobramycin
Negram (Antibacterial) see Nalidixic Acid
Neocon 1/35 (Contraceptive) see
  Contraceptives, Oral
Neo-Cytamen (Vitamin) see Vitamin B$_{12}$
Neogest (Contraceptive) see
  Contraceptives, Oral
Neo-Mercazole (Antithyroid) see
  Carbimazole
Neo-Naclex (Diuretic) see Bendrofluazide
Neoplatin (Cytotoxic agent) see Cisplatin
Neotigason (Vitamin A analogue) see
  Acitretin
Nephril (Diuretic) see Polythiazide
Nerisone (Corticosteroid) see
  Diflucortolone
Netillin (Antibiotic) see Netilmicin
Neulactil (Tranquillizer) see Pericyazine
Neulente (Insulin) see Insulin
Neuphane (Insulin) see Insulin
Neurontin (Anticonvulsant) see Gabapentin
Neusilin (Insulin) see Insulin
Nipride (Antihypertensive) see Sodium
  Nitroprusside
Nitrocine (Anti-anginal agent) see
  Glyceryl Trinitrate
Nitrocontin (Anti-anginal agent) see
  Glyceryl Trinitrate
Nitrolingual (Anti-anginal agent) see
  Glyceryl Trinitrate
Nivaquine (Antimalarial and
  anti-inflammatory agent) see
  Hydroxychloroquine
Nizoral (Antifungal) see Ketoconazole
Nobrium (Tranquillizer) see Medazepam
Noctec (Hypnotic) see Chloral Hydrate
Noltam (Anti-oestrogen) see Tamoxifen
Nolvadex (Anti-oestrogen) see Tamoxifen
Norgeston (Contraceptive) see
  Contraceptives, Oral
Noriday (Contraceptive) see
  Contraceptives, Oral
Norimin (Contraceptive) see
  Contraceptives, Oral
Norinyl 1 (Contraceptive) see
  Contraceptives, Oral

Normison (Hypnotic) see Temazepam
Noroxin (Antibiotic) see Norfloxacin
Norval (Antidepressant) see Mianserin
Nozinan (Anti-emetic) see
Methotrimeprazine
Nubain (Analgesic) see Nalbuphine
Nuelin (Bronchodilator) see Theophylline
Nuso Neutral (Insulin) see Insulin
Nutrizym (Pancreatic enzyme) see
Pancreatic
Nystan (Anti-fungal) see Nystatin

Ocufen (Anti-inflammatory) see
Flurbiprofen
Odrik (Antihypertensive) see Trandolapril
Olbetam (Lipid-lowering agent) see
Acipimox
Omnopon (Narcotic analgesic) see
Papaveretum
Oncovin (Cytotoxic agent) see
Vincristine
One-Alpha (Vitamin) see
Alfacalcidol
One-Alpha Hydroxy Cholecalciferol
(Vitamin) see Alfacalcidol
Opilon (Vasodilator) see
Thymoxamine
Opticrom (Anti-allergic agent) see
Sodium Cromoglycate
Optimine (Antihistamine) see Azatadine
Oradexon (Corticosteroid) see
Dexamethasone
Orap (Tranquillizer) see Pimozide
Orbenin (Antibiotic) see Cloxacillin
Orgaron (Heparin-like anticoagulant) see
Low molecular weight heparin
Orlest 21 (Contraceptive) see
Contraceptives, Oral
Ortho-Gynest (Oestrogen) see Oestriol
Ortho-Novin 1/50 (Contraceptive) see
Contraceptives, Oral
Orudis (Anti-inflammatory agent) see
Ketoprofen
Oruvail (Anti-inflammatory agent) see
Ketoprofen
Ovestin (Oestrogen) see Oestriol
Ovran (Contraceptive) see
Contraceptives, Oral
Ovran 30 (Contraceptive) see
Contraceptives, Oral
Ovranette (Contraceptive) see
Contraceptives, Oral
Ovulen 50 (Contraceptive) see
Contraceptives, Oral
Ovysmen (Contraceptive) see
Contraceptives, Oral

Pabrinex (Vitamin) see Multivitamins
Palfium (Narcotic analgesic) see
Dextromoramide
Panadol (Analgesic) see Paracetamol
Pancrease (Pancreatic enzyme) see
Pancreatin
Pancrex V (Pancreatic enzyme) see
Pancreatin
Pancrex V Forte (Pancreatic enzyme)
see Pancreatin
Panzyrat (Pancreatic enzyme) see
Pancreatin
Paraplatin (Cytotoxic agent) see
Carboplatin
Parlodel (Dopamine-like drug) see
Bromocriptine
Parnate (Antidepressant) see
Tranylcypromine
Partobulin (Immunoglobulin) see Anti-D
immunoglobulin
Parvolex (Paracetamol antidote) see
Acetylcysteine
Penbritin (Antibiotic) see Ampicillin
Penicillin G (Antibiotic) see
Benzylpenicillin
Penidural (Antibiotic) see Benzathine
Penicillin
Penmix (Insulin) see
Insulin
Pepcid PM (Ulcer healing agent) see
Famotidine
Percutol (Anti-anginal agent) see
Glyceryl Trinitrate
Periactin (Antiserotonin) see
Cyproheptadine
Peroidin (Antithyroid agent) see
Potassium Perchlorate
Persantin (Antiplatelet and anti-anginal)
see Dipyridamole
Pertofran (Antidepressant) see
Desipramine
Pevaryl (Anti-fungal) see Econazole
Pharmorubicin (Cytotoxic) see
Epirubicin
Phenergan (Antihistamine) see
Promethazine
Phyllocontin (Bronchodilator) see
Aminophylline
Physeptone (Narcotic analgesic) see
Methadone
Pipril (Antibiotic), see Piperacillin, Drug
Update section, p. 401
Piriton (Antihistamine) see
Chlorpheniramine
Plaquenil (Antimalarial and
Anti-inflammatory agent) see
Hydroxychloroquine

Platet (Antiplatelet drug) see Aspirin
Ponderax (Appetite suppressant) see Fenfluramine
Ponstan (Anti-inflammatory agent) see Mefenamic Acid
Pramidex (Hypoglycaemic agent) see Tolbutamide
Praxilene (Peripheral vasodilator) see Naftidrofuryl
Precortisyl (Corticosteroid) see Prednisolone
Prednesol (Corticosteroid) see Prednisolone
Predsol (Corticosteroid) see Prednisolone
Pregaday (Iron and vitamin) see Ferrous Fumarate
Premarin (Oestrogen) see Oestrogens, Conjugated (Equine)
Prempak C (Hormone replacement therapy) see Oestrogens Conjugated
Prepulsid (GI prakinetic) see Cisapride, Drug Update section, p. 401
Priadel (Antidepressant) see Lithium
Primalan (Antihistamine) see Mequitazine
Primaxin (Antibiotic) see Imipenem
Primoteston (Androgen) see Testosterone
Pripsen (Anthelmintic) see Piperazine
Pro-Actidil (Antihistamine) see Triprolidine
Pro-Banthine (Anticholinergic) see Propantheline
Progynova (Oestrogen) see Oestradiol Valerate
Proluton Depot (Progestational hormone) see Hydroxyprogesterone Hexanoate
Prominal (Anticonvulsant) see Methylphenobarbitone
Prondol (Antidepressant) see Iprindole
Pronestyl (Antidysrhythmic agent) see Procainamide
Proscar (Prostate shrinker) see Finasteride
Prostigmin (Anticholinesterase) see Neostigmine
Prostin E₂ (Prostaglandin) see Prostaglandin E_2
Prothiaden (Antidepressant) see Dothiepin
Provera (Progestational hormone) see Medroxyprogesterone Acetate
Pro-Viron (Androgen) see Mesterolone
Pulmadil (Bronchodilator) see Rimiterol

Pulmicort (Corticosteroid) see Beclomethasone
Pur-in Mix (Insulin) see Insulin
Puri-Nethol (Immunosuppressant) see Mercaptopurine
Pulmozyme (DNA specific enzyme) see Dornase alfa
Pyopen (Antibiotic) see Carbenicillin
Pyrogastrone (Ulcer healing agent) see Carbenoxolone
P.Z.1. (Insulin) see Insulin

Questran (Ion exchange resin) see Cholestyramine

Rapifen (Sedative/Analgesic) see Alfentanil
Rapitard MC (Insulin) see Insulin
Rastinon (Hypoglycaemic agent) see Tolbutamide
Razoxin (Cytotoxic agent) see Razoxane
Recormon (Erythropoietin) see Epoetin
Relifex (Anti-inflammatory agent) see Nabumetone
Retrovir (Antiviral agent) see Zidovudine
Rheumox (Anti-inflammatory agent) see Azapropazone
Rhinacort (Corticosteroid) see Beclomethasone
Rhinoplast (Antihistamine) see Azelastine
Ridaura (Antirheumatic) see Auranofin
Rifadin (Antitubercule) see Rifampicin
Rimactane (Antitubercule) see Rifampicin
Rinatec (Decongestant) see Ipratropium Bromide
Rivotril (Anticonvulsant) see Clonazepam
Roaccutane (Vitamin A analogue) see Isotretinoin
Robinul (Anticholinergic) see Glycopyrrolate
Rocaltrol (Vitamin) see Calcitriol
Rocephin (Antibiotic) see Ceftriaxone
Roferon-A (Antiviral/Antitumour) see Interferon
Rogitine (Vasodilator) see Phentolamine
Rohypnol (Hypnotic) see Flunitrazepam
Ronicol (Peripheral vasodilator) see Nicotinyl Alcohol
Rubidomycin (Cytotoxic agent) see Daunorubicin

Rynacrom (Anti-allergic agent) see Sodium Cromoglycate
Rythmodan (Antidysrhythmic agent) see Disopyramide
Sabril (Anticonvulsant) see Vigabatrin
Salazopyrin (Anti-inflammatory agent) see Sulphasalazine
Saluric (Diuretic) see Chlorothiazide
Sandimmun (Immunosuppressant) see Cyclosporin
Sanomigran (Migraine prophylactic) see Pizotifen
Saventrine (Cardiac pacer) see Isoprenaline
Scopolamine (Antimuscarinic, anticholinergic) see Atropine
Seconal (Barbiturate) see Quinalbarbitone
Sectral (Beta-blocker) see Acebutolol
Securon (Anti-anginal and antidysrhythmic agent) see Verapamil
Securopen (Antibiotic) see Azlocillin
Semilente (Insulin) see Insulin
Semitard MC (Insulin) see Insulin
Semprex (Antihistamine) see Acrivastine
Senokot (Laxative) see Sennoside
Septrin (Anti-bacterial) see Co-trimoxazole
Serc (Antihistamine) see Betahistine
Serenace (Tranquillizer) see Haloperidol
Serenid-D (Tranquillizer) see Oxazepam
Sinemat (Anti-Parkinson agent) see Sinemet
Sinequan (Antidepressant) see Doxepin
Sinthrome (Anticoagulant) see Nicoumalone
Slo-Phyllin (Bronchodilator) see Theophylline
Slow Fe (Iron salt) see Ferrous Sulphate
Slow Fe Folic (Iron and vitamin) see Ferrous Sulphate
Sodium Amytal (Barbiturate) see Amylobarbitone
Solu-Cortef (Corticosteroid) see Hydrocortisone
Solu-Medrone (Corticosteroid) see Methylprednisolone
Solvazinc (Mineral) see Zinc Sulphate
Soneryl (Barbiturate) see Butobarbitone
Soni-Slo (Anti-anginal) see Isosorbide Dinitrate
Sorbichew (Anti-anginal) see Isosorbide Dinitrate
Sorbid SA (Anti-anginal) see Isosorbide Dinitrate
Sorbitrate (Anti-anginal) see Isosorbide Dinitrate

Sotacor (Beta-blocker) see Sotalol
Sparine (Phenothiazine) see Promazine
Spiroctan (Diuretic) see Spironolactone
Sporanox (Antifungal) see Itraconazole, Drug Update section, p. 401
Staril (Antihypertensive) see Fosinopril
Stelazine (Phenothiazine) see Trifluoperazine
Stemetil (Phenothiazine) see Prochlorperazine
Stesolid (Tranquillizer) see Diazepam
Streptase (Thrombolytic drug) see Streptokinase
Stromba (Anabolic steroid) see Stanozolol
Stugeron (Antihistamine) see Cinnarazine
Suliptil (Neuroleptic) see Sulpiride
Sulfasuxidine (Sulphonamide) see Succinylsulphathiazole
Sulphamezathine (Sulphonamide) see Sulphadimidine
Suprefact (Gonadotrophin antagonist) see Buserelin
Surgam (Anti-inflammatory agent) see Tiaprofenic Acid
Surmontil (Antidepressant) see Trimipramine
Suscard (Anti-anginal agent) see Glyceryl Trinitrate
Sustac (Anti-anginal agent) see Glyceryl Trinitrate
Sustanon (Androgen) see Testosterone
Symmetrel (Anti-Parkinson) see Amantadine
Synalar (Corticosteroid) see Fluocinolone
Synandone (Corticosteroid) see Fluocinolone
Synflex (Anti-inflammatory agent) see Naproxen
Synkavit (Vitamin) see Vitamin K
Synphase (Contraceptive) see Contraceptives, Oral
Syntocinon (Uterine stimulant) see Oxytocin
Sytron (Iron salt) see Sodium Ironedetate
Tachyrol (Vitamin) see Dihydrotachysterol
Tagamet (Ulcer healing agent) see Cimetidine
Talpen (Antibiotic) see Talampicillin
Tamofen (Anti-oestrogen) see Tamoxifen
Tampovagan (Oestrogen) see Stilboestrol
Targocid (Antibiotic) see Teicoplanin, Drug Update section, p. 401
Tarivid (Antibiotic) see Ofloxacin

Tavegil (Antihistamine) see Clemastine
Taxol (Cytotoxic agent) see Paclitaxel
Tegretol (Anticonvulsant) see
   Carbamazepine
Temgesic (Analgesic) see
   Buprenorphine
Tenormin (Beta-blocker) see Atenolol
Tensilon (Anticholinesterase) see
   Edrophonium Chloride
Teoptic (Beta-blocker) see Carteolol
Terramycin (Antibiotic) see
   Oxytetracycline
Testoral (Androgen) see Testosterone
Theo-dur (Bronchodilator) see
   Theophylline
Thephorin (Antihistamine) see
   Phenindamine
Ticar (Antibiotic) see Ticarcillin
Tilade (Anti-asthmatic) see
   Nedocromil
Tildiem (Calcium antagonist) see
   Diltiazem
Timentin (Antibiotic) see Timentin
Tinzaparin (Heparin-like anticoagulant)
   see Low molecular weight
   heparin
Tofranil (Antidepressant) see
   Imipramine
Tolanase (Hypoglycaemic) see
   Tolazamide
Tonocard (Antidysrhythmic) see
   Tocainide
Topilar (Corticosteroid) see
   Fluclorolone
Toradol (Anti-inflammatory analgesic)
   see Ketorolac
TpA (Thrombolytic) see Alteplase
Tracrium (Muscle relaxant) see
   Atracurium
Trandate (Alpha and beta blocker) see
   Labetolol
Transiderm-Nitro (Anti-anginal agent)
   see Glyceryl Trinitrate
Tranxene (Tranquillizer) see Potassium
   Chlorazepate
Trasicor (Beta-blocker) see
   Oxprenolol
Tremonil (Anticholinergic) see
   Methixene
Trental (Peripheral vasodilator) see
   Oxpentifylline
Triadene (Contraceptive) see
   Contraceptives, Oral
Tridesilone (Corticosteroid) see
   Desonide
Tridil (Anti-anginal agent) see Glyceryl
   Trinitrate

Triludan (Antihistamine) see
   Terfenadine
Trimopan (Anti-bacterial) see
   Trimethoprim
Trinordiol (Contraceptive) see
   Contraceptives, Oral
Trinovum (Contraceptive) see
   Contraceptives, Oral
Tritace (Antihypertensive) see Ramipril
Tryptizol (Antidepressant) see
   Amitriptyline

Ukidan (Thrombolytic agent) see
   Urokinase
Ultradil (Corticosteroid) see
   Fluocortolone
Ultralente (Insulin) see Insulin
Ultratard MC (Insulin) see Insulin
Unihep (Anticoagulant) see Heparin
Uniparin (Anticoagulant) see Heparin
Univer (Anti-anginal and antidysrhythmic
   agent) see Verapamil
Uniphyllin (Bronchodilator) see
   Theophylline
Urispas (Antispasmodic) see Flavoxate
Uticillin (Antibiotic) see Carfecillin
Utinor (Antibiotic) see Norfloxacin

Valium (Tranquillizer) see Diazepam
Vallergan (Phenothiazine) see
   Trimeprazine
Valoid (Antihistamine) see Cyclizine
Vancocin (Antibiotic) see Vancomycin
Varidase (Fibrinolytic agent) see
   Streptokinase/Streptodornase
Vascace (Antihypertensive) see Cilazapril
Velbe (Cytotoxic agent) see Vinblastine
Velosef (Antibiotic) see Cephradine
Velosulin (Insulin) see Insulin
Ventolin (Bronchodilator) see Salbutamol
Vermox (Anthelmintic) see Mebendazole
Vibramycin (Antibiotic) see Doxycycline
Vira-A (Antiviral agent) see Vidarabine
Virazid (Antiviral agent) see Ribavarin
Visken (Beta-blocker) see Pindolol
Volmax (Bronchodilator) see
   Salbutamol
Voltarol (Anti-inflammatory agent) see
   Diclofenac

Welldorm (Hypnotic) see
   Dichloralphenazone
Wellferon (Antiviral/Antitumour) see
   Interferon

X-Prep (Laxative) see Sennoside
Xuret (Diuretic) see Metolazone
Xylocaine (Local anaesthetic) see
Lignocaine
Xylocard (Antidysrhythmic agent) see
Lignocaine

Yomesan (Anthelmintic) see Niclosamide
Yutopar (Uterine relaxant) see
Ritodrine

Zantac (Ulcer healing agent) see
Ranitidine
Zarontin (Anticonvulsant) see
Ethosuximide
Zestril (Antihypertensive) see
Lisinopril
Zimovane (Hypnotic) see Zopiclone

Zinacef (Antibiotic) see
Cefuroxime
Zinnat (Antibiotic) see
Cefuroxime
Zinamide (Antitubercule) see
Pyrizinamide
Zincomed (Mineral) see Zinc
Sulphate
Zithromax (Antibiotic) see
Azithromycin
Zocor (Lipid-lowering agent) see
Simvastatin
Zofran (Anti-emetic) see
Ondansetron
Zoladex (Anti-cancer agent) see
Goserelin
Zovirax (Antivital agent) see
Acyclovir
Zyloric (Urate lowering agent)
see Allopurinol